THE AUTH

Wong Kiew Kit, popularly known as Sifu Wong, is the fourth generation successor of Venerable Jiang Nan from the famous Shaolin Monastery in China and Grandmaster of Shaolin Wahnam Institute of Kungfu and Qigong. He received the "Qigong Master of the Year" Award during the Second World Congress on Qigong held in San Francisco in 1997.

He is an internationally acclaimed author of books on the Shaolin arts and Buddhism including Introduction to Shaolin Kung Fu (1981), The Art of Qigong (1993), The Art of Shaolin Kung Fu (1996), The Complete Book of Tai Chi Chuan (1996), Chi Kung for Health and Vitality (1997), The Complete Book of Zen (1998), The Complete Book of Chinese Medicine (2002), The Complete Book of Shaolin (2002), Sukhavati:The Western Paradise (2002) and The Shaolin Arts (2002).

Since 1987, Sifu Wong has spent more time teaching qigong than kungfu, because he feels that while kungfu serves as an interesting hobby, qigong serves an urgent public need, particularly in overcoming degenerative and psychiatric illnesses.

Sifu Wong is one of the few masters who have generously introduced the once secretive Shaolin Qigong to the public, and has helped many people to obtain relieve or overcome so-called "incurable" diseases like hypertension, asthma, rheumatism, arthritis, diabetes, migraine, gastritis, gall stones, kidney failure, depression, anxiety and even cancer.

He stresses the Shaolin philosophy of sharing goodness with all humanity, and is now dedicated to spreading the wonders and benefits of the Shaolin arts to people all over the world irrespective of race, culture and religion.

THE COMPLETE BOOK OF

CHINESE MEDICINE

A HOLISTIC APPROACH TO PHYSICAL, EMOTIONAL AND MENTAH HEALTH

WONG KIEW KIT
Author of the bestselling *The Art of Chi Kung*

COSMOS

© **WONG KIEW KIT 2002**

Published by Cosmos Internet Sdn Bhd
45C (3rd Floor) Jalan Pengkalan
Taman Pekan Baru, 08000
Sungai Petani, Kedah
Malaysia

Disclaimer

We caution all our readers to consult their primary health care provider or professional alternative health care practitioners as this publication should not be considered as medical advice to patients or readers. We encourage all our readers to consult and discuss both the advantages and disadvantages of alternative and complementary medicine, with their primary health care provider or professional alternative health care practitioners. By reading this publication, the reader agrees to the terms of this disclaimer and further waives any rights or claims he or she may have against the Publisher, Author and/or any other parties involved in the publication or the distribution of this publication.

Designed and layout by Saw Seng Aun

Printed in Malaysia by Sun Printers Sdn Bhd

ISBN 983-40879-0-X

Dedications

This book is dedicated to all great masters and other people throughout the centuries who have developed and passed on the philosophy and practice of Chinese medicine to us.

CONTENTS

PREFACE

(Ancient Wisdom for Modern Societies)

It may come as a surprise to many readers that the initial part of this book was first written more than twenty years ago! Western medicine was then at its height, in morale if not in accomplishment. Writing in 1955, Erwin H. Ackerknecht, a professor of the history of medicine, concluded that "as a whole, medical progress during the last fifty years has been stupendous. ... His (the modern doctor's) powers to prevent and control disease have grown out of all recognition."

Yet, even at such glorious time, Ackerknecht also lamented that "the elimination of so many infections, with the consequent prolongation of the average life by decades, has led to an unprecedented prevalence of cancer and degenerative cardiovascular diseases against which so far medicine's ability to fight successfully is rather limited. ... And those who boast of medical progress might well remember that even now no answer can be given to a question asked by Jakob Henle more than a hundred years ago: `Has anybody something better to offer than words when it comes to the proximate causes of rheumatism, hysteria and cancer?'"

There is so much Chinese medicine can offer not only to explain the causes of, but also to suggest treatment for these and other diseases which western medicine considered as incurable, that inspired me to start writing this book. The very few English books on Chinese medicine then, and even now, were grossly inadequate. They could be grouped into two types.

Firstly, they were written by western scholars who, albeit being experts in their own fields, knew little about the culture, language and medical philosophy of the Chinese. As a result, their books were superficial at best, and shamefully misleading at most time.

Most of these books dealt with acupuncture and herbal medicine, mainly listing energy points and herbs with brief descriptions of what they were supposed to cure, often giving the impression that what the Chinese did for healing was either inserting needles at odd places into patients' body, or making them drink mixtures boiled from wild grass and bark. The term "yin-yang" was always mentioned, but never explained, except saying that yin referred to whatever was feminine, shady, cold and so on, and yang its opposites, thereby adding to the reader's bewilderment. The even less accurate books described Chinese medical practice as superstitious and metaphysical, or based on social-political systems of the past!

The second group of English books on Chinese medicine, coming later than the first group, were written or translated from classical texts by authors well versed in Chinese medical knowledge, but unfortunately they did not have the linguistic ability to present their material in a form readily comprehensible to western readers. Such descriptions like "He is sick because he has no fire in his stomach" and "The physician cures the patient by using earth to give birth to metal" are not uncommon in such writings.

Because of the vast linguistic and cultural differences between the Chinese and the west, medical information that is meaningful and even poetic in the original Chinese language, if literally translated, may appear nonsensical or even foolish. The inevitable result was that the western public could not see anything worthwhile, besides perhaps a few good laughs, Chinese medicine could offer the west.

Nevertheless, because of other commitments, the English book on Chinese medicine which I started to write in the hope of overcoming these shortcomings, did not materialize until now, more than twenty years later. Meanwhile, as western medicine becomes more and more reductionist and mechanical in practice as well as research, and as degenerative and psychiatric disorders approach epidemic proportions in the west, the optimism of the 1950s has gradually changed into a growing sense of dissatisfaction and unease today, as reflected in Prof. James B. Wyngaarden's observation that "The list of human diseases for which there are no definite measures for prevention or cure is still formidable. Fresh insights into the nature of these diseases are needed." Hence, the need to write this book has become even greater and more urgent because there is much in Chinese medicine that can contribute to overcoming these problems.

At the same time, the experiences and knowledge I have gathered in using qigong to help many people to be relieved of rheumatism, hysteria, cancer and other prevalent disorders, like cardiovascular diseases, kidney failure, diabetes, asthma, insomnia, depression and sexual inadequacy, during these twenty years have given me much confidence and a sincere wish to share the benefits of the wonderful Chinese medical system with other people, especially those in the west. Indeed, almost without realizing it, the fundamental aim in writing this book has developed from the original intention of correcting misleading information on Chinese medicine, to the present objective of presenting invaluable Chinese medical knowledge to the west in the earnest hope that it may contribute to solving the pressing medical problems facing us today.

The term western medicine as used in this book refers to not just the medical system practiced in the west, but the orthodox, conventional medicine of virtually all urban communities. It is sometimes called modern, scientific or allopathic medicine, characterized by the use of chemotherapy and surgery. Chinese medicine refers to not just the medicine practiced in China, but the medicine traditionally developed by the Chinese in the past and is now practiced not only in overseas Chinese communities but also in western societies. Some people have the misconception that Chinese medicine is only acupuncture and herbalism.

Chinese medicine is actually a very wide field, comprising many other areas like external medicine, massage therapy, traumatology and qigong, which will be explained in this book.

The terms "western doctor" and "Chinese physician" are frequently used in this book as general terms referring to professionals practicing western medicine and Chinese medicine respectively, without any geographical, racial or specialistic connotation. A western doctor, therefore, can be a Chinese living in the east, and his speciality may be immunology or surgery, whereas a Chinese physician can be a westerner practicing acupuncture, qigong therapy or any aspect of Chinese medicine in western societies.

Although many of the concepts discussed here may appear exotic to many readers, no previous knowledge of Chinese medicine is needed to understand this book. Moreover technical terms are explained in clear simple language. In order to derive the best benefits, readers are requested to adopt an open mind, and not to impose western medical thinking on a system that uses a totally different paradigm, which is equally, if not more, coherent, meaningful and effective. In this way many incredible cures which may seem impossible or irrational from a western medical view-point, will become sensible and logical. It may be motivational to remember that Chinese medicine is the oldest continuous medical system ever known to humanity, and the one serving the world's largest population. Any medical system that has been successfully practiced for thousands of years by a great civilization certainly has something useful to teach us.

The material presented in this book is quite extensive, covering all important aspects, principles and practices of Chinese medicine. A short history of both world medicine, with special emphasis on western medicine, and Chinese medicine is provided for background information. Then the main principles of Chinese medicine are discussed, followed by explanation of different major therapeutic approaches. Next is a section on mental and spiritual health, and the book concludes with a chapter on suggestions on how Chinese medicine can contribute to the physical, emotional, mental and spiritual well-being of all humanity through western medicine.

Although some readers will be impressed with the profundity of Chinese medicine explained in this book, the material presented here is only an introduction. Hugh volumes can be written for each chapter, and it is hoped that relevant masters will do so, so that the wonderful benefits locked in the hitherto mysterious medical tradition can be shared with more people. More significantly, it is hoped that modern scientists will investigate into the claims or suggestions made in this book so that the great store of ancient wisdom can be applied for the benefit of modern societies.

LIST OF ILLUSTRATIONS

WISDOM FROM PAST MASTERS
(World Medicine in Classical Times)

Wherever the art of medicine is loved, there is also love of humanity.

Hippocrates.

Paleo-medicine and Primitive Medicine

We will be in for some surprise if we think that medicine is a modern discovery, or that ancient men, at best, were crude healers. Medicine is as old as life itself! Archaeological evidence shows that our earliest animals like the dinosaurs and the prehistoric crocodiles suffered from inflammation of joints, fractures and benign tumours. From fossils we discover that bacteria quite like those types found nowadays, already existed about 500 million years ago. And when the earliest men at last made their appearance a million years ago, they suffered from diseases that were not very different from the diseases of today — like common cold, fever, pneumonia and kidney stones.

Prehistoric men learnt from experience that certain herbs were effective in curing certain diseases. They probably began with trials and errors, but soon they gathered some valuable knowledge of medicinal herb lore. Trephining, that is drilling a hole in the head as a therapeutic measure, as modern men suppose, was a widespread practice in prehistoric times. Archaeological evidence shows that Neolithic men did trephining very successfully. They also had a surprisingly high standard of surgery, especially in bone-setting. This will surely impress some people who think that paleo-medicine was purely supernaturalistic, or at the best consisted of few crude drugs, and that surgery was a comparatively late development in the history of medicine.

But by the time paleo-medicine merged into primitive medicine, supernaturalism had become prevalent. Paleo-medicine refers to the medicine of the Stone Age, whereas primitive medicine refers to the medical practices of the primitive men, who were about to leave the Stone Age culture to enter the civilization era, and who may still be found in some remote areas of the world today.

To the primitive man, diseases were caused by an evil spirit or an offended person. The witch-doctor or faith-healer usually advocated sacrifices, rituals or amulets, and occasionally administered some simple but effective drugs to induce vomiting or purging. Sometimes he also recommended physical therapies like massage and bathing. On the whole he was successful; and we usually attribute his success to the effectiveness of his drugs and physical therapy, as well as the psychological values of his spiritual preponderance; though the faith-healer and the patients themselves believed that some force beyond the corporeal was involved.

Ancient Egyptian and Indian Medicine

Ancient Egyptian medicine was of a very high standard, and greatly influenced the medicine of the ancient Greeks.　Herodotus in his "History" spoke of the Egyptian physicians as the best in the world.

The Egyptians, from whom the Greeks probably inherited, had the notion of four basic elements, namely fire, water, air and earth, which they believed influenced the health of a person.　Their anatomical knowledge was quite similar to that of the Chinese in many ways, and their physiology was based on the existence of the heart, forty four vessels and the life-giving role of the breath — similar to the Chinese concept of qi (pronounced as "chi").

The Egyptians were very good at cosmetics, and produced excellent oil and cream to make their skin soft and smooth despite the desert sun.　The Egyptians preceded by a few thousand years the English, who even in Elizabethan time, believed that the liver was the central human organ.　One interesting feature of Egyptian medicine was specialization, but this was probably because of insufficient knowledge rather than profound scholarship.　If you think that plastic surgery is a modern facility possible only because of 20th century technology, you will be amazed to discover that the ancient Indians were some of the finest plastic surgeons in the world.

Classical Indian medicine can be classified into two periods: the Vedic Period before 800 BCE (Before the Common Era), whereby the Vedas, besides being great religious and philosophical books, also explained detailed medical treatment; and the Brahminic Period from 800 BCE to 1000 CE (Common Era), when the practice of medicine as well as all religious matters were in the hands of powerful Brahmin priests.

The Indian materia medica was extensive, but was chiefly consisted of vegetable drugs.　Two notable drugs adopted by the west from the Indians are cardamon and cinnamon.　The Indian pharmacopeia contained detailed descriptions of elixirs, aphrodisiacs, cosmetics and antidotes.　The five senses were used in diagnosis, and the patient's nature of breathing and alternation of voice were carefully noted.　The Indian physicians also employed the pulse theory in diagnosis — a theory that is fundamental to the Chinese.　The chief therapeutic methods were induced vomiting, purging, sneezing, and injecting water or oil into the bowel.

The two greatest masters of Indian medicine were Charaka (about 1st century CE) and Susruta (about 500 CE), and their books which were based on the earlier Vedic practice, were regarded as authoritative medical texts.　The basic theory of Indian medicine was founded on the concept of prana, which is similar to the Chinese qi or energy.

One distinguished achievement of the classical Indians was the exceedingly high quality of surgery. Hundreds of years ago, the Indian surgeons had successfully performed excision of tumours, removal of puss collection, extraction of foreign bodies, punctures of collected fluids in the abdomen, and stitching of wounds using ant heads as clamps. The operation for the removal of bladder stones was remarkable, and their plastic surgery was the best in the world.

In matters of public health, the Indians exhibited some excellent examples. In their ancient cities of Mohenjodaro and Harappa some 3000 years ago, there were public baths and elaborate underground sewage systems. And during the Maurya Empire in the 3rd century BCE the benevolent emperor Asoka the Great built not only hospitals but also animal infirmaries all over India, a thousand years before organized hospitals were known in the west.

Medicine of other Ancient Civilizations

The ancient Mesopotamians, Mexicans and Peruvians had a wide range of materia medica. The Azetecs from the Mexican Civilization knew more than a thousand medicinal plants, and their knowledge of narcotics was particularly rich.

Surgery was highly developed, especially by the Mexicans and the Peruvians, who, like the ancient Indians, used ant heads as clamps in sutures. The Peruvians practised the interesting magic rites of transferring diseases from humans to animals, especially to guinea pigs. Probably it was here that these poor creatures started their long faithful careers in experimental medicine. The Peruvians also had high standard of public health; they had medical provision for the aged and the crippled.

The Mesopotamians too had a very high standard of surgery. A huge stone document showing the Code of King Hammurabi about 1700 BCE, indicated that negligent surgical practices would be severely punished. But such penalty did not apply to non-surgical practices, as Mesopotamians considered the patient himself to be responsible for the cause of his own illness. The Mesopotamians also contributed to the world the conception of regular rest days, of contagion, and of quarantine of lepers. These ideas were transmitted to the west by the Jews.

Ancient Greek Medicine

The Greeks, who laid the foundation of western medicine, had two major trends, that of Asclepius and of Hippocrates.

Asclepius, a great physician living around 1200 BCE, was later deified as the god of healing. His main therapeutics were baths, rest and corrective exercises. Many temples were built in his honor, and the practice of incubation, or temple-sleeping, became prevalent. The patient would sleep in an Asclepius temple so that the god of healing would visit him in his dreams to provide remedies for his illness.

Many modern readers may find this practice ludicrous, and laugh at it as superstition. But the coming of New Age awareness nowadays, with the realization of deeper levels of consciousness and transcendental experience, makes us ponder whether there was really some greater force at work in temple-sleeping than what we superficially understand. We should also remind ourselves that incubation must have been effective, otherwise that practice would not be so widespread, nor would the intellectual Greeks refer to Asclepius as the god of healing. His staff with a serpent wound round it, is used by our modern doctors as the symbol of their profession.

The rise of Hippocrates (about 460 - 377 BCE) marked the start of scientific western medicine. Hippocrates is often regarded as the father of western medicine for his role in bringing medicine out of its supernaturalistic background, and putting it on a firmly scientific basis.

The two most important legacies of Hippocrates were the Corpus Hippocraticum, a voluminous collection of about seventy medical books, and the Hippocratic Code, which still acts as an ethical code for doctors today.

Hippocrates might have written some of the books in the Hippocratic Collection, but most were written by physicians who followed his tradition. The four principal characteristics of the Hippocratic tradition are that diseases were caused by natural, and not supernatural, agents; the emphasis of medicine was on prognosis, not diagnosis; the physician should treat the patient, not just the disease; and treatment should be of the whole person, not just any part of it. These characteristics were strikingly similar to those of the Chinese, except that the Chinese also placed great emphasis on diagnosis. It is also worthy of note that many modern doctors seem to have forgotten the last two Principles.

The Hippocratic Code, besides other things, forbade the physician to prescribe deadly drugs even if it was asked of him; nor to aid abortion, accept bribes and induce seduction of either male or female. The physician was also required to keep as secrets from public whatever particulars of the patient that might cause him embarrassment, and to practise his medicine according to his ability and judgment. By any standard, this code is certainly of admirably high moral values.

Alexandrian and Roman Era

With the expansion of the Hellenistic culture, medicine became focused at Alexandria. Two famous physicians of the Alexandrian era were Herophilus (about 300 BCE) and Erasistratus (about 330 BCE).

Herophilus made some important contributions to anatomy: he described the eyes, the vessels of the body, the genital organs, the brain, and the duodenum, which was actually named by him. In the clinic, his chief therapeutics were blood-letting and poly-pharmacy.

Erasistratus, on the other hand, opposed blood-letting and poly-pharmacy. He advocated corrective diet, massage and exercise. Erasistratus noted the existence of separate sensory and motor nerves, and made detailed descriptions on the anatomy of the brain and cerebellum, the heart, the veins and arteries. All these happened 2200 years ago, more than 1800 years had passed before Harvey's sensational discovery of blood circulation!

Later, there was a group of physicians known as the Empiricists, who opposed philosophical speculations as well as scientific experiments. They based their knowledge and treatment of medicine on their pure observations. These Empiricists made some valuable contributions to symptomatology, surgery and pharmacology.

Roman medical contribution, even at the height of its empire, was overshadowed by that of the Greeks, but their accomplishments in public health were excellent. There were impressive gymnasiums and public baths, efficient system for disposal of sewage and admirable domestic sanitation. Their water supply was without parallel and hospitals were strikingly modern. The Romans even appointed public physicians to look after the poor. Their prominent accomplishments in public health, as compared to the medical achievements of the Greeks, suitably reflect the different types of minds between the intellectual Greeks and the magnificent Romans.

One of the greatest physicians of this time was Asclepiades (about 130 BCE), who contented that disease was caused by either the constricted or relaxed condition of solid particles supposedly making up the body. His methods of restoring harmony of the particles were typical Greek remedies of massage, fresh air, corrective diet and carefully developed exercises. He was amongst the very first in medical history to release the insane from confinement in dark cellars, and prescribed occupational therapy, soporifics, soothing music and exercise to improve their attention and memory — a courageous move that preceded Pinel's famous removal of chains from the insane in Paris by about 2000 years!

A school of physicians called the Methodists insisted that the cause of disease was either excessive opening or excessive narrowing of internal pores. They wanted to reduce the principles and practice of medicine to a few simple methods. Another school, the Pneumatists, claimed that disease was caused by disturbance of pneuma, which is a form of energy similar to the Chinese qi (or chi). This significantly illustrates the fertility and creativeness of the Greek minds even under Roman rule, that refused to accept the old masters, despite their great contributions, as final authorities. This attitude contrasted sharply with that from the Middle Age, which accepted authorities like Galen without questions.

Galen of Asia Minor (130-200 CE) attempted to synthesize these various schools of thoughts before him, though he generally relied on the Hippocratic humoral pathology. His diagnostics as well as therapeutics were astonishingly similar to those of the Chinese. He emphasized the importance of pulse rate in his diagnostics, and used a system of "cold" remedies against "hot" diseases and vice versa.

However, it was in anatomy and physiology that Galen was best known. From his dissections of pigs and apes — dissection of humans were illegal then — Galen gave to medicine a knowledge of bones and muscles that the world had never known before. He gave an anatomical description of the brain, and demonstrated the functions of the recurrent nerves, the medulla and the arteries.

The Middle Age

Galen marked the zenith of Greek medicine, after which it became sterile, and the onus of medicine fell to the scholar-priests during the long Middle Age, which began with the fall of Rome in 476 CE and lasted till the 15th century.

The medical scholars were usually Christian priests cloistered in their monasteries. Illness was thought of as punishment for sin, possession by the devil, or the effect of witchcraft. The chief therapeutics were prayers, repentance and invocations of the saints. Cures were often regarded as miracles. The cult of saint-therapy developed, with the practice of entreating specific saints to aid in curing specific diseases. For example, St Erasmus was invoked for the disease of the abdomen, St Blaisius for lungs and throats, and St Vitus for twitching.

The main medical activities of these priests, however, were not in clinical practices but in writing medical texts inside the monasteries. Undoubtedly their medical writings were to a large extent colored by philosophy and religion; at best, they were reproductions of classical Greek authorities. The best known of such center of medical composition was Monte Cassino, where medical knowledge written in Arabic was translated into Latin.

Besides these Christian medical writers, the Arab scholars also held great medical influence. These Arab scholars wrote not in monasteries but in the newly founded universities, the most important of which was at Salerno, the first organized medical school in Europe. A great writer was a Persian named Avicenna (980 - 1037), whose chief work "The Canon of Medicine" remained the authoritative textbook for many centuries. Avicenna derived much from Chinese sources, as in pulse theory and the rich Chinese materia medica. As both Christian and Muslim beliefs forbade the shedding of blood, surgery dropped to its lowest ebb in this period.

Although the Middle Age was also the Dark Age of medicine, this period was not without its contributions. The Arabs greatly enriched medicine with their materia medica and their knowledge of chemistry. Since the initiation set by the Roman Emperor Constantine, hospitals were built on a large scale in Europe. Western medical practices were first legislated in 1140 by King Robert II of Sicily, making it obligatory to pass state examinations before one could practise medicine. The greatest contribution of the Middle Age, however, was the preserving and transmitting of Greek medical knowledge, without which the succeeding age would have to start from scratch again. We shall read about its revival and the birth of western medicine in the next chapter.

2

THEY LET US LIVE HEALTHIER, LONGER LIVES

(Medicine from Renaissance to Modern Time)

There are no such things as incurables; there are only things for which man has not found a cure.

Bernard M. Baruch.

The Renaissance

Anyone studying the history of world medicine will be impressed by the amazing medical wisdom the ancient masters possessed. However for a thousand years, this rich medical knowledge was virtually lost to Europeans during the dark Middle Age. The first germination of what we now know as scientific western medicine only emerged after the Renaissance.

The Renaissance, which began in 1453, signalled a return of medicine to the clinic and the sick bed, no longer cloistered in monasteries nor universities. Surgery, led by outstanding surgeons like Ambroise Pare, regained its former glory. This was also the period of disease isolation: individual diseases like chickenpox, syphilis and typhus, were first described and differentiated from the vague mass of "plagues" and "fevers".

Three great figures stood out prominently in this age, namely Fracastoro, Paraceleus and Andreas Vesalius — the three figures that not only represents three distinctive advances in medicine, but also characterized three cardinal lessons in the history of medical progress.

Fracastoro (1478 - 1552) of Verona expounded the notion of contagion, attributing the cause of disease to certain imperceptible particles carried by air or by contact. Had society been more sympathetic to Fracastoro's theory then, the progress of medicine would have been brought forward by four centuries and many more lives would have been saved! Not only pioneers were seldom well received, they were often severely abused and mocked by hostile conservatism. For example, when Michael Servetus (16th century) suggested the idea of pulmonary circulation, he was burnt to death as a heretic.

To reward Pierre Brissot (18th century) for his protest against excessive bloodletting, he was ostracized and died in exile. Looking at the history of medicine, or of any science or art for that matter, a reader with feeling could not help wondering when would mankind ever learn, and why couldn't we be just a little more kind to brave men and women who dare to be advance of their times.

Yet despite such hostility, truths remained triumphant. Paraceleus (about 1490 - 1541) started his professorship at Basel by burning the works of Galen and Avicenna in public, not as a protest against these two masters although some of their beliefs were found incorrect, but against the servile attitude and passive book learning during that time. Galen and Avicenna had for centuries been held as the final authorities whom no one dared to differ. Paraceleus' search for specific remedies for specific diseases also characterized the modern practice of chemotherapy.

It was Andreas Versalius (1514 - 1564) who broke the Avicenna tradition of book learning, and showed that even Galen was not the ultimate achievement in anatomy. His momentous work "On the Fabric of Human Body" illuminated many of Galen's errors like the five-lobed liver and the horned uterus, and laid the foundation for modern anatomy. Versalius's outstanding examples of abandoning speculation and replacing it by direct observation at the dissection table, dealt a final blow to bookish conservatism and placed medicine firmly on a progressive scientific basis.

The 17th and 18th Centuries

The scientific spirit began to bear fruit in the 17th and 18th centuries. With the discovery of the compound microscope, a new world of micro-organisms was open to mankind. For the first time, man could study disease-causing agents accurately from direct observation, rather than depended on speculation.

This was soon followed by the discovery of blood circulation by William Harvey (1578 - 1657), who published his "Movement of the Heart" in 1628. His work also illustrated significantly that his momentous discovery was the result of objective experiments, not of imaginative speculation. Harvey's discovery promptly initiated two important ideas, that of medicinal injection and of blood transfusion, which, however, were practiced successfully only later when certain complications like embolism and blood groups were overcome.

Other great accomplishments in the 17th century include the discoveries of ducts and glands, of the lymphatic system, of the sweetness of diabetic urine, of hysteria as a disease of the nervous system, and of brain haemorrhage as the cause of strokes. The physiology of respiration, digestion and nervous system became known. New fields in occupational ailments, tropical diseases, surgical pathology and obstetrics developed.

There were also some exotic attempts to search for a comprehensive system for all medical problems. The iatrophysicists regarded the human body as a machine, whereas the iatrochemists viewed life as a series of chemical processes. These attempts were not successful, and soon doctors returned to the ancient Hippocratic system of clinical observation, strongly advocated by Thomas Sydenham (1624 - 1689) who was aptly called the English Hippocrates.

Despite the outstanding achievements of this century, many peculiar practices were still rampant. Many people believed in the magnetic cures of Great-rake, the astrological medicine of Culpeper, and the sympathetic powder of Digby who claimed to cure wounds by placing the powder on the causative weapons. The cult of scrofulosis — mass healing by the touch of kings — was prevalent.

The search for a comprehensive system continued in the 18th century. Some viewed the body as a hydraulic machine, some considered a "nervous force" as the cause of disease, and others attributed illness to either under stimulation or over stimulation. The major therapeutic methods of this century, however, still consisted of excessive bloodletting, large doses of toxic drugs, induced vomiting and purging. Nevertheless eminent progress was also made.

Many new diseases like diphtheria, typhoid and pellagra were identified. With the publication of his work at the age of seventy nine, "On the Sites and Causes of Diseases", Giovanni Morgagni (1682 - 1771) established the science of modern pathology. The emphasis on the explanation of disease now shifted from deliberations on general conditions and humors to the study of localized changes in the organs.

One of the greatest medical scientists of the age was Lazaro Spallanzani (1729 - 1799). He swallowed a packet of food with a long string attached to it, and pulled out the food from his stomach for close study after every short intervals. He did this continually, not for a few days, but for many years! Spallanzani also practiced artificial insemination in animals, and illuminated the spectacle of tissue respiration.

Smallpox was a widespread killer especially among children. It was only in this century that Edward Jenner (1749-1823) demonstrated vaccination against smallpox, a method that had been practiced in China for many centuries. Meanwhile the new philosophy of Enlightenment helped to disperse superstitions, and mental patients were no longer considered possessed by the devil. The changing attitude was dramatized by Phillippe Pinel (1755 - 1826) when he liberated insane patients from their fetters and chains.

One controversial figure was Franz Anton Mesmer (1734 - 1815), who expounded a therapy using what he called "animal magnetism". Mesmer was previously a successful physician using orthodox methods; he was even more successful when he changed to his "magnetic" method, and his clients included nobility. Mesmer's therapy was in fact similar to the Chinese esoteric art of energy channelling. Yet he was severely attacked — mainly by other jealous physicians — not for his practice, which was undoubtedly successful, but for his theory.

Mesmerism later developed into medical hypnotism, which also had a very rough start. Much later, in 1829, when Cloquet reported to his medical academy about his use of hypnotism as the only means to induce anaesthesia in a successful operation to remove breast tumour, the academy was either naive enough or ridiculous enough to suggest that his patient was pretending to feel no pain! When great doctors like John Elliotson (who introduced the stethoscope into Britain) and James Esdaile (who performed more than 300 major operations in India using hypnotism as anaesthesia) reported the successful use of hypnotism in the 1840s, they were regarded as quacks and impostors!

The 19th Century

The 19th century was an eventful one with outstanding accomplishments in many fields like histology, epidemiology, endocrinology and pharmacology — accomplishments that set the pattern of present day clinical medicine. The pathological emphasis shifted from particular organs to particular tissues, which became the basic unit in physiology. The fundamental biological theory that the cell is the basic unit of all life, also originated in this century. This cellular theory, together with localistic pathology, marked the end of traditional humorism.

The two greatest achievements of the 19th century were made in bacteriology and surgery. Bacteria were first seen by Anton Von Leeuwenkoek (1632 - 1723) in the previous century, but bacteriology as a definite science was established by Louis Pasteur (1822 - 1895), who demonstrated that fermentation was the work of micro-organisms. Pasteur's greatness was enhanced by the fact that he was not a medical man by profession, but a chemist who set an unprecedented trend in medical matters amidst traditionally conservative scepticism.

The greatness of Ignaz Semmelweis (1818 - 1865), however, was tragic, even though his discovery was equally significant. One of the most fearful dangers at the surgeon's table during that time was not technical shortcomings of the operation itself, but infection caused by contamination. It is sad to reflect that surgery at ancient times, as shown in the previous chapter, was much safer than that in the 19th century. Semmelweis was shocked at the high mortality rate at the Vienna University obstetric clinic, and after careful study, he concluded that it was primarily caused by contaminated hands of doctors and medical students coming from autopsy rooms. His recommendation of routine hand-washing with chlorine solution vastly reduced the mortality rate. Semmelweis attempted to spread his life-saving discovery, but was ignored. Meanwhile thousands of people died unnecessarily because of stubborn conservatism. In his frantic and angry effort to save lives, Semmelweis was sneered and ridiculed by such hostile opposition that he became mad and died at a comparatively young age in an asylum.

But truth and goodness always triumphed. Struck by the big difference in mortality rate between simple and compound fractures, Joseph Listen (1827 - 1912) protected open wounds with carbolic acid. This principle of antiseptic was soon extended to all fields of surgery. After hearing the tragedy of Semmelweis' heroic fight, the great Lister generously accredited the honor of founding asepsis to Semmelweis.

Such selfless generosity, however, was not the salient quality of the founders of western anaesthesia. There was bitter controversy over who the actual founder was. Ether's role in surgery was confirmed in a famous trial operation in Massachusetts General Hospital in 1846. Chloroform was introduced the following year. But actually anaesthesia had been successfully used by surgeons since ancient times.

With the successful application of asepsis and anaesthesia, surgery rose to greater heights. Areas that were previously considered forbidden because of great risks, such as the abdomen, the head and the vertebral column (yet the ancients operated quite successfully on them), were now open to surgeons. Operations on the gall-bladder, the appendix, the kidney, the ovary and on tumours of the brain and of the spinal cord were soon accomplished.

Many new specialities like paediatrics, obstetrics, gynaecology, orthopaedics and ophthalmology were established. Neurology developed into an independent speciality. Later, as many widespread mental diseases provided no anatomical or physiological symptoms, psychiatry branched out as a separate science. The psychiatrist who expounded psychoanalysis was Sigmund Freud (1856 -1939), who regarded sexual repression as the central theme of psycho-pathology. However, the effectiveness and even the validity of Freud's method are now being questioned; and many psychotherapists nowadays prefer the behavioral or the humanistic approaches.

Much progress was also made in public health and preventive medicine, especially after epidemics of cholera, malaria and tuberculosis swept Europe sparring neither rich nor poor. The leading force for the new sanitary movements against over-crowded housing, bad sewage system, polluted water as well as child labor, was stimulated not by a medical man, but by a lawyer, Edwin Chadwick (1800 - 1890), who probably saved more lives with his sanitary proposals, than the total medicine of all the physicians of his time put together. Nursing, which was previously carried out by compassionate nuns or uneducated helpers became systematic and respectable after the admirable efforts of Florence Nightingale (1823 - 1910).

The 20th Century

Five major trends are noticeable in the 20th century, namely chemotherapy, immunology, endocrinology, nutrition and geriatrics. Chemotherapy, or the application of specific chemical drugs to known diseases, is perhaps the most remarkable medical development of this century. It was inaugurated by Paul Ehrlich (1854 - 1915) when he found a chemical compound for treating syphilis.

Soon sulfonamide, penicillin, streptomycin and other antibiotics were discovered.

While chemotherapy provided effective cures for many diseases, immunology helps to prevent them from occurring. After the discovery of viruses in the 1930s, the scope of immunology was extended to many viral diseases like yellow fever, influenza and poliomyelitis.

The most significant accomplishment in endocrinology was the discovery of insulin in 1921, which gave new hopes to diabetes patients. Earlier in 1902 Ernest Sterling (1866 - 1927) discovered the internal secretions of endocrine glands. These secretions he called "hormones", which, he theorized, controlled the physiological actions of our bodies; and this theory revived humoral pathology which was replaced by localistic pathology in the previous century.

As medicine progressed tremendously, its main purpose in the 20th century changed from saving lives to keeping fit. Nutrition, therefore, gained unprecedented importance. A definite direction was made in the last century when Justus Von Liebig (1803 -1873) classified basic foodstuff into proteins, fats and carbohydrates. A notable advance in this century was the discovery of vitamins, which helped to cure diseases like rickets, scurvy and beriberi.

The term "geriatrics" was first used in this century, although medicine of old age had been practiced since ancient time. The two major areas of geriatrics are cardiovascular diseases and cancer, the two top killers in the west today — even surpassing motor accidents.

The cause of cancer is not fully understood yet, and the three standard therapeutic methods are still chemotherapy, surgery and radiotherapy. At present much research work on cancer is being carried out, and we can be confident that soon this killer disease, like other killer diseases before it such as tuberculosis, cholera and diphtheria, will be conquered by man.

Actually many cases of cancer have been cured by unorthodox means, such as meditation and faith healing, both in the west and in the east. Personally, I have helped numerous patients to be relieved of their cancer through practicing qigong, an ancient Chinese art of energy development that has tremendous therapeutic value.

While cardiovascular diseases have caused much trouble to medical circles in the west, the preventive as well as curative methods of cardiovascular diseases have been practiced successfully for a long time in China in the form of qigong! The "Five-Animal Play" of Hua Tuo, the "Eight Embroidery Exercises" of the Taoist hermits, the pugilistic arts of Shaolin Kungfu and the calisthenics of Taijiquan, all have beneficial effects in preventing or curing cardiovascular diseases. Such successes are not just documented in classical Chinese texts, but are also real experiences of many cardiovascular patients who learnt qigong from me.

The growing dissatisfaction with conventional medicine in dealing with cardiovascular and many other ailments caused many people in the west to seek alternative therapies, such as naturopathy, homeopathy, acupuncture, chiropractic, shiatsu, reflexology and herbal medicine. Some of these alternative therapies, like acupuncture and herbal medicine, are actually conventional medicine in many eastern societies, and have been successfully practiced for ages. Andrew Stanway, a doctor turned writer, expressed the problem succinctly: "People have always wanted alternative forms of medical therapy to those which are readily available but today in the West the need is apparently greater than ever. . . . while we have almost eradicated infectious illnesses of childhood and adulthood, we have not succeeded in preventing degenerative processes and malignant growth, the two most common diseases of mid-life and old age."

Such statements are, of course, made in good faith. No conventional doctors should ever feel slighted. Nobody can deny that conventional western medicine has contributed greatly to the welfare of mankind. On the other hand, alternative therapies certainly have a lot to offer; and to deride them prior to any serious investigation, especially when there is much evidence to show that these alternative therapies work, is a clear sign of one's insecurity.

Happily many people in the west now favor alternative or complementary medicine. Fulder reported that according to a Gallup poll in 1985, 78% of the British population wanted complementary practitioners to be state registered. The trend is even more pronounced in other European countries. "A survey of GPs in the county of Avon found that no less than three-quarters referred patients to therapists. Above half of the 145 doctors wanted complementary medicine on the NHS and more than half felt that acupuncture and hypnosis were useful or very useful. Why are GPs *en masse* doing something that would be unthinkable 15 years ago? What made them change their minds? The answer, according to the Avon study, and as reported in *The Times* on 13 March 1985, is simple: the doctors themselves are receiving treatment from complementary practitioners, and they liked it."

Recently there is a frightening threat from AIDS, or acquired immune deficiency syndrome, which at present is incurable and fatal. But research has given us some glimpses of hope. Our hope to combat and eventually conquer AIDS will be much enhanced if we will also systematically look into the possibility of cure in alternative medicine. In theory, qigong is an effective means to counter AIDS, because qigong, as an art to develop our own intrinsic energy, is excellent in promoting immunity. In this connection it is useful to remind ourselves that many great discoveries, in medicine as well as in other fields, started as theories.

The history of medicine is a long, interesting one, illuminating man's various ideas of sickness and remedies through the ages. The next time our doctor prescribes a pill or any therapeutic methods, we know it represents some thousands of years of medical thoughts and experiments.

More importantly, history shows that the untiring efforts of great men and women, medical and otherwise, whose courage and devotion not only free us from many deadly diseases, but also make it possible for us to live healthier, longer lives. We cannot help but feel grateful; and the moral strength we derive from their greatness makes us feel inspired to emulate them, to build on the priceless foundation they bequeath us, so that we too will leave to our children an even healthier and brighter world. It is with such inspiration that I write this book to share the invaluable medical knowledge successfully practiced by the Chinese for many millennia, with the hope that great men and women will make further research into this knowledge. If only just one of the many medical facts in this book proves to be beneficial to mankind, then the time and effort spent in this sincere attempt will be amply rewarded.

3

FROM ACUPUNCTURE TO BODHIDHARMA

(History of Chinese Medicine to Tang Dynasty)

The system of healing whose theoretical principles transferred the socio-political conceptions of Confucianism to the medical sphere rested on a syncretic doctrine that was influenced, as already indicated, by concepts of demonic medicine, the theories of yin-yang and the Five Phrases, homeopathic magic, concepts of finest matter influences as the basis of life, as well as by structural elements associated with the unification of the empire.

Prof. Paul Ulrich, Medicine in China, 1985.

World's Longest Successful Medical System

Because of numerous factors, like philosophical, cultural and linguistic differences, as well as semantic distortion resulting from reading translated sources, it is easy for westerners to misunderstand the principles and practice of Chinese medicine. Stephan Palos, who has studied the subject more deeply, says:

> The achievements of China's ancient culture are known to everyone. ... A wealth of experience in the art of healing, accumulated over thousands of years, has enabled her to achieve notable results in that field as well, and their importance is gaining increasing recognition from modern medical science. ... It is only during the last decade that any modern medical source material has become available in Chinese ... there are frequently very great discrepancies between the Chinese and Western sources. The Western books often quote deductions or personal opinions which may represent a revaluation rather than an interpretation of the traditional Chinese art of healing.

A sensible approach to an understanding of Chinese medicine, and hopefully to derive some benefits from it, is to refer to the Chinese masters themselves, especially to those who are able to explain Chinese medical concepts using a vocabulary and an imagery that western readers can readily comprehend. This book is a modest attempt in this direction.

It is useful to remind uninformed readers who regard Chinese medicine as superstitious quackery, that though the Chinese medical system was not the oldest, it is the longest continuous medical system known to man, and for millennia has been successfully serving the world's largest population that have enjoyed a very high level of civilization.

As you read its history in this and the next chapter, you will find out that the Chinese cured contagious diseases long before antibiotics were discovered in the west, effectively performed major surgical operations before much of Europe and all of America and Australia were known on the map, and successfully treated psychiatric illnesses long before westerners thought they were caused by evil spirits. You will also discover that many medical discoveries hailed in the west as remarkable breakthroughs had been preceded by the Chinese often by a few centuries.

The mention of these facts, of course, were never meant to belittle conventional western medicine. Numerous people, including many in the conventional medical profession itself, may have voiced their dissatisfaction with certain aspects of conventional medicine, such as its extreme reductionist approach and its inadequacy in countering degenerative diseases; but as far as I know, not a single Chinese medical practitioner nor any alternative therapist has ever derided conventional medicine, for they all appreciate its value.

It is also noteworthy that throughout its long history, Chinese medicine has been distinguishably free from any control of a priestly class. Many Chinese did, and still do, seek help from divine powers in medical matters, but such practice belongs to the realm of religion and mysticism rather than that of Chinese medicine. In fact, if we were to say that Chinese medicine is superstitious because the people of the ancient Shang Dynasty (18th-12th century BC) consulted oracles regarding their illness, then western medicine would be more so, for the standard modes of therapeutics in the west were prayers, repentance and invocation during the Middle Age, or at best bleeding and cupping to let out evil blood as recently as the 19th century!

We need to be careful if we condescend to regard the ancient Chinese, or the ancient Egyptians, Mesopotamian, Indians, Greeks or Romans, as superstitious, because the ignorant party may turn out to be ourselves, as latest findings in physics, psychology and other sciences suggest that the divination and other metaphysical practices of these ancient peoples were actually means to tap into the deeper levels of intuitive wisdom. We should remember that those ancient people who consulted oracles were often not ordinary folk, but powerful men like generals and emperors, who were always advised by the wisest men of the time.

Another unique feature of Chinese medical history is its consistency of principal medical thinking throughout the ages. There have been no drastic, revolutionary changes in the philosophical, pathological or therapeutical aspects in Chinese medicine since ancient time till now! Whereas the notions of diseases caused by micro-organisms and of chemotherapy in this twentieth century are so drastically different from the notions of humours and of bleeding and cupping in the early phase of western medicine, the principles of yin-yang and of various therapeutic methods of the Chinese are practiced now as much the same way as before.

This does not mean that Chinese medicine does not progress or stagnant in thinking. On the contrary, medical progress and conceptual development have been remarkable, with many discoveries and theories well in advance of the west.

Prehistoric Medicine

The Chinese have the longest continuous history of medicine in the world. At least 500,000 years ago, men existed at the Hwang Ho Valley in China, and they have been existing continuously to the present day. As soon as there were people, there was medicine. Prehistoric medicine in China was of an amazingly high standard. Not only did the earliest Chinese established an extensive herb lore, they also accomplished much in surgery and acupuncture. It is not a comforting thought to reflect that only in this modern age, many thousand years after its successful application in China, the western world in general appreciates the effectiveness of acupuncture.

Archaeological findings in China revealed a vast number of expertly made bamboo and stone needles used for acupuncture, showing its widespread practice during prehistoric time. Another special and very effective aspect of Chinese medicine practiced by the prehistoric Chinese was qigong (chi kung) therapy, where qi (chi) or bio-energy is used to cure illnesses.

Though qigong is still comparatively unknown to the west, paradoxically it is probably the best aspect of Chinese medicine today that will help westerners to solve many of their health problems.

Some people thought that the two early emperors in Chinese prehistory, Shen Nong and Huang Di (or Hwang Ti), were the founders of Chinese medicine, and the authorship of the earliest Chinese texts on pharmacology and medicine — Ben Cao Jing (Great Herbal Classic) and Nei Jing (the Inner Classic of Medicine) — were often accredited to them respectively. Actually their names are only the personified representation of the collective effort of the whole prehistoric society.

Xia and Shang Dynasties

The beginning of the dynastic period of China with the Dynasties of Xia

(2205-1765 BC) and Shang (1766-1121 BC) marked the beginning of Chinese written history. Supernaturalism became rampant in this period, and medicine too became interwoven into the supernaturalistic patterns of the time.

But it is important to note that Chinese medicine since its beginning and throughout its history, is rational and scientific; and that this short, isolated stage of supernaturalistic influence during the Shang period was the outcome of its environmental consequences, not of its innate medical principles. Notwithstanding this, medical knowledge during the Shang period was of a surprisingly high standard.

By this time, Shang writing had been well developed, and its vocabulary showed the Chinese had such depth of medical knowledge as there are words during that period that means micro-organisms in the blood and parasites in the intestines! For example, the Shang word 蟲 (which is written 蟲 in modern Chinese) means micro-organisms in the blood. At a time thousands of years before the appearance of the microscope, such discoveries were certainly astonishing.

The early Chinese had high standards of personal hygiene and public health. The word 浴 (浴 in modern Chinese), which represents a person washing in a basin, means "having a bath"; and 牢 (牢), which means a sty or pen, shows their understanding of the need to separate their living quarters from that of their domesticated animals.

The Classical Age of Zhou

The succeeding Zhou Dynasty (1027-256 BC), often known as the classical age, witnessed the emergence of numerous schools of thoughts, including the philosophy of yin-yang and the five elemental processes. Many philosophical terms were adopted into Chinese medicine to represent certain medical concepts. The perfection of the lunar calendar enabled Chinese physicians to associate particular diseases to specific seasons; and they named six climatic conditions — cold, heat, wind, rain, dampness and sun — as the natural causes of diseases.

Personal hygiene and public health continued to be of high standard in the Zhou Dynasty. "The Rites of Zhou" mentioned many methods of destroying pests, and "The Book of Rites" recommended regular bathing, washing hands before meals, and forbade spitting on the floor. This book also recorded the classification of medical officers in this period into four groups, namely general physicians, surgeons, dieticians and veterinarians. This practice was several centuries ahead of the west.

During this time the two earliest and most revered Chinese medical classics appeared. They were *Huang Di Nei Jing* (the Inner Classic of Medicine of Hwang Ti) and *Shen Nong Ben Cao Jing* (the Great Herbal Classic of Shen Nong).

Actually, they were not written by an individual, but were the results of professional collections of all previous medical knowledge achieved by countless, nameless people since the beginning of man's existence in China. In their present revised editions, these two classics also contain medical achievements made in the later Qin and Han periods.

The Inner Classic of Medicine covers all fields of Chinese medicine, ranging from medical philosophy and ecology to therapeutic principles and acupuncture. Hence, it is a mistake, I believe, to translate the Nei Jing as the Classic of Inner Medicine, as is commonly done, because inner medicine is only one part of this extensive work.

It is startling that this Inner Classic recorded many medical facts that were discovered by the west only very much later. One notable example is its description of blood flow in the human body in an never-ending circle — a discovery at least 2500 years before William Harvey.

The Inner Classic is even more explicit. It described two different types of blood, the dark-colored yin blood, and the bright-colored yang blood. Another remarkable precedence over the west is the implication of the role autonomic nerves play in causing illnesses, and expressed the need to balance of yin-yang. This principle helped Chinese therapists cure many so-called incurable degenerative diseases.

The Great Herbal Classic, which provided the fundamentals of Chinese pharmacology, is probably the oldest pharmacopeia in the world, and has been continually revised and used until now! It described in detail 365 natural drugs, classified into three categories: the top category of 120 drugs of nourishing qualities, the middle category of 120 drugs of general therapeutic values, and the lowest category of 125 antitoxins and antibiotics.

The classic also discussed the four classes, five tastes and seven groups of medical drugs, and included valuable advice on drug collection, preparation and preservation. It prescribed 170 types of remedies for sickness that included internal medicine, surgery, gynaecology, ophthalmology and otology, and their therapeutic values have been found valid by modern science today.

One of the greatest physicians during this period was Bian Que (or Pien Chueh), who lived in the 5th century BC, probably a contemporary of Hippocrates. He excelled in many fields, like pulse theory, herbal therapy, acupuncture and massage therapy. One day as he was passing through the state of Fu, he cured the dying prince of a strange disease. The astonished public regarded Bian Que as a saint with miraculous powers, but the modest physician explained emphatically that it was rational medicine that cured the prince. His great work was "The Eighty One Difficult Topics of Hwang Ti", a treatise on diagnosis, anatomy and acupuncture.

Another great work of this period was "The Classic of Elixir" by a Taoist hermit, Wei Po Yang. Outwardly it resembles a book on alchemy, but actually it is a secret text written in symbolic language on qigong for health and longevity. The Taoists contributed greatly to preventive medicine, which the Chinese have always considered as superior to healing.

The Golden Age of the Han and the Tang

During the time of the Han (202 BC-AD 221) and the Tang (618-906), Chinese medicine reached its golden age, heralded in by two outstanding physicians, Hua Tuo and Zhang Zhong Jing, who were contemporaries of Galen.

Hua Tuo (c208-118 B.C.) was probably the first person known in the world to apply anaesthesia in surgery, about 2000 years ahead of the west! He is often depicted in a painting where he scraped the shoulder blade of Guan Yu, a renowned Chinese warrior who was later worshipped as the God of War, to remove infected flesh caused by a poisoned arrow, while Guan Yu played chess with a friend.

This picture was meant to demonstrate the bravery and stoic endurance of the warrior; but anyone who has experienced even a minor cut will know how painful it is! People now believe that the truth was Hua Tuo's effective application of anaesthetics. The Chronicle of Later Han also recorded that Hua Tuo successfully performed abdominal operations.

Hua Tuo was an exemplary doctor. The Lord of Wei, Cao Cao, offered him abundant gold to be his personal court physician, but Hua Tuo refused so that he could serve the common people. Later when he heard of Cao Cao's peculiar headache, he volunteered to attend to the lord without fees. Hua Tuo, whose thoughts and accomplishments were advanced of his time, suggested cranial surgery, but the suspicious Cao Cao, mistaking that Hua Tuo wanted to harm him, put the great physician in prison.

Hua Tuo also emphasized the indisputable importance of preventive medicine and health science. He devised a system of qigong exercises called "Five-Animal Play" which expresses the movements and spirit of the tiger, deer, bear, monkey and bird. His disciples who practiced these exercises daily, not only lived to ninety, but their teeth were strong and their senses keen even at old age.

Zhang Zhong Jing (150-219 B.C.), sometimes known in the west as the Eastern Hippocrates, insisted that illnesses are caused by natural, and not supernatural, agents. During his time an epidemic took away a high portion of the Han population. The people then resorted to superstition rather than rational medicine in their desperate attempt to fight the disease. Against such conservative background, Zhang Zhong Jing tirelessly strove to save lives and to educate the people in medical and hygiene matters.

His influential work was *Shang Han Za Bing Lun* (the Treatises of Epidemic

Colds and Fevers), which is China's first medical textbook based on actual application, not speculation, of medical theories. Zhang Zhong Jing formulated the Six Syndromes based on yin and yang as basic principles to explain infectious diseases. This concept is still being used today. He also wrote other treatises, including those on artificial respiration and women's diseases.

Many westerners are often bewildered by pulse diagnosis. One of the greatest texts on the pulse, *Mai Jing* (Pulse Classic), was written by Wang Shu He in the third century. He differentiated twenty four kinds of pulse and their significance. About the same time, the first book that specialized on acupuncture, "Fundamentals of Acupuncture", was written by Wang Po Yi.

The study of pathology was also prominent. At the end of the Six Dynasties period about the beginning of the 7th century, the Imperial Medical Professor, Chao Yuan Feng, and his colleagues edited the momentous "Pathology of Diseases" in fifty volumes. This huge collection discussed the pathology, symptoms, diagnosis and therapeutics of 1700 different types of diseases, which included internal medicine, surgery, gynaecology, paediatrics and medicine of the sense organs.

It pointed out that parasites and other micro-organisms are responsible for contagious diseases, that other diseases are not contagious, and that particular skin diseases are the result of certain deficiency in one's diet. It is amazing how much the Chinese were ahead of the west in such knowledge. But the most extraordinary thing is that the remedies he recommended in this great work to cure diseases were not in the form of medicinal herbs as was the practice, but in the form of qigong therapy exercises!

The Chinese were also the first to produce a governmental pharmacopeia. Commissioned by the Tang government, a group of dedicated physicians led by Su Jing edited fifty four volumes of the "New Herbal Pharmacopeia" in 657 — more than eight centuries before the Florentine Nuovo Receptaris, which is the first western pharmacopeia! Seventy years after its publication it spread to Japan, where the Japanese emperor decreed that no physician would be allowed to practice medicine if he had not thoroughly studied this pharmacopeia.

Surgery reached an exceedingly high level during the Tang Dynasty. "Magical Inherited Formulae" by Gong Qing Xuan, despite its supernaturalistic name, provided many rational and effective methods as remedies for gangrene and various skin diseases, stoppage of bleeding and elimination of pain, treatment for shock and detoxification of poisons. It is probably the world's earliest book that specializes on surgery.

Another great work from the Tang Dynasty that can easily be mistaken by the uninitiated as mystical medicine, was "Therapy for Injuries and Fractures as Taught by the Saints" by the Taoist Priest Lin. Despite its mention of "saints", this classic did not resort to religion nor supernaturalism, but dealt with injuries and fractures in rational, scientific ways.

It emphasized the constant movement of joints as precaution against stiffness after treatment, recommended the use of splints for immobilization *only* if necessary, and insisted on the thorough washing of open wounds before stitching to prevent infection. All these important measures were realized in the west only very much later.

Dentistry and ophthalmology also developed into specialities with outstanding achievements. The Tang dentists already accomplished remarkable results in the extraction and filling of teeth. In ophthalmology, it is awe-inspiring to learn that more than a thousand years ago, the Chinese already performed successful operations on the eyes to extract excessive fluid!

To maintain the high level of medicine, the Tang government established the Imperial School of Medicine, which was earlier than the first medical school of the west at Salerno by two hundred years. There were three major faculties with professional chairs: internal medicine, acupuncture and surgery (including massage therapy). There were also provincial schools following the same model. Nevertheless, the common mode of medical training and teaching was still the age-old master-disciple system.

It was during the Han and Tang Dynasties that Chinese medicine spread to other countries on a large scale. Chinese medical influence on Japan had been constant and significant. The Japanese emperors sent their royal physicians to China to study, while many Chinese physicians also went to Japan to teach. One outstanding example was the Buddhist Monk Jian Zhen who not only taught Chinese medicine but also spread Buddhism to Japan. His wooden statue is now kept in the Tokyo Museum as a national treasure.

The spread of Chinese medicine to Chosen (Korea) and Vietnam was just as significant. Principal Chinese medical classics, like Inner Classic, Great Herbal Classic, and Fundamentals of Acupuncture, were indispensable, authoritative texts in Chosen. In Vietnam, a noted Chinese physician named Shen Guang Xun employed Chinese therapeutic methods to cure countless Vietnamese of a chronic chest disease. Chinese medicine spread as far as India and the Arabic Empire. Chinese materia medica like dang gui (Radix Angelicae Sinesis), fu ling (Poria cocos), wu tou (Radix Aconiti), ma huang (Herba Ephedrae) and xi xin (Herba Asari) were adopted in India. The Arabs benefited much from Chinese pulse theory, alchemy and also materia medica. It was the Arabs who later transmitted alchemy into Europe in the eighth century.

On the other hand, the Chinese also learnt much from other countries. From Chosen, the Chinese acquired many herbs like wu wei zi (Fructus Schisandrae), ting hu su (Corydalis), kun bu (Thallus Laminariae seu Eckloniae) and wu yi (Macrocarpa); from Vietnam, ding xiang (Flos Syzygii Aromatici), chen xiang (Lignum Aquilariae Resinatum) and su he xiang (Resina Liquid-ambaris Orientalis); and from the Arabic Empire, mo yao (Resina Commiphorae Myrrhae), ru xiang (Resina Pistacia) and xue jie (Resina Draconis). Indian contribution to

China was closely related with Buddhism. Indian influence in ophthalmology was also substantial.

In 527 an Indian patriarch, the Venerable Bodhidharma, went to China to teach Buddhism. At the famous Shaolin Monastery he devised a system of exercise known as Eighteen Lohan Hands, which later developed into Shaolin Kungfu, a highly esteemed system of martial arts. Bodhidharma also introduced the Meditation School of Buddhism, or Chan Buddhism, which later spread to Japan and the world as Zen Buddhism.

Buddhist meditation has contributed greatly to preventive medicine, as well as to many alternative healing systems which have helped to cure numerous diseases regarded as incurable by conventional western medicine.

Chinese medicine, therefore, has a history of outstanding achievements. It learnt and benefited from other medical systems as well, and its influence was felt not only in neighbouring Korea and Japan, but as far as the Arabic lands and Europe. Why, then, is Chinese medicine still comparatively unknown in the twenty first century? This is because it also underwent a dark age, albeit a very short one, and is now experiencing a renaissance.

We shall read about this dark age and renaissance in the next chapter, as well as other startling accomplishments so that we can have some historical perspective when we study its fascinating principles and practices, which are so different form those of conventional western medicine, and which may provide alternative ways of thinking leading to solving present medical problems.

INSPIRATION AND HOPE FROM CHINESE MASTERS

(Chinese Medicine Since the Song Dynasty)

The Chinese anticipated modern biochemistry to such an extent that by the second century BC they were isolating sex and pituitary hormones from human urine and using them for medicinal purposes.
Robert Temple.

Medical Achievements Anticipating the West

Chinese medicine is the longest continuous medical system known to man. By the end of the Tang Dynasty in the 10th century, five centuries before the birth of western medicine, the Chinese had already developed a highly comprehensive body of medical knowledge and methods, many of which were far in advance of the west, as discussed in the previous chapter.

The succeeding Song (960-1279) and Yuan (1280-1368) Dynasties witnessed continued medical achievements. In 1026 Wang Wei Yi published his "Illustrated Classic of Bronze Statue Acupuncture" in three volumes. He also made two bronze statues of the human body expertly perforated with acupuncture points. Later many replicas were made. One of the original statue is now kept in a special underground chamber in Tokyo Museum.

Chinese orthopaedics is undoubtedly one of the best in the world. In the 14th century Wei Yi Lin mentioned the use of man tuo luo (Datura alba) and wu tou (Radix Aconiti) as anaesthetics, a practice still successfully used by Chinese traumatologists today. He was the first to apply aerial suspension as a therapeutic means for fractures of the spine. It was only in 1927, six hundred years later, that its usefulness was first suggested in the west by Davis.

Chinese theory of pathogenesis was enriched by the addition of "Seven Emotions" and "Six Evils" as causative agents of diseases, expounded by Chen Wu Ze in the twelfth century. These concepts show that the Chinese clearly knew the differences between internal causes of "emotions" and external causes of "evils". They also demonstrated the great importance the Chinese placed on psychological and environmental factors in their attempt to understand illnesses.

Another world's first by the Chinese is in forensic medicine. The earliest literature on autopsy was known as "Collection of Prison Suspects" and was published in 951. In 1247, Song Ci, a famous coroner, published his monumental "Records of Justice in Autopsy". This is the earliest comprehensive textbook on forensic medicine in the world, earlier than its western counterpart "De Morbis Veneficies" by 348 years.

It described the human anatomy accurately, gave professional accounts of postmortems, and expertly discussed the causes of death, indicating clearly the differences between murder and suicide. It is astonishingly comprehensive and professionally reliable. For example, it explained in detail how a coroner, by examining the colour, location and appearance of an injury, could tell whether a victim died from a cause directly inflicted by the murderer and with what causative agent, or from other subsequent causes indirectly affecting the victim.

Its revised edition in Japan was treasured not only by physicians, but also by samurai warriors, as it gave detailed descriptions of various death spots in the human body. This authoritative forensic medical text has been translated into Japanese, Korean, Russian, English, German, French, Dutch and other languages.

Long before tuberculosis held sway as a dreadful killer in the west, the Chinese had already found effective methods to control and cure the disease! The classic known as the "Ten Marvellous Cures", that specializes on tuberculosis, and which was published in 1348, recommended ten groups of tuberculosis therapeutics, like remedies for coughing and blood vomiting, and corrective diets to strengthen the body's resistance. Later in the Qing Dynasty a great physician Ye Tian Si applied these therapeutics to cure countless tuberculosis patients.

It is a disturbing thought to reflect that, had there been greater inter-change of medical knowledge between China and the west, this dreadful disease usually associated with poverty and slums, would not be a killer in Europe and in Asian countries that were under European rule as recent as the beginning of the twentieth century! Yet, as we move into the twenty first century, at a time we think western medicine has conquered tuberculosis, it is making a comeback, not only in developing countries but in advanced countries like the United States, with apparent immunity to orthodox antibiotics.

The World Health Organization reported that eight million people are infected by tuberculosis each year, out of which three million will die! Will western experts care to learn something from the Chinese to save lives? Or can people be so conceited that they always consider other medical systems inferior or suspect, despite massive evidence of their effectiveness?

Benefiting from Their Experience

Chinese medicine is even more beneficial in the area of degenerative diseases, the major medical problem in the west today. Some Chinese therapeutic methods, especially qigong therapy, have been successfully applied to degenerative diseases for ages; and this book will explain their principles and practices. Whether the west or any other people wish to use these proven methods to free themselves of degenerative diseases, or choose to bear them with conventional supportive medication, will of course be their own prerogative.

Chinese gynaecology and paediatrics also attained remarkably high standards. Perhaps the most influential book on women's medical problems was "Women's Medical Encyclopaedia" by Chen Zi Ming in 1237, which dealt with gynaecology as well as obstetrics. Amongst the striking accomplishments mentioned in "Canon of Children's Health" published in 1224, were descriptions of examining finger lines as a diagnostic method, and surgical operations to correct infant deformities.

Only in 1981, the western pioneer in this field, Dr James Miller of the Children's Hospital in Vancouver, Canada recommended that a fingerprint examination should be part of every child's routine medical examination because the information revealed by the hand may be critical in diagnosing physical and mental abnormality.

The Song period was also characterized by scholarly disputes among various schools of thoughts. There were four representative schools: cold remedies school, purgative school, nutrition school, and yin-nourishment school. They all agreed on basic medical philosophy; their difference was their emphasis on therapeutic approaches in internal medicine.

It is worthy of note that physicians of one school would not hesitate to use methods of another school if they found the methods appropriate in specific situations. The prominent principles of these contending schools have been found accurate by modern knowledge, and are still practised by Chinese doctors today. A rough analogy of the emphasis of the above schools in modern western terms is treatment by antibiotics, by naturopathic means, by food supplement, and by physiological strengthening.

The Song government regarded medicine as an essential aspect of its duties to the people. In 1057 the government set up an Imperial Medical Editing Center to revise and publish previous as well as new medical literature. In 1076 the Imperial Dispensary was set up to facilitate the preparation and distribution of medicines, and later Provincial Dispensaries were established. The Imperial University of Medicine was greatly expanded from three faculties to thirteen faculties, which included obstetrics, paediatrics, orthopaedics and ophthalmology.

Today anyone investigating into the medical systems of the Song and the Yuan must be impressed by the high "modern" standards of that period. At a time when Europe was being plundered by barbarians, the Chinese were enjoying such enviable health measures as efficient sewage and drainage systems, appropriate sanitation, and government street sweepers!

Numerous books from this period gave evidence of sound knowledge in respect of personal health. The "Essential Knowledge for Children", for example, mentioned the necessity of brushing teeth before and after meals, washing hands after toilet, and regular changing of clothing to check lice and bugs. The "Economic Manual" mentioned the importance of regular meals, the dangers of under as well as over eating, and the prevention of water contamination.

The records of prevalent hand diseases among miners, eye diseases among furnace attendants, and lung diseases among quarry workers, in the book "General Talks" are evident of their profound understanding of occupational medicine. It was also in the Song Dynasty at the beginning of the eleventh century that the Chinese discovered immunization against smallpox; only much later did this method spread to the west.

Chinese medical principles and practices continued to spread to other countries. Since 1103, imperial physicians from China were sent to Chosen to teach medicine at the request of the Chosen government. In return the Chinese learnt from Chosen important herbs like the wondrous Panax gingseng.

Chinese medical influence in the Arab world could be reflected in such works as Avicenna's "Canon of Medicine". During the Yuan period, acupuncture spread to the Arab world. Marco Polo in his "Travels" recorded that Chinese vessels carried Chinese medicine like da huang (Radix et Rhizoma Rhei), she xiang (Moschus moschi-ferus), and rou gui (Cortex Cinnamomi) from the Malabar coast to Aden, from where they were transported to Alexandria. The Arab, on the other hand, made valuable contribution to Chinese medicine. Many Arabic medical textbooks were translated into Chinese, resulting in a further enrichment of medical knowledge. ·

The Modern Period

During the Ming and early Qing period, 1368-1840, many outstanding medical works were published. "Medical Case Histories" (1549), the earliest book of its kind, reviewed 2000 years of curing and preventing diseases from the Han to the Yuan Dynasty. "The Encyclopaedia of Ancient and Modern Medicine" (1556) in 100 volumes described the thoughts and practices of all major medical schools. The "Classic of Surgery" by Chen Shi Gong in 1617, recorded all effective surgical methods from the Tang to the Ming Dynasty.

Syphilis, previously unknown in China, was brought in by foreigners through Canton. In the "The Secret Records of Syphilis", which is the first book written in Chinese that specializes on syphilis, Chen Si Cheng described various stages of the disease, and recommended the application of such drugs as pi shuang (arsenic), qing fen (calo-mel) and shui yin (mercury).

In ophthalmology, Chuan Ren Yu recorded 109 different eye diseases in his comprehensive book titled "Ophthalmology Encyclopaedia". In laryngology, the physiological, pathological and diagnostic aspects of throat diseases, including diphtheria, were explained, and many effective remedies including acupuncture and surgical operations, were recorded.

The greatest medical accomplishment during the Ming Dynasty is undoubtedly the publication of the "Great Herbal Pharmacopoeia" compiled by

Li Shi Zhen (1518-1593). To compile this monumental work, Li Shi Zhen reviewed over 800 relevant works, and travelled widely to the sources of the herbs so that he could study their habitat and properties more closely.   He interviewed countless people, including herb gatherers, farmers, fishermen and labourers, who became his friends and teachers.

Altogether he spent twenty seven years, including thoroughly rewriting his work three times, and finally in 1578 produced the finest work on Chinese pharmacology — perhaps of any pharmacology.

This masterpiece is a collection of 52 volumes which described in detail 1892 different kinds of materia medica with over 1000 illustrations and over 10,000 medical prescriptions or medicinal recipes. For each materia medica, he expertly explains its appearance, habitat, properties, collection, preparation, preservation, therapeutic values, possible effects, and relevant medical prescriptions. It has been translated into Japanese, Korean, German, French, English and many other languages. Li Shi Zhen was certainly one of the greatest medical scientists of all times.

His sincerity in serving mankind, his humility in his quest for knowledge, and his perseverance and devotion in his work, serve as an everlasting source of inspiration to all later generations.

Fevers became a speciality itself during the Ming period. The Chinese made fine distinctions between colds and fevers. In the "Recollections of Medical Classics", the author Wang Fu Dui explained that while colds derived their name from the pathological cause of the sickness, fevers derived their name from the symptoms. And whereas colds developed from external to internal in their prognosis, fevers developed from internal to external.

The Ming period was also an age where the Chinese explored overseas. Hence with many important herbs as well as ideas were exported. In the 16th century, many dispensaries in England sold Chinese tea leaves as a therapeutic agent for colds and fevers! Numerous foreign doctors arrived in China to learn medicine, and many Chinese medical books were brought back to Europe for translation. The Russians, for example, sent their doctors to China to learn immunization against small-pox. "Secrets of the Pulse" was translated by Hervien in Paris in 1735.

It was also during this period that Chinese acupuncture spread to the west. Rhyne (1684) and Kampfer (1692) were amongst the earliest to introduce acupuncture to Europe, but the initial reception was cold and met with suspicion. European knowledge of acupuncture was also inadequate, and their practice often inaccurate. Only much later, after determined effort by some brilliant French and German medical scientists, and after Morant Saulie returned from China in 1929 with genuine knowledge of Chinese acupuncture, that this useful medical practice became a significant therapeutic method in the west.

During the Qing Dynasty, Zhao Xue Min collected time-tested therapeutic methods used by travelling medicine men or barefoot doctors as they are called, and compiled them into eight volumes known as "Fine Collections" (1759). Because of environmental factors, barefoot doctors were generally illiterate, but their therapeutic methods, which had been passed down from generations by mouth, were not only effective but also economical.

The Opium War of 1824 marked the dark age not only of the Chinese dynastic history, but also of Chinese medicine. After the humiliating defeat at the hands of superior western firearms, the Chinese reverted from a close-door policy to blind worship of anything western.

Nevertheless, some outstanding works were produced, like Wang Meng Ying's "Dissertations on Fevers" (1852), Zhou Xue Hai's "Manual of Diagnosis" (1895), and He Lian Chen's "Case Histories of Famous Physicians of China" (1927). There were also many books that specialized on plague, dysentery, cholera and diphtheria.

Dark Age and Renaissance

Perhaps the greatest irony in the history of Chinese medicine was made in 1929 by the Koumintang government. The Central Committee for Health, which comprised entirely of physicians that were educated in the western tradition, recommended the abolishment of Chinese medicine in favor of western medicine!

The immediate protest from the public was vehement, and an appeal led by Chen Cun Ren caused the government to retreat its resolution; hence 17th of March is now celebrated as Chinese Medical Day. Indeed it is shuddering to think of the far-reaching consequences had the Koumintang government abolished Chinese medicine.

The medical policy of the Communist government was in direct contrast. While learning much from western medicine, the Communist government also encouraged the study and development of Chinese medicine in a progressive and scientific manner. Their success in the treatment of poliomyelitis, in attaching severed limbs, and in acupuncture anaesthesia were not only awe-inspiring, but, more importantly, promising a brighter future for the progress of Chinese medicine.

It is only in this generation, more significantly than ever before, that physicians from other countries see at first hand the successful combination of western and Chinese medicine. It is only in this generation, especially after President Nixon's historic visit to China, that acupuncture became popular world wide, and people from other countries, irrespective of race or religion, can benefit on a large scale, from the medical practice that was previously exclusively reserved for the Chinese for many millennia.

But acupuncture is only one aspect of Chinese medicine. Another noteworthy aspect, which is just beginning to emerge from behind the once secretive bamboo curtain, and which the west will certainly benefit tremendously, is qigong therapy — the ancient esoteric system that has proved effective in treating degenerative diseases.

It is indeed tempting, but justifiable, to believe that in the present century we can benefit from what ancient Chinese physicians had discovered, and that we can profitably continue to build upon and improve on their discoveries, so that we can bequeath to our children the rich medical knowledge that will enable them to live full and healthy lives. The history of Chinese medicine shows that there have been so many instances where the Chinese preceded the west in decisive discoveries.

We can rightly ask: are there other major Chinese discoveries in medicine that the west had not realized, but may be crucial to our health and well-being? Obviously, instead of groping about in haphazard experiments hoping to strike a lucky discovery that may solve pressing health problems like cancer, AIDS and degenerative diseases, it will be more meaningful as well as more economical to test or research into relevant traditional claims of Chinese medical achievements to see if they are valid, and if so, whether they can be rewardingly transferred to the west.

One promising area is the Chinese profound understanding of qi (chi) or energy, and its application in curing degenerative diseases for ages! This claim of employing qi to cure degenerative diseases, is not based on historical documents alone, but from my own experiences in helping literally hundreds of patients to be relieved of their so-called incurable illnesses.

It is in this spirit of sharing that I write this book, with the sincere hope that some readers may find in this humble presentation of Chinese medicine, materials that prompt further study and research which may one day prove beneficial to world medicine. Perhaps it is fitting to think of world medicine as one wholesome discipline; terms like Chinese medicine or medicine of any other peoples are mere convenient names to denote the contribution of these peoples towards world medicine.

5

TWO ASPECTS OF ONE REALITY
(Yin-Yang in Chinese Medicine)

Chinese medicine is not yet well known. Owing to the lack of technical glossaries certain classical works present difficulties of interpretation even to scholars of Chinese, and their translation into Western languages poses many problems.
Pierre Huard and Ming Wong.

Overcoming Preliminary Difficulties

It is a common misconception that a knowledge of Chinese philosophy is essential to an understanding of Chinese medicine. Knowing Chinese philosophy is helpful, but not indispensable, because the principles and practice of Chinese medicine are based on science and experience, not on philosophy nor metaphysics, as is often misconceived in the west, even by otherwise learned scholars. Many Chinese themselves have this misconception too.

Why are so many people mistaken? Let us look at the following basic principle in Chinese medicine, which may be laughable to the uninitiated:

Solitary yang does not permit life, solitary yin does not permit growth.

This is a statement on medicine, not cosmology nor metaphysics. Yin and yang are symbols. The expression means that if we have only one aspect of the two complementary aspects of reality, then health or natural development is not possible. For example, even if our physiological functions are working properly, but the respective organs are structurally damaged, then health is absent.

On the other hand, even if the organs are physically intact, but they are not functioning properly, then health is also not possible. In this example, structure is symbolized by yin, and function by yang. After you have read about yin-yang in this chapter, you would be able to think of other examples yourself.

The Concept of Yin-Yang

Yin and yang are the two most frequently used terns in Chinese medicine; they are also the two most commonly misunderstood! Virtually every English book on Chinese medicine mentions yin-yang; but, unfortunately, very few explains what they actually mean. Merely echoing that yin refers to what is feminine, dark, soft, retrogressive, etc.; and yang, the opposite, is not only inadequate, but further baffles the uninitiated reader as how all these relate to health.

The harmony of yin and yang is essential to health. Almost everyone has read or heard that. But what does it mean? Why and how is disharmony of yin-yang detrimental to health?

When I first studied Chinese medicine, I fancied that parts of our body were yin, and other parts were yang. It was not necessary, I thought, that exactly half the body was yin and the other half yang; it was not even necessary that the various yin and yang parts were symmetrically distributed over our body; but if health were to be maintained, a balance of some sort amongst these bodily parts must be achieved. All these, of course, are hilarious, and not true.

Yin and yang do not refer to any specific parts or aspects of the body. In fact, they do not have any specific meanings; they are not absolute terms. Yin and yang are merely convenient symbols to represent two opposing yet complementary aspects in medicine and in all other fields. The significance and manifestations of yin and yang may sometimes be profound and numerous, but in their simplest form, yin and yang refer to the concept of two opposing yet complementary aspects of reality, irrespective of whether the reality is expressed as objects or ideas.

In the field of environmental medicine, for example, Chinese physicians long ago realized the great importance of environmental conditions to health. Man must be able to harmonize himself to climatic changes, failing which sickness may occur. The Chinese physicians explain this relationship by using yang to represent all the subtle and myriad environmental changes, and yin to represent man and his adaptability. If a man fails to adapt himself to a sudden climatic change and becomes ill, it is described as a disharmony of yin and yang.

In anatomy and physiology, yin is used to represent the structural composition of man's organs, and yang their respective functions. Yin-yang disharmony occurs if, for example, an organ fails to function properly, though its structure may still be intact.

For the individual organs, yin and yang are also used to denote their respective location, appearance and other features. For example, describing the body as the whole, the upper body is yang, and the lower body yin; the dorsal side is yang, and the ventral side is yin. If, in an accident for instance, the upper and the lower part of an arm are out of proper alignment, then yin-yang disharmony is present.

Describing the internal organs, yin refers to the five organs that "store" — heart, liver, spleen, lungs and kidneys; while yang refers to the six organs that "transform" — intestines, gall bladder, stomach, colon, urinary bladder and "triple warmer". These organs are intimately connected by an elaborate set of meridians or energy pathways. If, for example, disease at the intestines disrupts the smooth flow of energy to the heart, then there will be yin-yang disharmony at the heart.

The differentiation of diseases into yin and yang is an important factor in Chinese diagnosis. Yin refers to diseases with symptoms like feeling cold, liquid faeces, clear urine, weak respiration and slow pulse rate. Yang diseases have symptoms like fever, constant thirst, hard faeces, yellowish urine, dark-colored tongue and fast pulse rate. This classification is a very useful and convenient way for the physician to understand the patient and his illness.

In prognosis, yin is used for sickness that exhibits weakness, retrogressiveness and internal development; while yang sickness shows excitability, feverish conditions and external development. If a physician has diagnosed his patient's illness as yin, but the prognosis shows yang features, then something is wrong, and the physician will have to review the case.

In pharmacology and therapeutics, yin medicine is generally cool, cold, salty, sour and bitter; while yang medicine is warm, hot, flat tasted, tart and sweet. If a patient's illness was caused by insufficient yang, for instance, then the physician will use yang type of medicine and therapeutic methods to restore the harmony.

For example, if a patient suffers from a dysfunction of the stomach (insufficient yang), then the physician will use therapeutic methods that will increase yang, and medicine that will "warm" the stomach. (How this can be done will be discussed in later chapters.)

Inter-Dependency and Inter-Changeability

Yin and yang are therefore abstract concepts; they are not, by themselves, material things. While yin and yang are each opposing the other, they are also complementary and inter-dependent — the two opposing aspects uniting into one entity.

For example, a person's lung is a substantial, structural organ, and thus is represented by yin. Its respiratory process is formless and functional, and is represented by yang. Its substance and its function are two complementary and inter-dependent aspects of the lung. If there is no yang function in the yin substance, then the lung is useless without its respiratory process. On the other hand, if there is no yin substance, then there is no form for its yang function to operate.

Yin and yang are also ever changing, and its changeability develops from its complementary nature and its inter-dependency. The food we take in has form, and is therefore expressed as yin. The yin substance depend on the yang function of the stomach to digest the food into suitable nourishment for our body. And in the yin structure of the stomach, this nourishment changes into yang energy to further the function of the stomach.

Harmony of Yin-Yang

The inter-changeability of yin and yang must be harmonious. Although at certain particular instances, either yin or yang may be more prominent than the other, its general, overall harmony must be maintained. If this harmony is constantly disturbed, then illness or poor health occurs.

In this section, you will read about some important terms frequently used to describe fundamental concepts concisely in Chinese medicine. Although these are basic terms, many readers not yet familiar with Chinese medical theory will probably find them — depending on their attitude — either very frustrating or very fascinating. In order to understand and enjoy this section better, it will be helpful to study the tabulated information below carefully:

Disharmony of yin-yang results in illness. This disharmony can be due to:

1. Yin deficiency, or
2. Yang deficiency.

Yin deficiency can be caused by
(a) insufficient yin, or
(b) excessive yang.

Yang deficiency can be caused by
(a) insufficient yang, or
(b) excessive yin.

The classification above is for the convenience of study. In practice, there are many overlapping of factors.

If there is too much yin, or too little yang, then yang deficiency occurs, and sickness results. For example, if there is too much food for the stomach to cope with — that is, too much yin; or if the digestive function of the stomach is not working properly — too little yang; then that person becomes sick, even if medical examination shows that there is "nothing wrong" with the (yin) structure of the stomach. This disharmony of yin-yang which causes sickness is due to yang deficiency.

Sickness can be caused by yin deficiency too. Yin deficiency can result from insufficient yin or excessive yang. A person's natural resistance is referred to as yin. For some reasons — such as excessive worry or fatigue — his resistance is weakened, and yin deficiency may occur, with the result that he cannot cope with the pathogenic micro-organisms around him. This disharmony of yin-yang which causes illness, is brought about by yin deficiency, which in turn is the result of insufficient yin.

Notice that in this case, the amount or potency of disease causing micro-organisms remains the same. In normal circumstances, these micro-organisms, which are represented as yang, cannot harm him. But in this particular situation, he becomes ill not because of any change in the amount or potency of micro-organisms, but because of a decrease of his own yin resistance.

On the other hand, yin deficiency can be caused by excessive yang. In other words, a person's yin remains the same, his natural resistance against diseases has not changed; but yang has become excessive, there is a tremendous increase in the amount or potency of disease causing micro-organisms.

This can happen if he has a wound which allows an excessive amount of bacteria to enter his body, or he has consumed contaminated food, or the strain of bacteria that he has breathed in is very powerful. Hence, he becomes ill because of yin deficiency, which, in this case, is brought about by excessive yang.

This principle of yin deficiency and yang deficiency applies to all types of diseases — contagious, organic and psychiatric.

In environmental medicine, for example, if someone travels to another country and experiences a sudden change of weather conditions, and if he cannot sufficiently adapt himself to this sudden climatic change, he may become sick, though a medical examination may show that he is physically well, and that there are no excessive pathogenic micro-organisms in his blood stream. Here is an example of yin deficiency as a result of excessive yang — inability to adapt himself to excessive changing environmental conditions (excessive yang).

Alternatively, he may be staying in his usual locality, and the weather conditions are normal. But for some reasons — such as excessive stress or anxiety — his adaptability is weakened. He may then become sick, in an environment which in normal situations he would be able to cope with. This is also an example of yin deficiency, but here it is brought about by insufficient yin, while yang remains constant.

Yin Deficiency and Yang Deficiency

In Chinese medicine, yin deficiency and yang deficiency are two important terms popularly used to explain and classify the causes of illnesses.

Yin deficiency is often manifested as feverish conditions, feeling of irritability and anxiety, heavy perspiration, fast metabolism and over-functioning of other physiological processes.

The manifestations or symptoms of yang deficiency are chilly conditions, nervousness, incessant perspiration, passiveness, slow metabolism and under-functioning of other physiological processes.

As sickness is the result of disharmony of yin and yang, the principal approach in healing is to restore harmony, making sure what yin and yang in that particular situation represents. Deficiency can be remedied by methods such as "enhancing" and "invigorating", whereas excessiveness can be reduced by methods such as "cleansing" and "dispelling". For example, if yin deficiency occurs, the harmony of yin-yang can be restored by enhancing yin and/or cleansing yang. More will be said about this in later chapters.

We must be remember that although this harmony of yin-yang is the general principle used for diagnosis as well as therapeutics, it was not meant to be the all-inclusive, all-embracing doctrine that simplifies the causes and remedies of all diseases into one easy method — a misconception many laymen and some misinformed students may believe. The yin-yang principle is comparable to a mathematical formula: it can express complex ideas concisely.

The disharmony of yin-yang that brings illnesses, has many different manifestations. It can be manifested as insufficient yin blood-defence against excessive yang viruses, as in measles and influenza. It can be manifested as excessive yang functioning of physiological processes, like the over-functioning of the thyroid glands resulting in goiter. The disharmony can be manifested as inadequacy of yin substance, like the structural defects of bodily organs. It may be the disharmony of "shen" (spirit) or of the "seven emotions", thus causing neurological or psychiatric disorders.

Conventional Use of Yin and Yang

The following table shows the convention in using yin and yang to refer to various aspects of phenomena. Can we, for example, use yang for "front" or "substantial", instead of yin as it is usually done. We can, but we are likely to cause a lot of misunderstanding, just like calling our spouse — out of endearment, perhaps — a monkey instead of wife or husband.

Position :
    Yin   : front, lower and internal.
    Yang : back, upper and external.

Anatomy :
    Yin   : substantial, structural, blood and the six "excreting" organs.
    Yang : formless, functional, qi and the five "storing" organs.

Diagnosis :
    Yin   : cold, not thirsty, liquid faeces, clear urine, passive, slow pulse
            rate, light colored tongue and weak respiration.
    Yang : feverish, thirst, hard faeces, yellowish urine, fast pulse rate,
            dark colored tongue and heavy respiration.

Prognosis :
> Yin   : slow, quiet, cold, apparent, controlled, functionally diminishing, weak, internal, lower and falling.
> Yang : fast, active, hot, real, irritable, functionally increasing, potent, external, upper and rising.

Pharmacology :
> Yin   : salty, sour, bitter, cool, cold, falling and sinking.
> Yang : flat-tasted, tart, sweet, warm, hot, rising and floating.

Do not worry if you find some of the terms puzzling. They will become clear as other chapters unfold.

Holistic Approach of Chinese Medicine

With some understanding of yin-yang, let us have some fun with the following quotation:

> Heaven has four seasons and five elemental changes; hence, there is germinating, growing, gathering and storing; giving birth to cold, heat, dryness, dampness and wind. Man has five viscera, generating five energies; hence, there is joy, anger, sorrow, worry and fear. Joy and anger injures spirit. Cold and heat injures form. Excessive anger injures yin, and excessive joy injures yang. Negative energies rise up; pulse rates lose their structures. If joy and anger is uncontrolled, cold and heat is excessive, then health is impaired.
> Nei Jing.

The above quotation is in fact one of the core passages of Nei Jing, the Inner Classic of Medicine, expressing in a very concise manner the essence of Chinese medical thought. But those not familiar with Chinese medical theory will be greatly puzzled, and it is not unreasonable if they think it is based on philosophy or metaphysics.

Much bewilderment can be avoided if we bear in mind that classical Chinese, with which much of Chinese medical knowledge was written, is very concise. For instance, in the above quotation, the term "cold and heat" does not refer to cold and heat only. It is an idiomatic expression for the "six evils", which are actually six generalized groups of external causes of illness, namely cold, heat, dampness, dryness, wind and fire. Of course, they must not be taken at their surface meanings only. Cold, for example, refers not only to a lowering of temperature, but also to the weakening of bodily functions.

The annotated meaning of the above quotation is as follows:

There are four seasons and five elemental processes in nature. The four seasons are germinating in spring, growing in summer, gathering the harvest in autumn, and storing supplies in winter. The five elemental processes that symbolically describe all phenomenal changes in nature, are the processes of metal, water, wood, fire and earth, and they can cause climatic conditions of dryness, cold, wind, heat and dampness.

Man has five internal "storage" organs, and six "transformation" organs. The five "storage" or "zang" organs are heart, liver, spleen, lungs and kidneys; and the six "transformation" or "fu" organs are small intestine, gall bladder, stomach, colon, urinary bladder and "triple warmer". These organs generate energies for their respective functions; for example, the heart generates energy for the functioning of the heart, the small intestine generates energy for the functioning of the small intestine, and so on.

Man also has seven emotions, namely joy, anger, sorrow, worry, fear, anxiety and shock. If "joy and anger" — which is a short form referring to all the seven emotions — are disharmonious, they injure a man's spirit. Thus the seven emotions are internal causes of illnesses. If "cold and heat" — a short form referring to the six evils of cold, heat, dryness, dampness, wind and fire, — are disharmonious, they injure the physical body. Thus the six evils are external causes of illnesses.

For example, excessive anger injures the liver, because when a person becomes excessively angry, the resultant disharmonious energy interacts against the liver. As the liver is responsible for regulating blood, this will subsequently affect our natural resistance provided by our blood against diseases. Natural resistance is symbolized as yin, in contrast with yang external pathogenic agents. Hence, excessive anger injures yin defence, thus resulting in yin-yang disharmony.

Excessive joy injures the heart, because the resultant disharmonious energy reacts against the heart, which in classical Chinese often means the mind. The heart, or the mind, controls various physiological functions, and as functions are symbolized as yang, excessive joy, therefore, injures yang functions, thus causing yin-yang disharmony too.

When disharmony of yin-yang occurs, various negative energies will result. This will disrupt normal energy and blood flow, and can be detected from irregular pulse rates. Hence, if man loses control of his seven emotions, or fails to contain the six evils, his health will be impaired.

You will notice how concise the original quotation is. You will probably be impressed by the profound knowledge the ancient masters had concerning man's health. Chinese medical terms like five elemental processes, six evils and seven emotions, and how they affect health, will be explained subsequently.

The Chinese approach to health is holistic; it involves not only the fight against invading micro-organisms, and the proper functioning of his organs, but also his harmonious relationship with himself, with other people, with climatic and environmental conditions and with the whole universe. And if illness occurs, the Chinese physician will examine the cause not from a localized, reductionist viewpoint, but attempt to relate it to all relevant factors, internally and externally.

ARCHETYPICAL INTERACTIONS OF MYRIAD PHENOMENA

(The Five Elemental Processes)

So much misinformation about Chinese medicine crowds the shelves of European and American bookshops that a Chinese account is badly needed.

Nathan Sivin.

Archetypical Processes, Not Ingredients

The next most widely used concept in Chinese medicine, besides yin-yang, is probably the "five elemental processes", which is usually translated into English as the "five elements".

These so-called five "elements" are actually not elements — vastly different from the four elements of air, water, fire and earth of the Greeks and the Indians. The Chinese classifications of wood, fire, earth, metal and water were not meant to describe the primordial ingredients that fundamentally constitute the universe; they were meant to describe archetypical processes or changes. Hence, I prefer to translate them as the five elemental processes. They are also known as the "five movements".

The "five elemental processes" concept is used not only in Chinese medicine, but also in such diverse disciplines as metaphysics, chemistry, and military strategies. Ancient philosophers noticed that the universe is made up of never-ending combinations of changes or movements. There are of course countless different types of changes or movements, but they all can be classified into five archetypes of processes, each with their own common characteristics.

Some processes have the quality of being pliable, yet in its myriad transformations are able to retain their original essential character. Ancient masters referred to this archetypical process as the "metal process".

Some processes have the characteristic of fluidity, and are often beneficial to other processes. The ancients called this elemental process the "water process".

The "wood process" is the archetype for those processes that have the quality of growing, are elongated in nature, and possess potentials for future development.

The "fire process" refers to the archetype of processes that consume or transform other processes. They have the character of rising, and are hot or active in nature.

Processes that are grounded, that exhibit features of confidence and stability belong to the archetype of earth process. It also has the quality of focusing or being central.

Hence, metal, water, wood, fire and earth are the symbolic terms used to describe the five elemental processes. It is not the substance of the five "elements", but the nature of their characteristic behavior, that is crucial in the conceptualization of these processes. In other words, when the ancient philosophers mentioned "wood", for example, they were referring not to the substance wood, but to a class of processes that had the quality or features of wood.

Inter-Creativity of the Five Processes

From their observations, the ancient philosophers discovered that these five archetypical processes endlessly inter-create and inter-destroy each other, and they generalized this everlasting cycle of actions and reactions of phenomena into the principles of inter-creativity and of inter-destructivity.

The inter-creativity principle refers to the mutual actions and counter-reactions of the elemental processes in creating subsequent growth or development. The usual analogy to explain this inter-creativity principle is as follows.

If we water a plant, it will grow into a sturdy tree. This is the principle of water creating wood. This wood can be used as fuel for burning; thus wood creates fire. Burnt material is nourishing to the soil; thus fire creates earth. From earth, we can get metal; hence, the principle of earth creating metal.

When metal is heated, it turns into liquid, symbolized as water; therefore, metal produces water. And when we water a plant, we get wood, and the inter-creativity principle continues endlessly.

For most people, including Chinese, the problem starts when this analogy ends. So what, they legitimately ask. How does this water-creates-wood-creates-fire concept explain the myriad changes in nature or in medicine? This will become clear if we examine some actual processes.

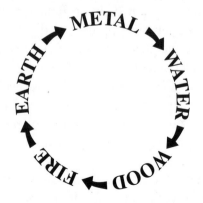

Fig 6.1 Cycle of Inter-Creativity

The blowing of a gentle spring breeze is an example of the water process. This will enliven our spirit, thus helping in our mental or spiritual development, which is of the wood process. This is the principle of water creating wood.

Hence, when we recommend a depressed person to stay in a mountainous, scenic environment, and if after being invigorated by the pure, fresh air, he gradually becomes cheerful, we can symbolically describe this curative process as water nourishing wood.

The process of wood creating fire is illustrated when well grown vegetables (wood process) is digested to give us more energy (fire process).

When a doctor shows love and concern to his patient (fire process), and this enables the patient to be calm and assured (earth process), it is an expression of fire creating earth.

When the patient is calm, his appetite improves (earth process), making him open himself to friends, environment and activities (metal process). This is the process of earth creating metal.

As a result his energy and blood circulation improves (water process), and this contributes to improving his health (wood process). These are the processes of metal creating water, and water creating wood.

It should be noted that the examples above may change, and the changes are limitless, but the essence is that processes of typical characteristics will produce archetypes of processes with their own special features.

Inter-Creativity and Inter-Destructivity

While the processes react on one another to inter-create, they also destroy one another in a continuous cycle. Wood destroys earth, like a tree absorbing the essence of the soil. Earth destroys water, as it absorbs water when it is thrown over the water. Water, in turn, extinguishes fire; hence water destroys fire. Fire can melt metal; hence fire destroys metal. Metal destroys wood, as in using an axe to chop down a tree.

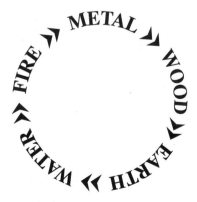

Fig 6.2 Inter-Destructivity of Five Processes

A growing child (wood) uses up a lot of food (earth), manifesting the process of wood destroying earth. After taking a heavy meal (earth), we become lazy and our blood circulation slows down (water), the process of earth destroying water.

Nevertheless, if you take a rest (water), you can overcome your anger (fire), manifesting the process of water destroying fire. When a person is angry (fire), he is not likely to open himself to others (metal), which is fire destroying metal.

A patient, expending his energy in too many activities (metal) instead of resting, hampers his recovery from his illness (wood), which expresses the process of metal destroying wood.

The principles of inter-creativity and inter-destructivity do not just operate between one elemental process and another; they operate in an inter-related metamorphosis of the whole range of processes. For example, while fire destroys metal; at the same time, it is destroyed by water. And metal, while undergoing destruction by fire, simultaneously destroys wood, which in turn destroys fire.

These twin forces of inter-creativity and inter-destructivity are necessary to maintain the continuous transformations going on all the time in man as well as in the cosmos. If there is only inter-creativity without inter-destructivity, or vice versa, then the harmony of man or the cosmos cannot be maintained.

The transformations are continuously occurring at the infinitely large scale of the universe, as well as the infinitesimally small scale of the subatomic particle. In health and medicine, these transformations can happen at any levels — environmental, bodily, organic, tissue, cellular and even at the "non-substantial" energy level.

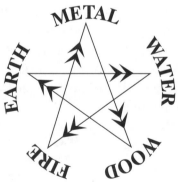

Fig 6.3 Inter-Creativity and Inter-Destructivity

Extraordinary Reaction and Mutual Correspondences

If any process is too little or too much, in potency or in amount, then its reactions with other processes may result in anomalous situations. For example, when our vital energy and blood are flowing harmoniously (water process), disease-causing micro-organisms (fire) that have entered our body will be destroyed by our own defence system. This is the process of water destroying fire.

If our vital energy and blood are plentiful, not only the destruction of harmful micro-organisms can be accomplished more easily (enhanced process of water destroying fire), and growth is better (enhanced process of water creating wood), we will not be drowsy after a heavy meal, instead the food will be digested faster (reversed process of water destroying earth).

The inter-creativity and inter-destructivity principles of the five elemental processes occur in all phenomena at all levels. Through long years of observation and study, ancient philosophers and scientists discovered that they could classify these archetypical processes in groups, and that there is a close relationship between groups. This relationship is known as the Mutual Correspondences of the Five Processes.

The Chinese masters were more interested in finding out how these correspondences of the five elemental processes could be put to practical uses, than in speculating why they happened. And the first step towards this end was to tabulate the correspondences to see their relationship, as shown in the diagram below.

Five Processes	Seasons	Directions	Storage Organs	Transformation Organs
Metal	Autumn	West	Lungs	Colon
Water	Winter	North	Kidneys	Urinary Bladder
Wood	Spring	East	Liver	Gall Bladder
Fire	Summer	South	Heart	Intestines
Earth	Long Summer	Center	Spleen	Stomach

Five Processes	Body	Openings	Emotions	Climate Conditions
Metal	Skin and Hair	Nose	Sorrow	Dryness
Water	Bones	Ears	Fear	Cold
Wood	Tendons	Eyes	Anger	Wind
Fire	Blood	Tongue	Joy	Heat
Earth	Flesh	Mouth	Worry	Dampness

Five Processes	Secretions	Tastes	Sounds	Colors	Houses
Metal	Mucus	Tart	Crying	White	Psyche
Water	Saliva	Salty	Sighing	Black	Intellect
Wood	Tears	Sour	Shouting	Green	Soul
Fire	Sweat	Bitter	Laughing	Red	Spirit
Earth	Lymph	Sweet	Singing	Yellow	Awareness

Fig 6.4 Mutual Correspondences

The knowledge concerning the five elemental processes is the result of experience and observation, not from imaginative speculation. This, incidentally, is another difference between the Chinese concept of five processes, and the Greek concept of four elements.

Harmony via the Correspondences

To achieve perfect harmony, the ancient sages believed, it is best to follow the correspondences closely. The Spring and Autumn Annuals records that even emperors adhered to these correspondences, wearing appropriately coloured clothings and staying in the appropriate sections in the palace during the different seasons. In spring, for instance, the emperors remained in the eastern chamber of his palace, dressed in green robes, and wore green jade jewellery.

If you are tempted to think that these correspondences are ridiculous or old-fashioned superstitions, be gently reminded that these correspondences were practiced by people who had achieved a very high standard of civilization at a time when much of Europe and all of America were not even known. And if you think the emperors were silly, do not forget that even if they were, they were advised by some of the wisest men during that time.

Recent discoveries by prominent western scientists show that our health, behaviour as well as our intelligence are greatly, but subtly, influenced by previously unknown cosmic forces from outer space. Professor Gino Picardi noticed that unknown cosmic forces affected identical chemical reactions carried out at different places. Dr Maki Takata discovered that blood index varied according to sun spot activities. Dr Kurt Koeller noted that the rate of industrial accidents rose by at least 10% on the day following solar eruptions. Dr Albert Abrams discovered that he would always elicit a dull note of percussion over a specific area of the abdomen of his cancer patient only when the patient faced west.

All these should spur us to ask at least two questions. Could the Chinese be right in their correspondences? Can we afford to miss such invaluable information if they were right? Actually it is not difficult to set up research to find the answers, if the right people feel strongly enough to discover the answers for the questions above.

Applying the Processes in Medicine

Chinese physicians have long discovered the answers. They had no need for formal, controlled research, because they have been using the correspondences of the five elemental processes successfully in their clinical practice for ages. The five elemental processes are used to explain the internal organs and their physiological functions. The function of the lungs is symbolized by metal, because of its resonance nature. The function of the liver is symbolized by wood, as the liver has the growing properties of wood in nourishing and regulating blood.

The function of the kidneys is symbolized by water, as the kidneys are responsible for spreading vital energy throughout the body. The heart function is symbolized by fire, as the heart is responsible for the physiological and psychological activities of the body. The stomach function is symbolized by earth, as it is the source from where food nutrients are derived.

Once again, it must be pointed out that Chinese terms like "fire" and "wood" are symbolic; and that should the above description appear ridiculous to you, it is because you have unwittingly but prejudicially use western medical paradigm on a totally different Chinese system.

Chinese physicians in the past noticed that the inter-relationship among the internal organs correspond closely to that of the five elemental processes. When a person is healthy, all the organs function properly in harmonious coordination. But when one organ is diseased, it will directly or indirectly affect other organs.

For example, anger and worry can harm the liver. The injured liver can affect the stomach, causing a loss of appetite. This is expressed as wood (liver) destroying earth (stomach). Thus this sequence of cause and effect from anger or worry to loss of appetite is a manifestation of the inter-destructivity principle.

On the other hand, when one organ is diseased (yin deficiency) or is not functioning properly (yang deficiency), it can be restored to normal by nourishing its related organ. Let us take tuberculosis for illustration. As a tuberculosis patient is usually very weak, and the tuberculosis bacteria are highly resistant, thus giving a course of antibiotics is not recommendable.

So the Chinese physician uses a different approach, making use of the inter-creativity principle. He nourishes his patient's stomach with appropriate food that is rich in nutrients, increases his appetite and improves his digestion with appropriate medical prescriptions.

This will help the patient to build up a better supply of energy that can then flow to the lungs and strengthen them, thus enabling the natural resistance of the lungs to overcome the invading bacteria. This is employing the principle of earth (stomach) creating metal (lungs).

In fact a team of Chinese physicians sent by the emperor, used this inter-creativity principle and saved thousands of lives during a tuberculoses epidemic in Vietnam, which was then under the suzerainty of the Ming Dynasty.

The use of the five elemental processes in diagnosis is a concise, symbolic way of explaining complicated symptoms and changes. For example, giddiness, watery eyes, irritability, anger and incessant flow of tears are "wood symptoms" related to diseases of the liver meridian. Reddish face, fiery feeling and excessive perspiration are "fire symptoms" related to the heart meridian. (Meridians will be explained in a later chapter.)

Of course while diagnosing a patient, the physician does not depend on these classifications alone, nor are these classifications rigid and compartmental. Nevertheless, they serve as helpful guidelines.

A patient suffering from a disease of the heart meridian, often loses his appetite — that is, his stomach functions are affected by the diseased heart-meridian. This condition can be expressed as fire (heart) failing to create earth (stomach).

Please note that in this case, there is nothing physically wrong with the stomach, though the symptoms seem to be located there. If we treat the stomach, we cannot remove this problem; we may probably aggravate it. The problem lies with the disharmony at the heart meridian.

Once harmony is restored, fire will be able to create earth, and the patient's appetite will return.

Treating Psychosomatic and Psychiatric Diseases

The role of emotional factors in medicine has been recognized by Chinese physicians since ancient times. The Chinese were in fact excellent in the treatment of psychosomatic and psychiatric diseases. Perhaps our modern psychiatrists could learn a thing or two from them. However, psychiatry was never a speciality in Chinese medicine, because Chinese physicians have always believed that the mind and body are one inseparable unity.

The inter-creativity and inter-destructivity of the five processes are frequently used to express the interrelations of emotional factors. For example, people who are usually sorrowful generally have weak lungs. The Chinese physician expresses this as sorrow affecting the lungs, as both belong to the metal process. How then can we cure a patient suffering from weak lungs?

A mediocre physician may prescribe medication that will strengthen the lungs. A more informed physician would strengthen the stomach instead, so that greater appetite will provide more energy to nourish the lungs, using the inter-creativity principle of earth creating metal. However, a master physician will do neither. Why? Because the real problem is not at the lungs; it is an emotional problem.

Strengthening the lungs with medication will create new problems. The lungs are structurally weak (inadequate yin); if we strengthen its performance (increase yang), we will create a yin-yang disharmony at the lungs. This type of strengthening is yang-strengthening, i.e. strengthening its function, which is not suitable in this case. The yin structure of the lungs now cannot cope with its excessive yang functioning. (If you are wondering what yin and yang mean, you probably have missed some important information found in the previous chapter.)

Strengthening the lungs indirectly through the stomach is better, but does not remove the root cause of the illness. Here it is yin-strengthening, i.e. rebuilding the lung tissues that have been worn away by the negative energy of sorrow. This approach may relieve some of the patient's suffering — at least his lungs are not so weak; but as soon as he stops taking good food, the symptom of weak lungs will relapse.

A master physician treats the cause, not the symptom. How to treat sorrow? There is a Chinese saying that "emotional illness is best overcome by using emotions." The principles of the five processes are exceedingly useful when treating sicknesses caused by emotions.

Sorrow corresponds to the metal process. Metal can be destroyed by fire, and the emotion that corresponds to fire is joy. So if the physician can make the patient joyful, his sorrowful emotion would be overcome, and the symptom of his weak lungs will gradually disappear. This is applying the inter-destructivity principle of fire destroying metal. The theorist supplies the principle; how well can the practitioner make his patient joyful will depend on his skill.

Emotional problems often manifest themselves as real physical ailments. By applying the principles of the five elemental processes, physicians can often help patients recover from their sickness without the use of any medical prescriptions. There are many interesting recorded examples of such cases in Chinese medical history.

Here is an illuminating story of how successfully — from the viewpoint of the patient, not the physician — a practitioner used the theory described above. The emperor was ill, and his imperial physicians could not cure him. (With the advantage of hindsight, we may wonder whether they *could* not, or they *did* not, cure the emperor!) Despite the most delicious delicacies prepared by the best chefs in the land, the emperor could not regain his lost appetite.

Then one day, a distinguished physician, who had earlier refused to work in the palace so that he could serve the common people, offered his services to the emperor.

"I'm glad you have finally decided to serve in the palace."

"It'll be my last chance to show my loyalty to Your Majesty," the physician replied mournfully. "But I would beg Your Majesty to grant me one wish."

"I can grant you a thousand wishes if you can cure my ailment."

"Just one wish, Your Majesty, and Your Majesty's ailment will be cured. May I be allowed to wander freely in your palace?"

"No problem," the emperor said, "the palace, I presume, is extensive enough for your wandering."

(Actually the last statement was my addition. It was unlikely for the emperor, to have said that. You can probably guess the reason behind the physician's unusual request, by the time you have finished reading this story.)

But when the emperor visited his favorite concubine at his favorite time, he found, to his unbearable fury, the physician trying to rape his little darling.

"Drag him out to be beheaded immediately," the emperor raged in uncontrollable anger.

Soon after the emperor was cured! The emperor's loss of appetite was due to excessive worry. Worry corresponds to the earth process, and is destroyed by the wood process. The emotion that corresponds to wood process is anger. Hence employing the principle of wood destroying earth, the loyal physician used excessive anger to overcome worry, thus curing the emperor of his seemingly queer illness.

Chinese psychiatry will be discussed in greater detail in Chapters 25 and 26. Meanwhile, if you want to use the interplay of the five elemental processes to solve your own emotional problems or your patients' emotional problems, the following relationship of processes will be helpful. Anger hurts the liver, but sorrow overcomes anger; joy hurts the heart, but fear overcomes joy; worry hurts the spleen, but anger overcomes worry; sorrow hurts the lungs, but joy overcome sorrow; fear hurts the kidney, but worry overcomes fear.

If you find the above confusing, as it often is, the following diagram will be helpful. Drawing the diagram to show the relationship of emotions or other factors, is actually quite easy. Link the five processes in a continuous circle, draw the lines to indicate the direction of inter-creativity and of inter-destructivity (Fig 6.3), then place the relevant factors at their appropriate processes (Fig 6.4) to produce a diagram like Fig 6.5.

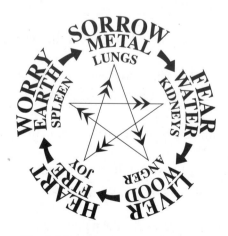

Fig 6.5 Relationship of Emotions

The concepts of the five elemental processes and yin-yang not only have enabled medical scientists and philosophers to express complex and profound ideas concisely, they also have provided a useful theoretical framework for much research and development in the long history of Chinese medical thoughts and practices.

With some basic understanding of these concepts, we are now better prepared to study and appreciate the system of medical thoughts and practices that has successfully served the largest population in the world for millennia. Hopefully we can also derive some insight and inspiration that can be beneficial to our own societies.

In the next chapter, we shall examine how the Chinese view the workings of internal organs. But if you think this is a revision of what you have learnt in anatomy and physiology, you will be in for some surprises. The Chinese physicians view the workings of man's internal organs very differently. You will find out, for example, why by looking into a patient's mouth, the physician can have a good idea of the condition of his heart. So turn the page and treat yourself to a whole new dimension of man's internal cosmos.

7

MAN'S INTERNAL COSMOS

(Chinese Anatomy and Physiology)

> *The classics say that man derives energy from grains. Grains enter the stomach, then energy is transmitted to five storage organs and six transformation organs. The pure is known as glory, the unfiltered as defence. The glory is transported inside vessels, the defence outside. The circulation is never-ending. Fifty times they meet. Yin and yang is complementary in endless cycles. Hence glory and defence are mutually operative.*
>
> *Bian Que (5th century BC).*

Organs for Storage and for Transformation

The above quotation from Bian Que, one of the greatest Chinese physicians of all times, is likely to baffle many readers. The quotation is purposely translated literally, so as to illustrate two common problems in studying such writing.

First, the writing is in classical Chinese, many centuries away from us in time. Therefore, even modern Chinese scholars may have difficulty with the language.

Secondly, the information was conveyed in extremely concise medical terms, which even classical Chinese scholars may not understand, unless they are also well versed in Chinese medical philosophy.

Luckily we have its commentary, which explained the quotation as follows:

Medical classics say that man's vital energy is derived from various types of food and drinks. Food and drinks enter the stomach, where the process of digestion, with the help of the spleen system, transforms food and drinks into vital energy. This vital energy is then transmitted to the five storage organs of heart, liver, spleen, lungs and kidneys, and the six transformation organs of intestines, gall bladder, stomach, colon, urinary bladder and "triple warmer". The lighter, purified energy consisting of microscopic nutrients, is known as "glory energy" and is carried by blood in blood vessels. The heavier, unpurified energy is known as "defence energy", and it flows outside blood vessels, bathing and protecting every cell. The circulation of this vital energy (which includes both "glory energy" and "defence energy") is never-ending in every part of our body. After making fifty complete, continuous rounds in a day, the vital energy accumulates at the "hand major yin lung meridian".

The function of the "glory energy" is nourishing the body. Therefore it is internal, and symbolized by yin. The function of the "defence energy" is defending the body against exo-pathogenic agents. Therefore it is external, and symbolized by yang. Yin and yang are complementary in their endless flow, meaning that the actual location of "glory energy" and of "defence energy" is not necessarily inside or outside the blood vessels. They are two aspects of vital energy: where there is "glory energy" there is also "defence energy", and vice versa. The mention of inside or outside the vessels is relative, referring to their functions of internal nourishment and external defence.

After this lengthy explanation, we can see the profound understanding of ancient Chinese physicians regarding human physiology. It is more impressive that they had this knowledge as early as the 5th century BC. More significantly, it shows how easily many modern scholars, western as well as the Chinese themselves, may misinterpret such knowledge, and mistakenly think that Chinese medicine pays little attention to physiology.

A similar misconception can easily happen in the study of Chinese anatomy. Most Chinese medical books do not illustrate the shape or structure of human organs. The very few diagrams that are available looked elementary and out of shape, when compared to the detailed illustrations of the anatomy that are available in the west.

Actually the Chinese had advanced anatomical knowledge even in ancient times. For example, Bian Que's "Classic of Eighty One Difficult Topics", from which the above quotation was taken, gave accurate descriptions of the size, weight and volume of internal organs.

Moreover, the Chinese were dissecting human bodies for detailed study when western anatomists had to draw inferences from animal dissections, as human dissection was forbidden for a long time in the west.

Why then are detailed illustrations of internal organs seldom found in Chinese medical books? This is probably because Chinese physicians are usually more concerned with their functions than with their structures, as revealed by the study in this chapter on how Chinese physicians view the internal workings of man, which is vastly different from western anatomical and physiological knowledge.

Anatomy and Physiology from another Perspective

It is helpful to bear in mind the following points when studying Chinese anatomy and physiology. When Chinese physicians refer to an organ, they do not just refer to the structure of that organ, but also to the whole organ system, including its functions and other related organs.

Hence, terms like "heart", "spleen" and "kidney" have different meanings in Chinese than in English. Technically, it may be more proper to use their respective Chinese terms like "xin", "pi" and "shen". For example, when Chinese physicians mention "xin", which is generally translated as "heart", they refer not just to that tough organ in your chest that pumps blood, but also to the circulatory system as well as the nervous system, as "xin" also means "mind".

However, to avoid the difficulty in remembering these Chinese terms, their English translations are used in this book.

It is a mistake to think that such semantic variation would cause much problem in Chinese. To those who understand the Chinese language, it is as easy to know whether "xin" means "heart" or "mind", as English readers know whether "man" means "male adult human being" or "human being who can be male or female, young or old".

It is useful to view the following description of man's internal cosmos from the Chinese medical point of view, without imposing, consciously or unconsciously, western medical viewpoints, at least for the time being.

As the purpose of this chapter is to get some idea on the Chinese concept of human anatomy and physiology so that we can better appreciate Chinese medicine, and hopefully derive some benefits from it, we will have a better understanding if we study their explanation as if we had no previous anatomical and physiological knowledge.

In this way, having temporarily set aside, for example, western concepts that the kidneys and the urinary bladder are mere filters, we will not be puzzled to find that Chinese physicians since ancient times have considered, and successfully applied the knowledge, that the kidneys are vital organs for sexual vitality, and the urinary bladder can directly affect muscle functioning!

Once we are prepared to put aside cultural blinkers, and our arrogance that the western medical way of viewing health and illnesses is the only correct way, we will find that many of the explanations offered by Chinese medical philosophy for incredible cures are logical and sensible after all.

Chinese physicians classified the viscera into two main groups, namely five "zang" and six "fu". Classical medical literature defines "zang" as organs that store energy, and "fu" as organs that transform food and drinks into energy. The five "zang" or storage organs are heart, liver, spleen, lungs and kidneys. The six "fu" or transformation organs are intestines, gall bladder, stomach, colon, urinary bladder and "triple warmer".

The triple warmer, which the Chinese regard as a "fu" or transformation organ, refers to the three levels of bodily cavities at the chest, the upper and the lower abdomen, responsible for respiratory, digestive and urogenital functions. The triple warmer is a major source of supply for most of the body's energy. If we find it odd that the Chinese consider it an organ, we are probably prejudiced by prior western medical thinking.

Indeed, from both the anatomical and the physiological viewpoints, the triple warmer has more claim to be called an organ than many other body parts that western medicine traditionally call organs, such as the skin and the appendix.

The Emperor and his Ministers

Let us start our tour of Chinese anatomy and physiology with what the Chinese usually regard as the most important organ — "xin" or the heart. The heart controls the spirit as well as the blood vessels. Being the seat of the human spirit, the heart is the source of consciousness and intelligence. It is also the source providing the energy for blood circulation. Because of its utmost importance, the heart is often figuratively described as the "emperor", controlling all other organs.

When the spiritual aspect of the heart is ill, symptoms like the following are common: heart beating fast, shock, anxiety, insomnia, loss of intellectual ability, and loss of emotional control. On the other hand, symptoms caused by the heart's "blood-flesh" aspect (i.e. the heart as a physical organ) include greenish or darkish face, dull complexion, lacklustre hair, pale-colored tongue and weak, sunken pulse. These two aspects of the heart are interconnected.

Have you ever wondered why Chinese physicians do not need elaborate instruments to examine the internal organs of patients? The reason is because they have simpler yet better ways to do so. For example, by looking at a patient's face, skin and tongue, a Chinese physician has a good idea of the actual condition of the patient's heart.

If the heart and the circulatory system are normal, a person's face is bright and rosy. If the heart or circulatory system is yin-deficient (structurally ill), the face becomes yellowish and lacklustre. If they are yang-deficient (functionally ill), the patient's face becomes dark and dull.

Classical masters described this relationship between the heart and the face as "The heart inside the body is the circulatory system; its glory is on the face."

The heart's condition can also be revealed by examining the tongue. If heart energy (physiological function) is excessive, his tongue will be bright red; if it is lacking, the tongue will be pale red. If the spiritual aspect of the heart is ill, the tongue will be sluggish and tired, and the patient does not like to speak. Classical masters described this relationship as "The heart manifests in the tongue."

Covering and protecting the heart is the "xin bao" or pericardium, which ancient masters figuratively described as the "ambassador", representing and serving the "emperor". As the heart is the most important organ, it must not be attacked by "external evil" (exo-pathogenic agents); any attack will be intercepted by the pericardium, which will bear the illness on behalf of the heart. When this happens, the patient may be semiconscious, unconscious or delirious. The pericardium is also regarded as the sixth "zang" or storage organ.

The heart is directly connected with "xiao chang", or small intestine, in the meridian system, which will be described in the next chapter. The main function of the intestine is to receive digested food and drinks from the stomach, and separate the "pure" from the "impure". Hence the intestine is figuratively described as the "receiving minister". The "pure essence" is absorbed and sent to the five "zang" for storage. Liquid impurities are sent to the urinary bladder, while solid impurities are sent to the colon.

Excessive "heat" (to be discussed in another chapter) in the intestine is manifested as sour tongue and ulcers in the mouth, sometimes accompanied with short or painful urination. This excessive heat may originate from the heart, as the heart and the intestine are directly connected by a primary meridian. It is interesting to note that while western medicine is unclear about the cause of oral ulcers, and treats them symptomatically, Chinese medicine understands that their root cause is found at the intestine or heart systems. Besides localized treatment, Chinese physicians also remove excessive heat at the source.

The pericardium is directly related to "san jiao" or triple warmer, which will certainly be novel and illuminating to English readers astonished to find such an organ. While the pericardium protects the heart, the triple warmer protects all the viscera.

The triple warmer is an extensive and exceedingly influential organ, figuratively described as the "transport minister". Its structural area covers the whole sphere occupied by all the "zang" and "fu", and its operation affects all their physiological functions.

The triple warmer consists of three levels. The first level or top warmer extends from the base of the tongue to the top of the stomach, corresponding to the chest cavity. Its main functions are to facilitate transmission of vital energy and nutrient essence, warm the body, nourish the skin, regulate the right amount of fat, and enable the harmonious spread of "defence energy".

The middle warmer extends from the diaphragm to the waist, corresponding to the upper abdominal region. Its main functions are digesting food and drinks, absorbing their essence, producing blood and other fluids, and facilitating the transportation of nutrients to the whole body.

The bottom warmer extends from the waist to the anus, corresponding to the lower abdominal region. Its main functions are to separate the pure from the impure, to excrete impurities, and to facilitate urination and defecation. Hence, ancient masters said, "The top warmer mainly receives, the middle warmer mainly processes, and the lower warmer mainly excretes".

The General, the Judge and the Quartermasters

Let us now meet the "general" inside our body. In our bodies, the "gan" or liver is also known as the "general". If we laugh at this Chinese imagery of internal organs as preposterous or "unscientific", let us not forget that this Chinese analogy is actually more profound than the western concept of the heart as a pump, the lungs as air sacs, or the gall bladder as a storage bag.

Why is the liver called the general? Because it controls the defence system, and is tough, diligent and endurable. Ancient masters said, "in the body the liver supervises muscles and tendons, its glory lies in nails, and its expression is shown in eyes." So, if you want beautiful eyes, a positive step is to have a healthy liver.

The main function of the liver is to store and regulate blood supply to every part of the body. When we are asleep or at rest, a lot of blood is stored in the liver. When we are active, the liver regulates the amount of blood flow according to our needs. If the blood flow is healthy, our muscles and tendons are well nourished, and the nails at our fingers and toes are strong and lustrous. By examining the strength, thickness, color and degree of lustre of a person's nails, a Chinese physician has a good idea of the condition of person's liver.

If your eyesight is failing, you should examine the condition of your liver, for they are intimately connected by meridians. The abundance or lack of a person's liver energy is shown in the sparkle or otherwise of his eyes.

A person who is impatient, intolerant, aggressive, and easily prone to anger will cause excessive liver energy to rise, which may result in headaches, poor eyesight and hypertension. You can now understand why a person who has perfect eyesight, may not see clearly when he is angry. On the other hand, symptoms of insufficient liver energy include giddiness, ringing sound in the ear, dryness of mouth, sore throat, reddened face and bad sleep.

The counterpart of the liver in the meridian system is "dan" or gall bladder, which is figuratively described as the "judge". In Chinese medical philosophy, the gall bladder is much more than a small sac for storing bile and secreting mucus. It is regarded as the seat of courage. In Chinese idiomatic language, "to have a big gall bladder" means to be very brave.

The main functions of the gall bladder are to further purify the essence of nutrients and then store it in the liver, and to regulate the amounts and types of essence for use in various parts of our body. The gall bladder and the liver are closely related, and symptoms of their illness are quite similar.

While western biology considers the main functions of the spleen as manufacturing, storing and destroying blood cells, in Chinese medical philosophy, the "pi", which corresponds to the spleen as a structural unit, is closely concerned with the digestive system. When a patient complains of poor appetite, the Chinese physician usually attends to his spleen rather than his stomach.

Medical records show that when tuberculosis affected large portions of the population during epidemics, Chinese physicians successfully saved countless of lives by nourishing the patients' spleen to improve their appetite and strengthen them so that they could overcome tuberculosis by their own self-resistance.

An astounding and sad, fact is that this happened a few centuries *before* tuberculosis became a widespread killer in western societies.

The main function of the spleen, nevertheless, is to receive and store nutrient essence from the stomach, and transmit nutrient energy (known as glory energy in ancient medical literature) to every part of the body. Hence the spleen is figuratively described as the internal quartermaster.

When the spleen is healthy, the person's flesh is well formed, and his lips are full and rich. On the other hand, lips that are undernourished and lacklustre indicate inadequate spleen energy. This is further manifested as having poor appetite, and finding food tasteless.

The spleen is also very important in controlling the quality and supply of blood. According to Chinese medical philosophy, the ingredients that form blood come from nutrient essence derived from food and drinks. If spleen energy is lacking, the quality and supply of blood will be affected.

Inadequate spleen energy may result in the inability to regulate harmonious blood flow in the blood vessels. This may cause blood to escape from the vessels, a condition known as "disorderly flow because of blood heat". Patients may vomit blood, cough out blood, nose bleed, pass out blood through defecation or urination, excessively discharge blood through menstruation or childbirth, which unfortunately is often fatal.

While western medical thinking is puzzled by these problems, the Chinese have understood their cause and have developed effective methods to check as well as cure them. Hopefully, western medical scientists may research into this invaluable medical knowledge discovered by the Chinese (but rarely known to the west due to linguistic and cultural differences), and make startling breakthroughs that will help them in saving lives.

The spleen is directly connected by a primary meridian to "wei", or stomach. The main function of the stomach is to receive food and drinks, and transform them into nutrient essence. It is man's "external quartermaster".

The nutrient essence is transmitted to the spleen for storage and distribution, while the remaining "heated paste of food and drinks" is passed onto the intestine for further purification and absorption. As the stomach is the principal organ where food and drinks are digested to produce nutrients for man's daily needs, it is sometimes called the "post-natal source of energy". For the production of nutrients the stomach works closely with the spleen.

It is worthy to note that Chinese physicians have successfully cured many chronic diseases, like liver infections, liver hardening, lung infections and kidney swelling, not by treating the affected organs respectively or diseased parts directly, but by way of the spleen-stomach systems. The fundamental principle is to strengthen the patients by improving their appetite so that their own body systems can overcome the diseases. The western parallel is food supplement or curative nutrition.

Nutrient and Energy, Work and Waterways

The lung, called "fei" in Chinese, is the "prime minister", controlling the body's vital energy and blood. According to Chinese medical thinking, life is sustained and operated by vital energy. Vital energy is produced from the combination of "heaven energy", which is derived from the fresh air we breathe in, and "earth energy", that is derived from the essence of food and drinks.

The lung is where "heaven energy" or cosmic energy is taken into our body as fresh air, and waste products in a gaseous state are exchanged as stale air. The lung is closely connected with the heart, where "earth energy" in the form of nutrient essence is found.

When vital energy is abundant, the skin is radiant and healthy, indicating that the lung is functioning properly. Dry and wrinkled skin shows that the lungs are not functioning inefficiently.

Lung diseases are manifested through the nose, such as blocked nose, running nose and loss of smelling sense. These diseases are caused by the deficiency of lung energy, with symptoms like shortness of breath, weak voice, being afraid of the cold, easily tired, dry skin, pale-colored tongue, and weak pulse; or by "lung heat", meaning the lung system is being attacked by exo-pathogenic agents, with symptoms like fever, cough, yellow phlegm, dark yellow urine, solid faeces, redness at tip of tongue, and yellow fur covering the tongue.

In the meridian system, the counterpart of the lung is "da chang", or colon, which is figuratively described as the "conductor", as its main function is to conduct the waste product it has received from the intestine out of the body through the anus, absorbing water in the process. For its operation, the colon derives its energy from the lungs. Hence, if the colon does not function properly, it is often because of weak lungs.

Diseases of the colon may be caused by "wetness" and "heat", which means it has been attacked by exo-pathogenic agents. Common symptoms include abdominal pains, feeling hot at the anus, short and reddish urine, weak pulse, purging and fever.

According to Chinese medical philosophy, the most important organ for a person's vitality is "shen", or kidneys. Many sexual problems, like men's sexual impotency and women's infertility, which have baffled western doctors, have been successfully treated by attending to the patients' kidney system. Here is a rich area where western medical science can benefit much from Chinese medical knowledge.

Besides carnal pleasures and physical activities, the kidney is also responsible for mental performance. Ancient masters figuratively refer to the kidney as the "work minister" — responsible for both physical and mental work.

The most important function of the kidney is to store and regulate essence and energy. There are two types or aspects of essence, namely nutrient essence for daily activities, and sexual essence for procreation.

There are also two types or aspects of energy, namely pre-natal energy and post-natal energy. Pre-natal energy is the primordial energy which first developed the person, and was derived from the father's sperm cell and the mother's egg.

Therefore, it was from the kidney that the rest of the foetus developed, and the initial energy (or whatever that remains of it) is still located there. The kidney is sometimes called the "pre-natal source of energy". Post-natal energy is the vital energy produced from the reaction of "heaven energy" (fresh air) and "earth energy" (food).

The kidney is also connected with memory, intelligence and other mental activities. This is because kidney energy is used for the production of "sui", which is marrow. According to Chinese medical thought, marrow circulates continuously in the hollows of the bones, through the vertebrae into the brain to nourish the brain, like blood circulation that nourishes other parts of the body. Hence, kidney energy directly affects the quantity and quality of marrow, which in turn affects the performance of the brain.

Again, if readers find this information odd, this is because of biased western medical perspective, which has not acknowledge such information yet. Chinese clinical experiences shows that Chinese physicians have been successful in applying this knowledge to improve patients' memory, cure giddiness and overcome insomnia by means of nourishing their kidneys to enhance marrow.

The condition of a person's kidney is reflected in his bones. If the bones are dry and brittle, for example, his kidney has not been function properly. Luckily, you do not necessarily have to take out somebody's bones to know the condition of his kidneys, because "the kidney's glory is manifested in his hair, and expressed in his ears." So, by the lustre or otherwise of a person's hair, you may have some idea of his sexual and general vitality. Deficiency in kidney energy often results in hard of hearing, or ringing noise in the ears. If you start hearing noises, the problem may not lie with your ears, but with your kidney.

The kidney is closely associated with "pang guang", or the urinary bladder. The main function of the urinary bladder is to extract nutrient essence from body fluid, and discharge the impure liquid as urine. The nutrient essence is sent to the kidney, from which it derives its energy for its operation. Weakness at the urinary bladder, therefore, may indicate weakness at the kidney. Ancient masters described the urinary bladder as the "waterways minister".

The meridian supervised by the urinary bladder covers an extensive area, stretching from the head down the back to the legs. The urinary bladder meridian is particularly connected to the muscle system. Deficiency of urinary bladder energy, therefore, directly affects the muscles, with the result that toxic wastes at the muscles may not be effectively disposed off.

Extraordinary Organs

The Chinese concept for internal organs is "five zang, six fu", meaning the five storage organs of heart, liver, spleen, lung and kidney, and the six transformation organs of small intestines, gall bladder, stomach, colon, urinary bladder and triple warmer.

A "fu" is where food and drinks are transformed into nutrient energy and waste products are excreted. A "zang" is where the nutrient energy is stored, regulated and dissipated to all parts of the body for various uses.

The pericardium is also regarded as a "zang", hence making twelve internal organs. All these twelve organs are linked by an intricate network of twelve primary meridians, which will be explained in the next chapter.

Besides these primary organs, there are "ji-heng-zhi-fu" or "extraordinary organs", which include brain, marrow, bones, vessels, gall bladder, and womb. They are called "extraordinary" because although they resemble "fu" structurally and geographically, they function like "zang". Except for the gall bladder, these "extraordinary organs" are not directly linked to the twelve primary meridians.

The gall bladder is special. Although it is regarded as a primary organ, and is connected to a primary meridian, it is also included as an extraordinary organ, because it is the sole "fu" of the six "fu" organs, that only transforms but does not excrete.

Some readers may be surprised that Chinese physicians do not accredit to the brain the kind of special attention western doctors normally give it. The brain is not even regarded as a primary organ. It is, nevertheless, considered as the "sea of marrow", where marrow of the whole body is accumulated. Marrow, which is very rich in nutrient energy, flows in bone hollows and its production depends on kidney energy.

Bones form the skeletal structure of our body. They also store and regulate marrow to nourish the brain. There are two types of "mai" or vessels, namely blood vessels and energy vessels, which are called meridians. These vessels bring blood and energy to every part of the body and remove waste products for disposal.

The two main functions of the womb, found only in female, are to supervise the menstrual cycle, and to prepare for pregnancy. The womb is connected by the "du mai" (conceptual meridian) and the "chong mai" (rushing meridian), which regulate the menstrual cycle before conception, and nourishes the foetus after it is formed.

Women whose menstrual cycle is not regular, or who have difficulty conceiving (despite confirmed to be clinically normal by gynaecologists) may have their problems solved by cleansing any blockage in the two meridians and nourishing the energy in them.

It is not uncommon nowadays for western doctors to find nothing clinically wrong with their patients, though both are aware that the complaint or illness is not imaginary. Instead of blaming it on stress or any other psychological factors, and merely advising patients to relax, it is worthwhile to re-examine these cases in the light of the new information (though it has been known and successfully put into practice by Chinese physicians since long ago) mentioned in this and other chapters.

All the interesting relationships among the various organs are possible because of vital energy. Indeed, vital energy, or qi, is the most important factor in Chinese medicine — irrespectively of whether we view from the perspective of physiology, pathology, diagnosis, prognosis or therapeutics. In the next chapter we shall study the intricate network of energy flow in our body, and discover that many hitherto incredible things in Chinese medicine are sensible after all.

LIFE IS A MEANINGFUL EXCHANGE OF ENERGY

(Qi in Chinese Medicine)

The idea of biological energy is developed to a greater or lesser degree in different therapies, but probably finds its most sophistical expression in traditional Chinese medicine where the energy is termed chi. ... It comes as something of a surprise to realize that conventional medicine is the only medical system ever known to man which has no concept of biological energy.

Julian N. Kenyon, M.D.

The Amazing Wisdom of the Ancient Chinese

Long before western scientists discovered that the stuff which constitutes the atomic particle as well as the infinite universe is energy, the Chinese have known this fact! Lao Tzu, the Taoist patriarch living in the 6th century BC, said:

Tao creates one. One creates two.
Two creates three. Three creates all phenomena.

What Lao Tzu meant was:

Tao, which is a convenient name for the Supreme Reality, creates
the cosmos. There are two aspects of the cosmos, namely yin and
yang. From yin and yang are derived positive energy, negative energy
and neutral energy. These three fundamental types of energy react
endlessly to form all phenomena.

It is a mistake to think that such profound knowledge was limited to only a few philosophers. In fact, the concept of energy as the ingredient of both the sub-atomic particle and of the universe, *has* all along been an important aspect of Chinese philosophy, and is known as "the theory of primordial energy". The great Neo-Confucianist of the Song Dynasty, Zhang Dai (1020-1077), explicitly said:

The cosmos is a body of energy. Energy has yin and yang. When it
disperses it permeates all things; when it unites it becomes nebulous.
When this settles into form it becomes matter. When it disintegrates
it returns to its original state.

Before our modern astronomers and nuclear physicists rediscovered these facts, many people thought Zhang Dai was talking nonsense.

Modern scientists must be astonished at what a classical Chinese scientist, Fang Yi Zhi, said in his "Understanding Physics":

> When energy integrates, it becomes form; when radiates, it becomes light; when vibrates, it becomes sound. All these are various forms of energy. Most of the energy exists in the pre-integration, pre-radiation and pre-vibration states. Hence, energy, form, sound and light are fundamentals.

Energy is the all-important aspect in Chinese medicine. In modern romanized Chinese, energy is "qi", which is pronounced "ch'i". It is not an exaggeration to say that all considerations in Chinese medicine — in physiology, psychology, pathology, pharmacology, diagnosis as well as therapeutics — involve qi or energy.

Indeed, the whole of Chinese medicine is to ensure man's meaningful and harmonious flow of energy — right from the cellular and tissue levels through the organ and system levels to the ecological and cosmic levels.

This is only logical if we remember that energy is not only the basic ingredient of man, but also of the infinitesimal particle and the infinite cosmos.

What the Classic Says about Energy

Let us see what the Nei Jing, or Inner Classic of Medicine, the oldest and still considered by many as the most authoritative Chinese medical test, has to say about health and energy. Regarding physiology, the Classic says:

> Man is born of the earth; derives his life from heaven; heaven and earth unite to produce energy; the resultant life is man.

As mentioned many times in this book, both the classical Chinese language and Chinese medical terms are extremely concise. It is very easy for English readers, including medical scholars and experts in other fields, to misunderstand the wisdom hidden in the often poetic description. The above quotation may be expanded as follows:

> Man's proper place is on the surface of the earth, upon which he depends for many things, including food. But the supplies from the earth, though essential, are not sufficient; he still needs cosmic energy (generally translated as fresh air for simplification) for the processes of life. This

energy from the cosmos reacts with the energy he gets from earth (from his food) to produce vital energy. This vital energy is essential for all the internal and external activities of a man's life.

Is the above explanation a matter of interpretation? Would some other persons interpret the concise terms in the quotation differently, like interpreting "born of the earth" as "made from the same elements that make the earth", and "derives his life from heaven" as "is able to live because of the grace of God or some heavenly beings"? No, it is not a matter of personal interpretation.

Any Chinese physician with a sound knowledge of Chinese medical philosophy, will interpret the quotation the way it is explained above, because this meaning is unmistakably expressed in other relevant parts of the Classic.

The concise nature of classical Chinese medical writing is two-fold: not only are the terms compact, information found in other parts of the book which informed readers are expected to know, is often not mentioned. Hence, in the above quotation, it is sufficient to mention "energy"; informed readers will know it is vital energy, and not other types of energy, and this meaning is confirmed in other parts of the book.

Many misconception of Chinese medical knowledge among western scholars are due to the fact that many works by Chinese writers, such as the above, are quoted out of context or without the essential background information.

This is illustrated in what the Classic says about energy and pathogenesis. Have some fun interpreting it, before reading the explanation below.

When energies are appropriate, there will be no cause of illness.
If evil enters, energy is certainly weak.

The expression above sums up the whole of Chinese pathology! But we shall be grossly mistaken if we think that the Chinese are very simplistic in their philosophy on the causes of diseases. Briefly, the above quotation may be expanded as follows:

The energies that flow inside our body and are responsible for all our physiological and psychological functions, are classified into six types according to our six "zang" organs, namely heart energy, liver energy, spleen energy, lung energy, kidney energy and pericardium energy. They also include their "fu" counterparts, namely intestine energy, gall bladder energy, stomach energy, colon energy, urinary bladder energy and triple warmer energy. When these energies are luxuriant and flowing harmoniously, physiological and psychological functions operate efficiently. Causes of illness will not occur. If evil energy, which is a figurative and collective term for all external agents causing diseases, enters the body, it is certain that the vital energy of the body has become weak. If the vital energy is strong, which is normal in a healthy person, the body's own self-defence, regenerative, immune and other systems will overcome the evil energy. Therefore, if a person is ill, his illness can be cured by restoring the flow of his vital energy. If his vital energy is flowing harmoniously along each and every meridian, then, he will not be ill.

The Inner Classic of Medicine asks rhetorically, "If energy flows harmoniously in all meridians, where can illness come from?"

Heart energy and pericardium energy are similar. Hence, the energies of the six "zang" organs and their corresponding six "fu" organs correspond to the five elemental processes, and is expressed in the principle "five movements and six energies." This principle is also applicable to the cosmos, as the different energies in the cosmos can be generalized into six main kinds. Man, therefore, is a microcosm of the universe.

Different Types of Energy

The Chinese have classified energy as used in medicine in many ways. Cosmic energy is derived from the sky while earth energy is derived from the earth through food and drinks. They react to form vital energy which is essential for life. The original energy from one's father and mother that formed the foetus, as well as the energy provided by the mother in the womb, is called pre-natal energy; while all the energy the child gets after birth is post-natal energy.

Energy that is good for the body is righteous energy (often referred to as vital energy), while energy that is detrimental to health is evil energy. Energy found in internal organs (like operating as physiological functions) is called organ energy, which is divided into "zang" energy and "fu" energy, and can be further classified according to the respective organs, such as liver energy, stomach energy, etc.

Energy that nourishes the body is known as nutrient energy, while that that defend against any external interference is called defence energy. Energy flowing in meridians is known as meridian energy, while energy that was transmitted out to another person by a master is called external energy.

This classification is for convenience, and there is often overlapping of terms. For example, nutrient essence travelling along a meridian is called meridian energy; when it enters the colon to aid in its operations, it becomes part of colon energy; but if it nourishes cells in the colon, it is termed nutrient energy.

If you find terms such as "righteous energy" and "evil energy", which are direct translations from the Chinese language, rather unusual or unique, it is because of the linguistic differences between the two languages. In the Chinese language, these terms are not only meaningful but poetic as well.

The flow of energy in man, as well as in the universe, is systematic and orderly. The twelfth century scientist, Zhu Xi (Chu Hsi), concluded that all phenomena are based on li and qi, i.e. principle and energy. Long before William Harvey demonstrated to the west in the 16th century that blood flow is systematic, the Chinese have known and made use of the intricate meridian system of energy flow (including blood) in man.

The Theory of Meridians

Even up to the beginning of the 20th century, many people laughed at concept of acupuncture, asking how could inserting needles into patients' body cure their sickness.

Then in the 1970s, western medical scientists were simply amazed to witness Chinese doctors successfully using acupuncture, and nothing else, as anaesthesia while performing major surgeries, and the patients were conversing with their surgeons during the operations, and they recovered faster.

Even more astonishing was the fact that in abdominal surgery, for example, the acupuncture needles were placed not at or near the abdomen, but far away at the patients' elbows and knees, to provide the anaesthetic effects!

After you have read about the meridian system in this and the next chapter, you will understand why this incredible feat is possible.

The theory of meridians is one of the most important theories in Chinese medicine. It is difficult to understand acupuncture and all other branches of Chinese medicine if one does not understand this theory. Yet, for various reasons, many westerners as well as the Chinese themselves are unfamiliar with it.

It is worthwhile to put in some effort to study the meridians and their significance, not only for a better appreciation of Chinese medical principles and practices, but the meridian theory may open some unsuspected avenues leading to crucial medical breakthroughs in man's noble effort in saving and prolonging lives irrespective of the medical philosophies or practices of the researchers.

The term "theory" is used here to mean an explanation, not a speculation. The meridians are not mere speculative ideas; they are facts that have been put to successful use by the Chinese since ancient time.

In 1960 a conference of Soviet doctors at Gorki reported that their experiments showed the existence of meridians and energy points at precisely where the Chinese had known them for centuries.

In 1963 Dr Kim Bong Lan of North Korea won an international award for discovering that the skin cells along the meridians are structurally different from other skin cells. The knowledge of Chinese physicians, since ancient times, are much more profound and useful than these "discoveries".

It is indeed a great pity if, because of a communication gap or other reasons, such profound knowledge is not widely used for the benefit of all humanity.

Meridians are pathways of energy flow inside our body. In Chinese, meridians are known as "mai", which also refers to blood vessels. But while blood vessels resemble pipes, as they have fixed boundaries, meridians are like streams, their shapes being formed by the actual flow of energy.

The boundaries and locations of meridians change according to the volumes and directions of energy flow, but in practice the changes are so minute that meridians virtually retain their fairly permanent shapes and locations, though over a period of time, meridians may become bigger in volume as the person's health improves.

Meridians (or more correctly, the energy of the meridians) flow deep inside our body, normally inaccessible to the touch of a finger. There are, however, certain points on the skin, where we may reach this energy flow with a finger, and these points are called energy points or vital points, or "xue" in romanized Chinese.

As these points are used in acupuncture and massage therapy, they are also called acupuncture points and pressure points.

In romanized Chinese, blood is also written as "xue". "Xue" meaning vital points is pronounced in the second tone, whereas "xue" meaning blood is pronounced in the fourth tone; but since tonal values are not usually indicated in writing, readers would have to be watchful of the differences.

Channels, Collaterals and Extensions

The intricate network of internal energy flow which connects literally every part of our body is called the meridian system, which consists of the following:

1. Twelve primary meridians.
2. Eight secondary meridians.
3. Twelve meridian-extensions.
4. Twelve muscle-meridians.
5. Fifteen branch meridians.

The twelve primary meridians, the most important in the system, are the major energy pathways that flow from hand to feet, and vice versa, through the twelve internal organs of the body, and they are named after the respective organs, such as the lung meridian, the colon meridian, etc. They are like main highways connecting major regions in a country. These primary meridians will be discussed in greater detail in the next chapter.

Actually the main meridians are called "jing", or channels; and branch meridian are called "luo", or collaterals. The lung meridian and the colon meridian, for example, are called the lung channel and the colon channel. But many English books have traditionally used the term "meridian" for "channel"; to avoid confusing English readers, the conventional use of the word "meridian" is also followed in this book.

The eight secondary meridians or channels do not flow through internal organs. They resemble vertical "energy grids" that protect the body, and they also act like reservoirs for reserving energy. They resemble trunk roads running the whole length of the country at the boundary, without touching any major regions. Two of the eight meridians are very important; they are the ren meridian (or conceptual meridian) and the du meridian (governing meridian), which flow the whole length of the front and back of the body.

The twelve meridian-extensions are extended from the primary meridians, and are named after them, such as lung meridian-extension, colon meridian-extension, etc. They flow long and deep into the body, and are important for connecting a primary meridian to another primary meridian, or to an internal organ. They are like connecting roads linking one highway to another, or to a major region.

The twelve muscle-meridians are continued extensions from the twelve primary meridians and the twelve meridian-extensions. Because they usually flow to muscles and tendons, they are called muscle-meridians. They are found mainly in the limbs and the head, and is located at the body surface, never deep into the internal organs. They are like smaller roads branching from highways or trunk roads to the countryside.

The fifteen branch meridians, or collaterals, are issued from each of the twelve primary meridians, and from the ren and the du meridians, as well as include a network of collaterals at the spleen. They are named after their parental meridians, like the lung meridian-collaterals, the ren meridian-collaterals, etc.

The collaterals at the spleen are known as "big collaterals of the spleen", which are different from the spleen meridian-collaterals. Collaterals may go deep into the body reaching internal organs. They are like country-roads. Collaterals subdivide into smaller and smaller collaterals known as "sun lou", or sub-collaterals, which reach every cell in the body. They are like small paths leading to every house in the country.

Chinese medical thought has always insisted that health and life are possible only if vital energy is flowing harmoniously. Illnesses occur because of energy blockage; and if the flow stops, life ceases. It is interesting to note that many modern biologists, after being disappointed with numerous past definitions, now define life as a meaningful exchange of energy.

We shall read more about this meaningful energy exchange and its inevitable effect on health in the next chapter.

9

THE UNIVERSE INSIDE YOU
(Network of Energy Flow)

Once you have attained the small universal energy flow, you will eliminate hundreds of illnesses; once you have attained the big universal energy flow, you will live a hundred years.

A qigong saying.

Universal Energy Flow

The "small universal energy flow", or the "small universe" is a qigong term meaning a continuous flow of vital energy round the ren and du meridians. Qigong, pronounced as "ch'i kung", is the once-esoteric art of developing vital energy, and the relevant aspects of qigong have been used to promote health and cure illnesses. The ren and du meridians are the two main meridians running along the whole length at the front and back of our body respectively.

The "big universal energy flow", or the "big universe", refers to a continuous flow of vital energy throughout all our twelve primary meridians. The twelve primary meridians are those that flow through our twelve major internal organs.

The above quotation is not an over-statement; it is a record of observation made through the ages.

If you want to eliminate hundreds of illnesses and live a hundred years — who doesn't? — you have to practise qigong from a master. It is not advisable to learn advanced qigong by reading a book, though learning simple qigong exercises, from a book for health, as we shall be doing later, is acceptable.

The purpose of this chapter, therefore, is not to provide instruction for practising the small or the big universe, but to provide information regarding the meridian systems along which their energy flows, information that will reveal some of the puzzling secrets of Chinese medicine.

Meridians are classified into two groups, namely "zheng jing" or primary meridians, and "ji jing" or secondary meridians. Primary meridians flow directly to major internal organs, secondary meridians do not. They are twelve primary meridians and eight secondary meridians, from which are derived meridian-extensions, muscle-meridians, collaterals and sub-collaterals.

The Twelve Primary Meridians

To some readers, the names of the primary meridians, like "hand tai yin lung meridian", can be quite daunting, and when they see the locations of these meridians in diagrams, they may wonder why a particular meridian that is named after a particular organ, is located in a totally different section of the human anatomy. For example the lung meridian is also found at the index finger or the colon. This section will answer these and other intriguing questions.

The short form of these twelve primary meridians are named after the six storage organs and the six transformation organs as follows:

1. heart meridian.
2. pericardium meridian.
3. liver meridian.
4. spleen meridian.
5. lung meridian.
6. kidney meridian.
7. small intestine meridian.
8. triple warmer meridian.
9. gall bladder meridian.
10. stomach meridian.
11. colon meridian.
12. urinary bladder meridian.

The meridians listed from number to 1 to 6 above are known as yin meridians, because they are directly related to the yin "zang" organs; and those from 7 to 12 as yang meridians, directly related to yang "fu" organs. Yin meridians generally flow along the anterior side of the body or limbs, while yang meridians on the posterior side.

All the primary meridians are in pairs, and they are arranged symmetrically in the body. So, there are actually twenty four primary meridians; but for convenience, only one of the pair is described.

The extremities of the primary meridians are found in the hands or legs. There are six (pairs of) hand meridians and six (pairs of) leg meridians. In each hand and leg, three yin meridians flow along the anterior side, and three yang meridians along the posterior side. Therefore, the twelve meridians may be classified as follows:

1. Three hand-yin meridians.
2. Three hand-yang meridians.
3. Three leg-yang meridians.
4. Three leg-yin meridians.

Figure 9.1 show the positions and the normal directions of flow of the twelve primary meridians diagrammatically.

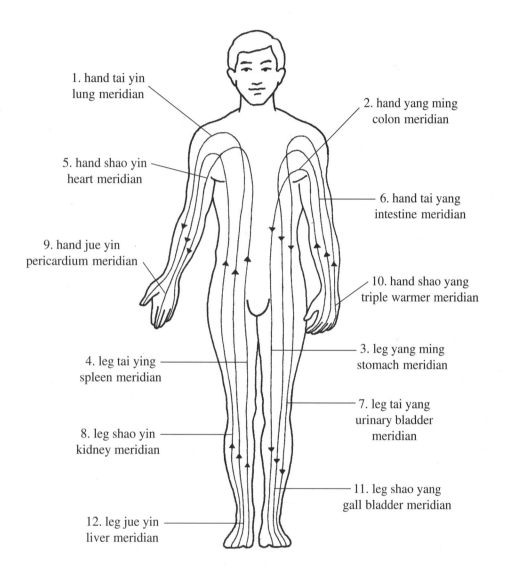

Fig 9.1 Positions and Directions of Flow of the
Twelve Primary Meridians (Diagrammatic)

Notice that the three hand-yin meridians flow from the internal organs to the fingers, where they join the three hand-yang meridians. These three hand-yang meridians flow from the fingers to the head, with their meridian-extensions branching off to link their respective organs. For simplicity, the organs and the meridian-extensions are not shown in the above diagram, but they will be shown later in diagrams illustrating the meridians individually.

At the head, the three hand-yang meridians join the three leg-yang meridians, which flow down the body, through their respective organs, down the legs to the toes. At the toes, these three leg-yang meridians join the three leg-yin meridians, which flow up the legs into the body to their respective organs.

Their respective meridian-extensions link these yang organs to the yin organs which continue the flow to the three hand-yin meridians, thereby repeating the never-ending cycle. The normal direction of flow is therefore as follows: hand-yin to hand-yang to leg-yang to leg-yin back to hand-yin.

So, on each arm and leg, and on the anterior as well as the posterior sides, there are three primary meridians, as illustrated diagrammatically in Fig 9.2 below.

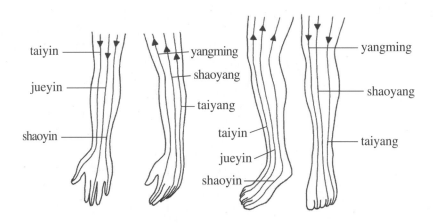

Fig 9.2 Positions of the Three Yin and Three Yang

Let us look at the three yin meridians at the arm and at the leg. The interior yin meridian (at the small finger or toe) is called "shao yin", or minor yin, meaning that the yin energy is just beginning. The external yin meridian is called "tai yin", or major yin, meaning that the yin energy is at its peak. The middle yin meridian is called "jue yin", or final yin, meaning that the yin energy is at its final stage, and is about to change into the first stage of yang.

Please note that the positions of the yin meridians shown in the diagram are simplified. In reality, while the three yin positions of the hand meridians are clear, those of the leg meridians are quite complex.

Now let us look at the yang meridians at the arm and legs. The interior yang meridian (at the thumb or first toe) is called "yang ming", or bright yang, meaning that the yang energy is at its final stage. The external yang meridian is called "tai yang", or major yang, meaning that the yang energy is at its peak. The middle yang meridian is called "shao yang", or minor yang, meaning that the yang energy is beginning.

So, if someone mentions "hand tai yin meridian", we know it is the meridian located at the external position of the anterior side of the arm. We also know the energy flowing in this meridian comes from a yin storage organ, and the energy is very strong. "Leg shao yang meridian" is the middle meridian at the posterior side of the leg. Its energy comes from a yang transformation organ, and is just beginning to generate force.

Nevertheless, if you are still puzzled by their names and locations, take consolation that even Chinese medical students have difficulties with them.

Lung and Colon Meridians

An easier way is to refer to the twelve primary meridians by their controlling organs, such as lung meridian, colon meridian, etc. The following is a simplified description of the twelve primary meridians; but it is sufficient to give us some idea of our fascinating internal energy flow. The important energy points of the meridians are also shown in the illustrations below.

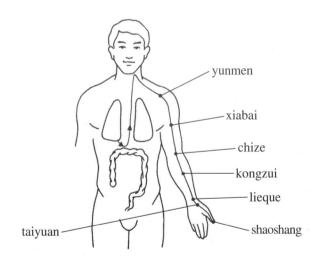

Fig 9.3 Hand Tai Yin Lung Meridian

The lung meridian, Fig 9.3, originates at the triple warmer where it receives energy from the liver meridian. Its meridian-extension flows down to the colon, while the main meridian flows up to the throat. At the chest, its extensive collaterals spread over the lungs.

At the throat, the lung meridian flows beneath the collar bone to the arm, down the arm along the tai yin side (external-anterior side) to the tip of the thumb. At the wrist, a branch meridian flows to the tip of the index finger, where it joins the colon meridian.

The lung meridian is the same as the "hand tai yin meridian". In fact the full name of this meridian is "hand tai yin lung meridian". So, we now know that the lung meridian is at the index finger to pass vital energy to the colon meridian; while far away at the colon itself, the other end of the lung meridian transmits lung energy to the colon for its operation. The lung and the colon are, therefore, closely related.

Please remember that the lung meridian and all other primary meridians are in pairs, and are symmetrical.

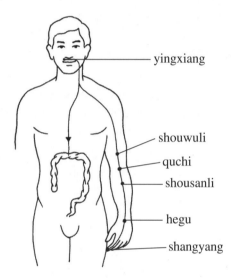

Fig 9.4 Hand Yang Ming Colon Meridian

If you have headache, sore throat, hearing difficulty or swollen face, you may have your problem relieved by working on the "hegu" energy point on the colon meridian.

Many people may wonder how does the colon meridian, of all the meridians, affect these ailments. The following description of the colon meridian will suggest the answers.

The "hand yang ming colon meridian" starts at the tip of the index finger where it continues from a collateral of the lung meridian. The colon meridian flows up the arm at the yang ming side (internal-posterior side), and at the collar, its meridian-extension turns downwards through the lung into the colon, where its collaterals cover the colon. Another meridian-extension flows down from the colon to the leg where it meets the stomach meridian.

At the collar, the colon meridian flows up the neck and terminates at the base of the nose. Collaterals from the colon meridian link with other collaterals related to many parts of the head. Hence, by stimulating the colon meridian appropriately, a healer can affect various parts of the head; and a convenient energy point where such stimulation can be performed is the "hegu". At the base of the nose a meridian-extension links the colon meridian with the stomach meridian.

Stomach and Spleen Meridians

The "leg yang ming stomach meridian" starts near the nose where it receives energy from the colon meridian. The stomach meridian flows round the face to the inner corner of the eye, where it joins the urinary bladder meridian, and where its collaterals flows into the brain.

At the neck the stomach meridian flows down the body into the stomach and the spleen, then down the leg at the yang ming side (internal-posterior side), terminating at the big toe where it joins the spleen meridian. Before the big toe, two collaterals branch out to the second and the third toes.

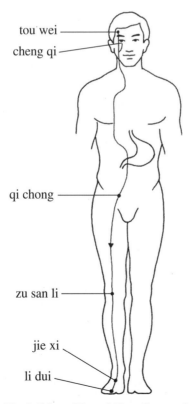

Fig 9.5 Leg Yang Ming Stomach Meridian

If you wish to turn off some lights in a big hall, of course you do not have to climb up the ceiling where the lights are; you merely have to turn off the switches, which are often some distance from the lights. Similarly, when surgeons want to operate on a patient's stomach, a master acupuncturist turns off the "switches" by manipulating relevant energy points at the legs, thus stopping energy impulses along the relevant meridians from reaching the patient's consciousness as pain.

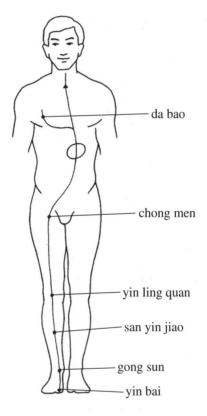

da bao

chong men

yin ling quan

san yin jiao

gong sun

yin bai

Fig 9.6 Leg Tai Yin Spleen Meridian

The "leg tai yin spleen meridian" flows from the big toe, where it receives energy from the stomach meridian, up the leg at the tai yin side (external-posterior side), enters the body into the spleen, stomach and pancreas, up again through the chest where it joins the heart meridian, and continues upwards to the throat and tongue.

So, if you complain of bowel disorder or any gastrointestinal diseases, and your Chinese physician massages your legs, don't imagine he is trying to loosen your leg muscles. He is probably stimulating better energy flow along your spleen or stomach meridians by manipulating certain energy points located at your legs.

Heart and Small Intestine Meridians

Continuing from the spleen meridian, the "hand shao yin heart meridian" flows in three directions. One meridian-extension flows downwards to the small intestine, supplying heart energy for the functioning of the small intestine.

Another flows up through the throat into the eyes and the brain, bringing nutrient essence to these regions. The main meridian flows through the lungs, then down the shao yin (interior-anterior) side of the arm, terminating at the small finger.

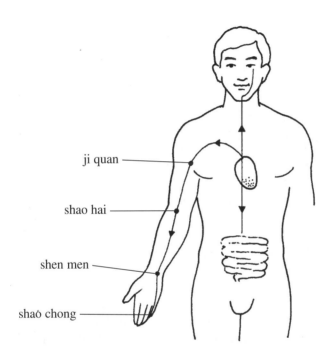

ji quan

shao hai

shen men

shaŏ chong

Fig 9.7 Hand Shao Yin Heart Meridian

The meridian system is not only for acupuncture and massage therapy; all branches of Chinese medicine use the meridian network. In internal medicine, for example, if the illness is related to the heart system, the physician will prescribe herbal decoction that enhances energy flow at the heart meridian.

The meridian system is very important in diagnosis. Why oral ulcers or reddish urine indicates disorder at the small intestine? An understanding of the meridian system will show that since the intestine meridian derives directly from the heart meridian, which in turn is connected to the mouth, illness of the intestine can be reflected in the mouth. This is the principle of "internal organ reflected in its corresponding external organ". And once we know that the intestine meridian flows directly to the urinary bladder meridian, it is not difficult to see that intestine disorder can be reflected as reddish urine.

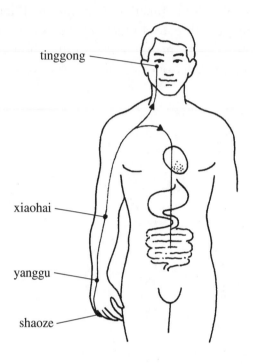

Fig 9.8 Hand Tai Yang Small Intestine Meridian

The "hand tai yang small intestine meridian" receives energy from the heart meridian at the small finger. The intestine meridian flows up the arm at the tai yang (external-posterior) side, and at the shoulder it turns downwards where its collaterals cover the heart. The main meridian flows through the stomach into the intestine, subdividing into many collaterals.

At the shoulder a meridian-extension flows up the neck to the outer corner of the eye, then into the ear. A collateral flows from the outer eye corner to the inner corner where it links with the urinary bladder meridian.

Urinary Bladder and Kidney Meridians

You will probably be surprised that the urinary bladder meridian is an exceedingly important meridian, frequently employed in the treatment of headaches, muscular pains, eye ailments, nervous disorders, high fever, and disorders of internal organs.

What is the connection between the urinary bladder and these seemingly unrelated complaints? Actually, they are intimately connected, as a brief study of the urinary bladder meridian will show.

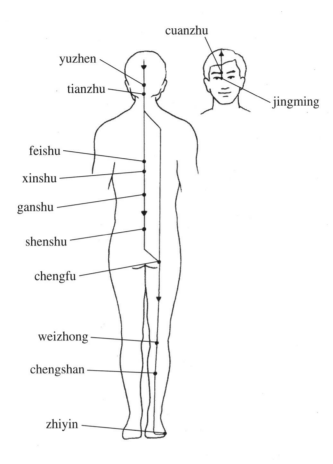

Fig 9.9 Leg Tai Yang Urinary Bladder Meridian

The "leg tai yang urinary bladder meridian" continues from the small intestine meridian near the eye. It flows up the scalp, with a branch going to the ear, from where its collaterals enter the brain.

The main urinary bladder meridian flows down the neck, and subdivides into two (making four altogether, as the meridian is in pair), flowing down the full length of the back, from where an extensive collateral network covers the muscle system of the body. The "shu energy points" of all "zang" and "fu" organs are found along this meridian. (A "shu energy point" is where the energy of an internal organ is focused.)

This gives an indication of how important the urinary bladder meridian is, as the energies of the viscera are focused all along this meridian.

At the waist, it enters the kidney, from where it flows to the urinary bladder. At the buttock, the two subdivisions unite into one meridian again, flows down the full length of the leg at the tai yang (external-posterior) side, terminating at the little toe.

Many Chinese pay much attention to the kidney system because they know it is directly related to their sexual pleasure and procreation, though they may not know why. Almost always, a patient with sexual problems is deficient of kidney energy.

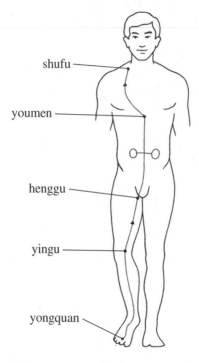

shufu

youmen

henggu

yingu

yongquan

Fig 9.10 Leg Shao Yin Kidney Meridian

Do not underestimate your little toe, for there is where your vital "leg shao yin kidney meridian" starts. It flows to the sole where a major energy point called "yongquan", or gushing spring, is located. A convenient way to test how strong your kidney energy is, is to stand upright and relax, and feel how strong (or otherwise) your gushing spring is.

The kidney meridian flows up the leg at the shao yin (internal-anterior) side, enters the sex organs, then the urinary bladder and the kidney. A collateral joins the ren (or conceptual) meridian, which links to the sex organs. Another collateral joins the chong (or rush) meridian, which flows to the sex organs in one end, and on the other end to the "niyuan" energy field, corresponding to the pineal gland. A meridian-extension continues flowing upwards to the liver, lung and heart.

Pericardium and Triple Warmer Meridians

Have you ever wondered why practicing internal exercises like Taijiquan and qigong can improve a person's emotional health, like making him calm and tolerant? There are many reasons, and one of them involves the meridian system.

According to Chinese medical thought, negative emotions are caused not so much by external stimuli, but by blockage of negative energy that results from the external stimuli. Hence, if energy is flowing smoothly in your meridians, it is unlikely that anyone can irritate you easily.

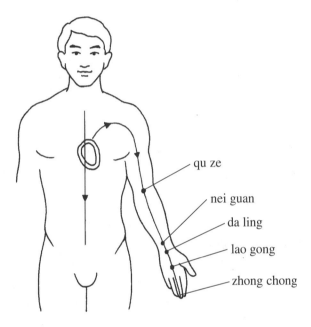

qu ze

nei guan

da ling

lao gong

zhong chong

Fig 9.11 Hand Jue Yin Pericardium Meridian

The heart is the most important organ concerning emotions. The organ that protects and often acts for the heart is the pericardium. You do not have to massage your heart or pericardium directly to effect their harmonious energy flow; this can be achieved by suitable gentle hand movements, as in Taijiquan and many qigong exercises, because the heart and the pericardium meridians flow right to your finger tips.

The "hand jue yin pericardium meridian" starts at the chest where it receives energy from the kidney meridian. Its collaterals covers the pericardium and the heart. A meridian-extension flows downwards and its collaterals spread over the triple warmer region. The main meridian flows to the armpit, then down the arm along the jue yin (middle-anterior) position to the middle finger. A collateral branches to the fourth finger where it joins the triple warmer meridian.

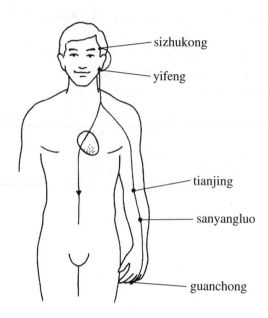

Fig 9.12 Hand Shao Yang Triple Warmer Meridian

The "hand shao yang triple warmer meridian" starts at the fourth finger, and flows up along the shao yang (middle-posterior) side of the arm. At the collar, it turns into the body, and its collaterals link with the pericardium, while the main meridian flows through the triple warmer region, subdividing into a network of collaterals.

At the chest a meridian-extension flows up along the neck to the back of the ear, where a collateral enters the ear, while the meridian-extension goes round the ear to the outer corner of the eye, where it joins the gall bladder meridian.

Once you understand the meridian system, you will appreciate why Chinese physicians always emphasize that health is holistic. When your triple warmer is full with energy, not only you will be emotionally stronger (as the triple warmer meridian and the pericardium meridian are directly related), even your eyesight is clearer, and your hearing sharper.

Gall Bladder and Liver Meridians

Health exercises are an important branch of Chinese medicine. There is a crucial difference between Chinese and western health exercises. While western exercises are mainly physical, loosening joints and muscles, the Chinese includes and go beyond this. The physical movements of Chinese health exercises are often not ends themselves, but means to induce internal energy flow, so that recovery works from inside out.

For example, when a patient complains of frequent stiffness at his neck, the cause of the problem may not be at the neck but at the gall bladder, especially if he also hears unusual noises!

So, when the therapist teaches him some neck and leg exercises, the purpose is not just loosening the joints, but a more thorough approach is to cleanse his gall bladder meridian, from where his problem originates but transmitted to the ears and neck. A study of the gall bladder meridian will further clarify this concept.

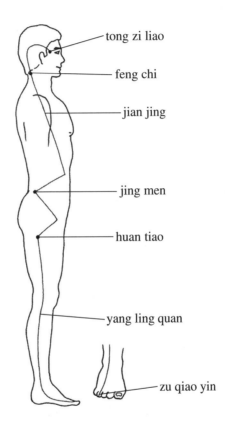

Fig 9.13 Leg Shao Yang Gall Bladder Meridian

The "leg shao yang gall bladder meridian" begins at the outer corner of the eye. There are two divisions, one flows round the ear where it meets the triple warmer meridian-extension at the "yifeng" (meaning "covering against wind") energy point, and enters the ear.

The other division flows down the neck, to the armpit, then down the body to the liver and the gall bladder, then around the pubic hair region, and down the leg along the shao yang (middle-posterior) side, terminating at the little toe, while at the ankle, a branch flows to the big toe.

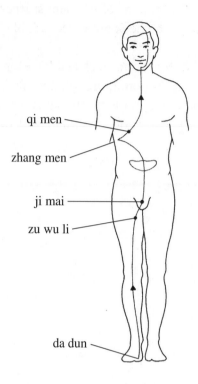

qi men

zhang men

ji mai

zu wu li

da dun

Fig 9.14 Leg Jue Yin Liver Meridian

The Chinese physician can have a good idea of the conditions of his patient's internal organs by examining the corresponding external organs. For example, by looking at the patient's eyes, the physician can diagnose the liver condition. This is the principle of "internal organs reflected by their corresponding external organs". How is this possible? By means of the meridian system. The liver, for example, is linked to the eyes by meridians.

The "leg jue yin liver meridian" receives energy from a collateral of the gall bladder meridian at the big toe, and flows up the foot to above the ankle where it meets the other two leg-yin meridians (spleen meridian and kidney meridian) at an energy point, which is appropriately called "sanyinjiao" (meeting of three yin meridians). The liver meridian flows up the leg at the jue yin (middle-anterior) side, and after entering the body, flows to the genitals.

Then it flows up to the liver, with a collateral to the gall bladder, up to the ribs, up again to the back of the throat, to the cheek and nose, and then to the eye system. From the eye, the liver meridian flows up the forehead to the back of the head to link with the du (governing) meridian.

A collateral flows from the eye to the mouth and goes round the lips, while at the liver another collateral goes into the lung, linking the liver meridian with the lung meridian, thus continuing the endless cycle of the meridian system.

Lakes and Seas of Energy

Chinese medical philosophers often refer to primary meridians as streams — along which vital energy flows; and secondary meridians as lakes — where reserved energy is stored.

There are eight secondary meridians, as illustrated in Fig 9.15:

1. Ren or conceptual meridian. (see Fig 9.16)
2. Du or governing meridian. (see Fig. 9.17)
3. Chong or rushing meridian.
4. Dai or belt meridian.
5. Yin qiao or in-tall meridian.
6. Yang qiao mai or out-tall meridian.
7. Yin wei or in-protective meridian.
8. Yang wei or out-protective meridian.

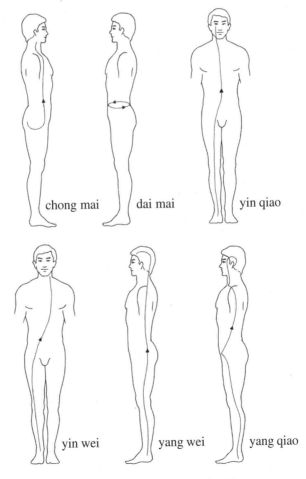

Fig 9.15 The Eight Secondary Meridians
(ren mai and du mai, see Fig. 9.16 and Fig. 9.17)

Of all the meridians in the body, the most important are the ren meridian and the du meridian. While the other meridians are considered streams and lakes, these two principal meridians are seas. The ren meridian is the "sea of yin energy", where all yin meridians flow to; while the du meridian is the "sea of yang energy", receiving all yang meridians.

The ren meridian flows from below the lower lip along the center of the frontal body, pass the navel, right to just before the anus, Fig 9.2. Numerous energy points (xue) and energy fields (dan tian) are found along the ren meridian.

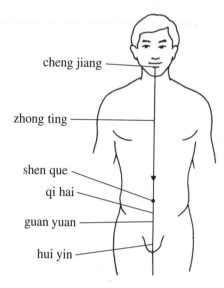

cheng jiang

zhong ting

shen que

qi hai

guan yuan

hui yin

Fig 9.16 Ren Mai or Conceptual Meridian

By stimulating an energy point with an acupuncture needle, or even with our finger, we can affect the energy flow along that meridian. An energy field is where much vital energy accumulates. It is a magnified energy point.

There are three major energy fields along the ren meridian: "tanzhong" or "middle of chest" found above the heart; "qihai" or "sea of energy" found about two inches below the navel; and "huiying" or "meeting of two yin" just before the anus.

This description of the ren meridian from the lips to the anus is according to the qigong paradigm where the "small universal qi flow" flows from the lips to the anus, then up the spine to the top of the head, and down again to the lips in a continuous cycle. In acupuncture books, however, the listing of the energy points along the ren meridian is from the anus up the lips.

Just after the anus, found at the tip of the spine, is the "changqiang" (long and powerful) vital point, from where the du meridian starts. The du or governing meridian, which is long and powerful, flows up the spine to the head, then down the front of the face to just above the upper lip, Fig 9.17.

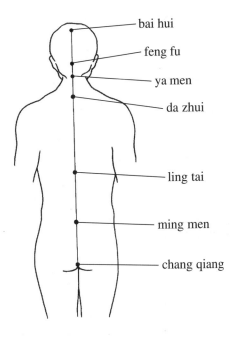

bai hui

feng fu

ya men

da zhui

ling tai

ming men

chang qiang

Fig 9.17 Du Mai or Governing Meridian

There are two important energy fields along the du meridian: "mingmen" or "gate of life" found at the center of the back waist; and "baihui" or "meeting of hundred meridians" found at the crown of the head.

There are two gaps separating the ren and the du meridians — the upper gap at the mouth, and the lower gap at the anus. If you can bridge these two gaps, and achieve a continuous flow of vital energy along the ren and the du meridians, you will have attained the "small universe", with the time-tested reward that you will never be ill.

If you can achieved the "big universe", having a continuous flow of vital energy throughout your twelve primary meridians, your reward is living to a hundred years. Obviously, many readers may find this claim ludicrous; but the claim was not made in jest, and it has been amply substantiated in Chinese qigong history.

On a personal note, while you have to wait another fifty years before I can tell you whether the big universe works for me, I am grateful to say that I really cannot remember the last time I was sick — thanks to my small universe.

10

DISCOVERING SEVEN EMOTIONS AND SIX EVILS

(The Principles of Chinese Pathology)

Much of the recent fundamental information in science has been
obtained by the process of reductionism — the exploring of details,
and the details of details, until all the smallest bits of the structure,
or the smallest parts of the mechanism, are exposed to scrutiny.

James B. Wyngaarden, M.D.

Different Philosophical Perspectives

A fundamental difference between western medicine and Chinese medicine is their attitude. When studying the cause of diseases, western medical scientists have progressed from organs and tissues to cells, scrutinizing in minute details the agents responsible for the sickness, and devising means to overcome these agents.

Chinese medical scientists are not so worried about such details; they are more concerned with the patient as a whole person, rather than the particular tissues or cells that are diseased.

Chinese physicians, for example, are not bothered whether an infected disease is caused by spiral-shaped spirochetes or obligate intracellular parasites, or whether asthma is caused by IgE-mediated external allergens or by alternation in airway temperature and humidity, so long as the infected disease or asthma is cured.

They do not know such ear-teasing pathogens like Haemophilus influenzae, Staphylococcus aureus, and Histoplasma capsulatum; or enzymes with tongue-twisting names like phenylalanine dehydroxylase, crystathionine B-synthase, and galactose-1-phosphate uradyl transferase.

This does not mean that when Chinese physicians are faced with ailments caused by such microscopic organisms, or disorder due to the deficiency of such enzymes, they would not know what to do. In fact the Chinese knew that microscopic organisms were found in our blood long before the Christian era!

How do Chinese physicians treat infectious diseases if they do not know in detail the exact causative agents? What specific drugs do they use to overcome the pathogens or the defective metabolic processes?

Chinese medical scientists are as interested in the cause of diseases as western medical scientists. But their approach is different.

While the western scientists emphasize the diseases, to the painstaking extent of studying the life-history of individual pathogenic cells or the molecular structure of enzyme reaction, the Chinese conveniently lump them together as evil energy and spleen energy respectively! Aren't the Chinese interested in which of the countless pathogens or enzymes that are responsible for the illnesses? No! But they are seriously interested in their patients getting well, and they accomplish this through treating their patients, not the disease.

Most, if not all of, the disease causing micro-organisms are already in our body. Yet, we are not sick because our natural systems can contain them. Western medical scientists, for example, find that the meningo-coccus bacteria may be present in the body but not effecting it, or they may cause life-inhibiting illnesses.

While western scientists try to solve this puzzling problem by investigating more deeply into the bacteria, the Chinese forget about the bacteria and analyze the changing conditions in the patient that caused him to succumb to the disease.

Prof. James Wyngaarden reflects the opinion of many western medical scientists when he says, "The list of human diseases for which there are as yet no definitive measures for prevention or cure is still formidable." What do the Chinese say? All great Chinese medical literature insists that if your yin-yang is in balance, and your vital energy is flowing harmoniously, you do not have to be sick in the first place!

In Chinese medical thinking, to be healthy is our birth-right. Sickness — whether contagious, organic or psychiatric — occurs *only* if certain parts of the body are not functioning naturally. Should a person be sick, as it sometimes happens, the logical approach is to restore his natural functions, and this can be done by restoring his yin-yang balance and harmonious energy flow.

The whole range of Chinese therapeutics is channelled to this purpose. Hence, there is no such term as "incurable diseases" in the Chinese medical vocabulary.

If the adjective "incurable" is used, it always refers to the patient, not his disease, such as when he has allowed his disease, which is curable in normal circumstances, to deteriorate to such an extent that recovery is difficult.

A Brave Attempt?

Perhaps a change of perspective from "treating the disease" to "treating the patient", if some western pioneers are brave enough to attempt, may have far reaching consequences in the future of western medicine. Many diseases are considered "incurable" from the western medical viewpoint, because western medical scientists have not found the root cause of these diseases. New diseases surface as soon as cures for old ones are found.

Moreover the western pathological conceptual framework is such that the same types of disease-causing agents are presumed to behave similarly even if they operate in different environments. It is not unreasonable to ask if such a premise is valid, as frequent reoccurrence of drug-resistant infections has often prompted the question.

The Chinese approach is different. They believe that the same pathogenic agents may work differently in different patients, just as the patients will react differently to the agents. Influenza viruses of the same amount and potency may harm one person but not another, because the latter has better flow of vital energy.

Taking a certain amount of rich food may cause hypertension in a sedentary worker, but not in an athlete whose effective body systems turn the rich food to better use. A stressful environment may bring psychiatric problems to some people.

Nevertheless, to those who practice meditation regularly, a similar environment may have minimal effects or none at all. It is not the pathogenic agents, but the failure to react effectively to the agents, that causes sickness.

Hence, because Chinese physicians look at the causes of illnesses according to the conditions of the patients, such as their energy flow, metabolic processes and emotional response; instead of according to the types of pathogenic agents, diseases which western medical thinking regards as the same because they are caused by the same agents, may be treated differently by Chinese physicians, though the generalization into convenient types of diseases is possible.

It is tempting to ask whether the cul-de-sac faced by western medical scientists concerning "incurable" diseases is due to their pathological approach. Since their therapeutics depend on their pathological discoveries, and since it is near impossible (if not actually impossible) to find the causes of some diseases because there are so many uncertain variables, it logically follows that cures have not been found — not because there are no cures, but because of faulty premise.

A philosophical shift from disease-emphasis to patient-emphasis in our pathological approach may open unsuspected avenues. It is worthy of note that the same pathogenic agents in different persons, or in the same person at different times, will produce different effects.

Western cancer experts believe that every person has cancer thousands of times in his life time, yet the same thousands of times he cures himself without his own knowing. "It is because of immune system errors and failures that we get the flu or cancer or even atherosclerotic plaques." What caused the immune system errors and failures that cause the flu or cancer or atherosclerotic plaques?

When we have decisively defined the disease as cancer, then we start looking for what caused the immune system to fail, it is difficult to pinpoint the unknown causes because they vary from persons to persons, as well as spatially and temporally.

But the same case will become a different situation if we adopt a different perspective, if we avoid predetermining the name of the disease and concentrate on the known conditions of the patient to find out in what ways these conditions are different from when he was healthy.

These pathogenetic conditions of the patient, which represent the patient's inability to react effectively to known or unknown diseases, are therefore the causes of the disease. Only when we have found the causes, we designate a name to the disease — but not before — because its designation depend on the causes, not on the agent.

We should remember that the same agent in a healthy environment will not cause the disease: that is why a healthy person can have cancer thousands of times without being sick, or harbour millions of deadly gems in his body without succumbing to its diseases.

If he ever becomes sick, it is not due to the agent, but due to his inability at that time to react effectively against these agents. Our job as healers, therefore, is to find out the causes of that inability, which is temporary and unnatural, and correct or remove the causes to restore the patient to his natural ability.

Internal Causes of Seven Emotions

There are of course countless individual factors that cause a person to temporarily lose his natural ability to overcome diseases, but these countless factors can be generalized into types. Chinese physicians have classified the types of causes that affect man's natural functioning, thus resulting in illnesses, into three groups: internal causes, external causes, and neither-internal-nor-external causes.

The importance of psychological factors in Chinese pathology is reflected in their naming the seven emotions as the internal causes of illnesses. These "Seven Emotions" are joy, anger, melancholy, anxiety, sorrow, fear and shock.

Joy is a healthy factor, but an intense and prolonged experience of overjoy harms the heart, and thus becomes an endogenous pathogenic cause. Overjoy drains away heart energy. This is a good example of moderation in everything. Negative joy, like pleasure derived from harming others, is similarly pathogenic.

Anger injures the liver. When a person is angry, he excites his liver fire (i.e. his liver over functions), his face becomes pale and his limbs tremble. Anger causes energy to rise, which may result in distorted eyesight, headaches, giddiness and vomiting blood. In Chinese medical thinking, the liver regulates blood flow and is related to the heart. Hence, a person who becomes angry easily is prone to heart diseases.

Melancholy injures the lung. When a person worries too much and is excessively melancholic, he may lose his appetite, cough and vomit, develop constipation and insomnia, and have sexual difficulties. His spirit is dejected and his energy flow is blocked. Melancholic people or those suddenly exposed to great worry easily succumb to lung diseases.

Anxiety injures the spleen. When a persons thinks too much or is excessively anxious, his spleen and stomach systems will be affected. His energy becomes congested, and his digestive and absorptive systems malfunction, resulting in loss of appetite, chest or abdominal flatulence, headaches and dizziness, insomnia and amnesia (loss of memory). Hence, when you are anxious, you lose your urge for food.

Sorrow injures both the heart and the lungs. Excessive sorrow makes a person lose his spirit and hope in life. It stresses the heart and drains away energy. The patient has no appetite, may cough, suffer from insomnia and may urinate blood. This explains why unrequited love often results in consumption.

Fear injures the kidneys. It causes energy to sink and be drained, and may result in losing control of faeces and urine excretion, involuntary diarrhoea, nocturnal emission, convulsions and mental disorder. It may cause sexual problems.

Shock injures the spirit and the heart. It scatters the spirit and disperses energy, and may result in severe palpitation, insomnia, loss of concentration, convulsion, loss of consciousness, and mental disorder. Shock also injures the gall bladder and the kidney.

These "seven emotions" clearly show the profound knowledge of the Chinese concerning the close relationship between physiological and psychological factors in health and medicine. Western medical scientists who wonder why psychosomatic and degenerative diseases are becoming widespread in modern living, may derive some insight and inspiration from this ancient Chinese wisdom.

The Chinese regard these physiological and psychological factors as endogenous pathogenic causes. The relationship between these seven emotions and psychiatric disorders will be explained in Chapters 25 and 26.

An interesting and effective technique employed in Chinese medicine is the use of the appropriate emotion in treating emotional or psychiatric illnesses.

According to Chinese psychology, sorrow overcomes anger, fear overcomes joy, anger overcomes worry, joy overcomes melancholy, and worry overcomes fear. For example, a person suffering from nocturnal emission as a result of fear, may have his sickness cured by making him worry.

A dejected lover suffering from tuberculosis — often caused by sorrow that weakens the self-defence system of his lungs — will soon recover if his lover agrees to marry him. There are many cases of such successful interplay of emotions, without using medication, recorded in Chinese medical case histories.

Some readers may be surprised that Chinese medicine is very advanced in psychiatry. Actually, psychiatry was never separated from other aspects of

Chinese medicine, as in conventional western medicine, because the Chinese have always regarded that the physical body, the emotions and the mind are intimately related.

External Causes of Six Evils

Besides physiological and psychological considerations, environmental and climatic factors are also very important in Chinese pathology. Since ancient times, Chinese physicians have recognized that even if a person is not subjected to microscopic organism attacks, organic dysfunction or psychosomatic disturbances, he can still be sick if he fails to adjust to climatic or environmental changes.

Perhaps western doctors, neurosurgeons and psychiatrists who find nothing clinically wrong with their patients, may find some useful information in the following paragraphs.

Chinese physicians classify climatic and environmental changes, as well as disease-causing microscopic organisms and all other external agents, as exogenous pathogenic causes, which are figuratively referred to as the "Six Evils". These six evils, which have no ethical or religious connotation, are wind, cold, heat, dampness, dryness and fire.

These terms, of course, are symbolic, and should not be interpreted literally. These causes are forms of energy. In their normal situations when they do not cause illnesses, they are refereed to as Six Energies, and may be beneficial to our body.

Wind is regarded as a primary evil, and it often combines with other evils to bring about illnesses. The chief features of wind are its changeability and fluidity. Wind brings about symptoms related to the common cold, like headaches, running nose, sore throat and cough.

Cold is brought about by agents causing contagious diseases, resulting in symptoms of feeling cold, pain at the limbs, no sweating, no thirst, sour limbs, headaches, fever, whitish fur on the tongue, and weak pulse rate.

Heat is caused by exposure to high temperature. This results in the draining energy and dehydration. The symptoms are fever, thirst, sweating, shortness of breath, tiredness, congested chest, loss of appetite, swollen abdomen and purging.

Dampness is related with pathogenic microscopic organisms in contaminated drinks and food. Its symptoms are heavy head, congested chest, painful limbs and joints, slight fever, and purging. It often takes some time to develop into illnesses.

Dryness is caused by dry, hot surroundings, and frequently affect the skin and the respiratory system. Its symptoms are dried lips, dried mouth, sore throat, little phlegm, dry cough, dry skin, fever, thirst, solid faeces, no sweating and blocked nose.

Fire is excessive heat, and brings about illnesses quickly. The patient's reaction is rapid and varied. Its symptoms are fever, deficiency of body fluid, various forms of bleeding, swelling, pain, rashes, irritability and coma.

The above evil energies, with the exception of heat, can also be internal. Internal wind affects the nervous system, with symptoms like giddiness, numbness of limbs, and spasms. Internal cold indicates the weakening of the body's metabolic processes, with symptoms like feeling cold, loss of appetite, clear urine, liquid faeces, and weak pulse rate.

Internal dampness suggests the dysfunction of the digestive system, and its common symptoms are yellowish face, little urine, purging, and swollen appearance.

Internal dryness points to the deficiency of body fluids, including lack of blood flow, with symptoms like fever, sweating, purging, thirst and dry skin. Internal fire refers to the over-functioning of internal organs. The symptoms vary according to which internal organ is involved, but some common symptoms are thirst, reddish face, feeling warm, and hard of sleep.

Readers used to western pathology may find the above pathological explanation of disease by the Chinese, odd or even ridiculous. To say that "wind causes running nose" may be tolerable, but headaches and coughing, and more imponderably, numbness of limbs and spasms? And what has dampness to do with heavy head, congested chest and purging?

A New Way of Viewing Disease

The following points will be helpful to puzzled readers. We are now viewing pathology with a different paradigm, and from a different perspective. Imposing western concepts onto it, is not appropriate.

The question as whether the western or the Chinese paradigm is correct or better, does not arise here; though readers may form their own judgment after they have understood the Chinese version. "Wind" here is used symbolically; of course it does not mean a flow of air as used in normal language.

If a patient experiences some pain at the shoulder, and later this pain "flows" to the elbow, the Chinese physician symbolically calls this particular syndrome "wind". (You may call this special pathological feature x, y or z, but then you will miss the benefit of sharing a vast amount of knowledge on "wind" gathered over the centuries.)

It is important to note that while the "six evils" may sometimes be applied to exogenous pathogenic agents, they are basically used to describe the conditions of the patient that cause his illness. For example, when a Chinese physician says that the cause of his patient's sickness is "dampness", he was not referring to the disease-causing micro-organisms, but the patient's conditions of having a heavy head, congested chest and purging.

If you ask, "How does a Chinese physician cure a patient suffering from diarrhoea caused by Staphylococcus aureus?", the answer is "He does not know." But if such a patient consults the Chinese physician, he will treat the patient (not the disease) according to the paradigm he is trained in, and be able to cure the patient easily.

He will diagnose that the disease was caused by "dampness" and "heat", and probably say that the patient's spleen energy and kidney energy are weak. He will prescribe the appropriate therapeutics to eliminate fever, thirst, purging, heavy head, congested chest and other related symptoms.

He will also, if he is a competent physician, follow up with nourishing the patient's spleen and kidney energy, though the lack of energy in these organs may not be an immediate problem.

What happened to the Staphylococcus aureus, which western doctors regard as the cause of the diarrhoea, but which Chinese physicians neither know nor are interested in? We do not know for sure. They may have been killed by the medicine the patient took, or by his own defence system, which has improved as a result of the treatment; or they may be involved in activities that modern scientists have not discovered, such as doing some useful work for their host!

What we know for sure is that these Staphylococcus aureus, dead or alive, no longer give their host any trouble.

If this patient suffers from diarrhoea again, he may not be given the same treatment. Why? Because, though the main causes are still "dampness" and "heat", there may be other changes in the patient's conditions. He may, for example, have improved his spleen and kidney energy; or he may have other complications like "wind" or "fire", or affected by some of the "seven emotions".

The physician, we should remember, treats the patient, not the disease.

Neither-Internal-Nor-External Causes

All other causes that do not fall into the internal causes of "Seven Emotions" nor the external causes of "Six Evils" are considered "Neither-Internal-Nor-External Causes". They include inappropriate food and drinks, insufficient exercise and rest, excessive sex, injuries caused by animals, and injuries from hits and falls.

In western medicine, dietetics is a 20th century development. Readers would be astonished to find that as early as the Zhou Dynasty, more than 2000 years ago, dieticians existed as a separate professional group in China.

A Chinese dietician does much more than advising people on how to keep slim; he plans elaborate programs for curing illnesses through food (not medicine), enhancing vitality (often applied by the rich for their sexual pleasure), and promoting longevity.

In pathology, too rich or too poor food, irregular meals and an unbalanced diet cause illnesses. The ancient Chinese also knew much about the prevention and cure for food poisoning.

Chinese physicians have long considered exercise and rest as important as food for maintaining good health. The great 2nd century physician, Hua Tuo, said that "just as a door which is not frequently used will rot, a person who does not regularly exercise will be sick."

The exercises for health recommended by Chinese physicians are gentle and graceful, different from the vigourous physical exercises in the west. The aim of Chinese exercises is to enhance energy flow, rather than exhaust it.

Insufficient as well as excessive rest is detrimental to health. A good guideline to show that a person has the proper amount of sleep is that he would jump out of bed fresh and alert the moment he wakes up. Irregular sleeping hours is unhealthy.

Excessive or inadequate food, exercise, rest or sex is harmful. While the Chinese believe that moderate and regular sex is healthy, excessive and licentious sex is one of the surest ways to drain away energy. Moderation should also be extended to other desires, such as pastimes and interests.

Diseases may result from a great variety of other causes, such as injuries from insect and animal bites, from occupational hazards and accidents, from sharp and pointed objects, and from hits and falls. Injuries sustained from hits and falls constitute a major branch of Chinese medicine, known as "die da" (pronounced as "t'iek t'a"), which is unique in the world. It will be explained in some detail in the chapter on Chinese Traumatology.

A Challenge for the Brave

Our conceptual framework on how illnesses happens, has a direct influence on the methods we devise to overcome it. The western approach, which many of its own experts lament as becoming over reductionist and mechanical, offers only one of the numerous possibilities, with the obvious and urgent setback that it cannot satisfactorily explain the cause, and consequently cannot suggest the cure, for many of today's pressing diseases.

The Chinese pathological approach is strikingly different. Concordant with the latest, startling scientific discovery that the universe is a body of energy rather than a big machine, Chinese medical philosophy postulates that health results from a harmonious flow of energy.

Distinctively in contrast with the reductionist and mechanical approach of the west, the Chinese approach is holistic and organic, insisting that health is natural, and that illnesses occur because of some unnatural interference, which can definitely be rectified.

This medical philosophy, which has been proven valid by practice since ancient times, rightly provides us with the hope and inspiration that cures are not found for many diseases in western medical thinking, not because these cures are not possible, but because it is technically inappropriate to expect what works for an isolated minute part in a machine, works equally well for a comparatively gigantic, ever-changing living organism.

Another striking difference worthy of note is that while western pathology relates the disease to the pathogenic agent, Chinese pathology relates the disease to the patient. The western doctor first defines the disease, then he prescribes the appropriate treatment based on this definition. If he does not understand the pathogenic agent sufficiently, he is helpless in his treatment.

Until recently, when faced with diseases such as non-fatal viral infections and organ dysfunction, he could afford to continue with the current practice of providing supportive medication. But with the increasing threat from cancer and AIDS, perhaps it is time to consider other alternatives to complement or improve on the current practices.

It is reasonable to ask whether a philosophical shift of pathological approach can help to solve the present pressing problems. The Chinese physician is less concerned about the exactness of the pathogenic agent; he transfers his full attention to the patient, seeking why the patient has failed contain the disease which he could successfully contain in the past.

The Chinese physician firmly believes that health is a natural birthright, that the present disease occurs because certain natural functions fail to operate as they should. His job is to define where this failure of natural functions lies, and in his paradigm the term "incurable" becomes irrelevant.

Cancer occurs in every person thousands of times, yet for the same thousands of times, his own natural systems overcome the cancer. When one or some of these systems fail to function naturally, cancer surfaces. Dedicated researchers have spent so much time and effort trying to pinpoint the cancer-causing agents, but so far to no avail. Isn't it sensible to try the alternative approach, at least for some of the research, transferring our attention from the elusive pathogenic agent to the patient, who has until recently successfully fought cancer throughout his life, finding out why he cannot do so now? Once we know the reasons, it will not be difficult to restore his natural functions.

While many patients may think the placebo cures them of their viral infections, all doctors know that the patients cure themselves. It is therefore a blatant mistake to say that viral infections are incurable.

Technically, probably the only difference between AIDS infection and other non-fatal viral infections is that AIDS is fatal.

As long years of research have shown that chemotherapy is ineffective against viral infections, and we know that viral infections can be cured by the patients' natural systems themselves, wouldn't it be advisable to focus on the patient instead of the agent in at least some of the research to find a cure for AIDS?

Chinese medical scientists have amassed a rich body of knowledge concerning their patient-orientated approach to medicine. In the past, because of linguistic, cultural and other difficulties, such invaluable knowledge is generally not accessible to the west.

This book is a modest attempt to overcome this problem, and to share in a vocabulary and imagery easily comprehensible to English readers this Chinese medical wisdom, with the hope that some courageous researchers, ready to bear the inevitable mockery of their conservative and mediocre colleagues, may take up the challenge to study present pressing problems from a different perspective so as to come out with some startling medical breakthroughs for the benefit of all humanity.

Some of this wisdom regarding what principles Chinese physicians use in diagnosing their patients, will be explained in the next chapter.

WHAT'S WRONG WITH THE PATIENT, NOT THE DISEASE

(The Principles of Chinese Diagnosis)

Care more for the individual patient than for the special features of the disease.

Sir William Osler.

The Chinese Perspective

The Chinese have a very elaborate procedure for diagnosis, because it is very important in Chinese medicine.   Only when we know what the patient is suffering from, can we prescribe the correct therapeutics. This truth is so obvious that the statement appears like a platitude.

Yet it is not infrequent that even specialists in western medicine openly admit they are not sure of the disease they are treating, and that they have to try out a few types of medication before they can narrow down to the correct type! These doctors should be admired for their honesty and efforts despite the shortcomings, which are not their faults.

The faults lie with the western pathological perspective, which presumes that all diseases, known and unknown, can be categorized into specific types, given specific names, and that treatment for a particular disease type for one patient is basically the same as for all patients.

Chinese physicians certainly know much less about diseases than their western counterparts. But this does not matter much, because Chinese physicians do not treat diseases; they treat patients! In other words, when a patient consults a Chinese physician, the physician's objective is to restore the patient to health, and not just to eliminate his disease.

Superficially, restoring health and eliminating diseases look like two roads to the same goal; but on closer study, there are some crucial differences. The Chinese physician is usually sure of the road, for it is relatively easier to find out what is wrong in the patient's health, which is working with known variables, than what causes this wrong, which is working with the unknown. But the western doctor is sometimes uncertain whether such a road exists when he fails to define the disease.

Moreover, the goal may not be the same, because eliminating the disease may not necessarily restore the patient to health! The disease may be eliminated but the patient is often weakened by the treatment or by the side-effects of the treatment; and sometimes other ailments arise. In the case of cancer, this problem is saddening.

Western treatment of cancer may eliminate the disease by killing all the cancer cells, but it can be so drastic that it also kills the patient. Even if he survives, his quality of life has deteriorated to such an extend that it is difficult to say his health has been restored.

One even wonders whether it is better to let the patient carry on his normal life despite his cancer, than to subject him to drastic treatment which many honest doctors know has a very low chance of success, but which will transform the patient into a physical and mental wretch.

The criteria for measuring recovery are different too. Western doctors usually insist on quantitative measurement (especially when claims of recovery are made by other healing systems), and they only admit of a cure when no relapse is recorded for a certain period. Chinese physicians measure qualitatively.

If the patient can reasonably carry on with all the activities he normally does when he is healthy, he is considered to have been restored to health. Chinese physicians do not even have the instruments for sophisticated measurements, as they have never considered them necessary.

My own experiences with Ron, a heart patient who is about seventy years old, typically illustrates that what concerns a patient most is his health, and not technical measurements of his disease which often confuses him. Ron's condition was so bad that literally he was unable to walk ten steps without falling.

The hospital he was staying in, asked him to go home "instead of wasting expensive fees". Yet, after six months of qigong therapy, he was well enough to walk alone to town to enjoy breakfast.

I told him to return to his former hospital for quantitative measurements for his heart's condition so as to confirm he was cured. His reply was illuminating. "I know I am cured," he said. "I can do most things I used to do, though now with extra care and caution. Why should I seek confirmation from those who could not cure me in the first place? It may start my problem all over again!"

This happened a few years ago; he is still sound and healthy — irrespective of what the technical readings of his heart's conditions may be.

There is a saying in Chinese medicine: "It is easy to prescribe medicine, but it is difficult to diagnose a patient," To help the physician in his diagnosis, past masters summarized their experiences into a simple verse:

> The formula of eight words should be used
> The practice of four methods must be sound
> The findings be analyzed and compiled
> The causes of all diseases can then be found

It is interesting to note that Chinese physicians believe that the causes of all diseases can be found; therefore there is no such thing as "incurable diseases" in Chinese medical vocabulary. If a physician fails to cure a patient, it is not because the disease is incurable, but because the physician fails to diagnose the right causes, or fails to prescribe the correct therapeutics, or the patient has become so severely sick that recovery is difficult.

The Chinese physician seeks the causes of the disease in the patient, not in the disease itself, because the "same" disease would operate differently in different patients or in the same patient at different times. Hence, the physician sets to find out not what exactly the disease causative agents are, but what exactly went wrong in the patient that permits the disease to happen.

In other words, the physician's job is not to define the disease nor its agents — like whether a kidney problem is acute tubular necrosis or prerenal azotema, or whether the pathogens are Bacte-roides fragilis or Clostridium difficile; but to define disease-causing conditions — like what aspects of the patient's yin-yang are not balanced, or where his energy flow is not harmonious.

In short, the Chinese physician does not diagnose the disease as western doctors do; he diagnoses the patient.

This does not imply that Chinese physicians deny the crucial role of microscopic pathogens. The Chinese certainly recognize that microscopic organisms can cause diseases. In fact, long before the west they have devised special systems to classify diseases caused by exogenous pathogens, as we shall see in the next chapter.

Eight Diagnostic Principles

The "formula of eight words" mentioned in the above verse refers to eight principles used by Chinese physicians to understand illnesses. These eight words, which work in pairs, are cold, hot, empty, solid, internal, external, yin and yang. The words are meant to summarize syndromes exhibited by the patient, not characteristics of pathogenic agents.

We must also bear in mind the linguistic and cultural differences between the English and the Chinese: as in other medical terms translated from Chinese to English, the words should be interpreted symbolically, not literally.

Whether the disease is classified as cold or hot depends on the nature of the disease. Cold diseases show the following symptoms: deficient in body warmth, afraid of being cold, not feeling thirsty, clear urine, liquid faeces, slow and feeble pulse rate, cold limbs, pale face, and whitish fur on tongue. Cold diseases are related to weakening of physiological functions and low energy level.

In other words, when a Chinese physician diagnoses a disease as cold, it suggests that one, some or all of the patient's internal organs are under-functioning.

The following are the symptoms of hot diseases: feverish, warm limbs, feeling hot and stuffy, thirsty, thick and short urine, solid faeces, red face, dried lips, red or yellowish tongue, and rapid and strong pulse rate. Hot diseases are related to activated physiological functions and increased metabolic processes.

They are often found in contagious diseases. "Cold" and "hot" here are different from, but related to, "cold" and "heat" as two of the six evils mentioned in the previous chapter.

Whether the illness is "empty" or "solid" refers to the relationship between the natural physiological functions and body resistance on one hand, and the effects of pathogenic agents on the other. Generally, empty diseases are the result of the weakening of the bodily functions, whereas solid diseases are caused by the increasing potency of pathogenic agents.

The cause of an empty diseases is not obvious, like energy blockage or hormonal imbalance, whereas the cause of a solid disease is obvious, like a viral attack or a structural defect.

When a physician diagnoses a patient as having a solid disease, for example, it suggests that he is not reacting effectively to some exo-pathogenic agents.

Common symptoms of empty illnesses are sweating, slow and feeble pulse rate, shrunk tongue, feeling weak and tired, and failing physiological functions. Common symptoms of solid diseases include strong pulse, swollen tongue, bodily swelling, pus, phlegm and other secretions.

When your conventional doctor cannot find any clinical cause of your sickness, though both you and your doctor realize that the ailment is not imaginary, it is likely to be an empty disease.

External or internal diseases refer to the depth or developmental stage of the illness. External diseases are found at the skin and flesh levels, whereas internal diseases occurs inside the body or in internal organs.

However, the crucial factor in determining whether the disease is external or internal, is not so much the location of the disease, as the state of the patient's reaction against it. An infection, for example, may be found at the skin level, but if its effect threatens the internal organs, it can be regarded as at the internal stage.

The main symptoms of external diseases are being afraid of cold or wind, fever, blocked nose, whitish fur on the tongue, "floating" pulse, headaches, sour limbs and body pains.

The main symptoms of internal diseases are very high fever, solid faeces, thick and yellowish urine, yellowish tongue, "sunken" pulse, congested chest, swollen abdomen, delirious, dejected, and semiconscious.

Yin and yang refer to the two primary guidelines that can summarize the other six factors mentioned above. Diseases that are internal, cold and empty are generally termed as yin illnesses, whereas diseases that are external, hot and solid are yang illnesses.

Yin illnesses shows the following main symptoms: pale face, feeble voice, afraid of cold, clear urine, liquid faeces, not thirsty, and weak pulse rate. Yang illnesses includes the following main symptoms: red and bright face, fever, loud voice, solid faeces, thick and yellowish urine, fast breathing, and strong pulse rate.

These eight principles are useful guidelines enabling the physician to understand his patient's symptoms systematically. These principles, however, must never be taken as rigid rules.

In his diagnosis, the physician must also be aware of "false symptoms". For example, the patient may be feverish, thirsty and have a clear pulse rate, thus giving an appearance of a yang illness. On closer examination, we may find his metabolic processes not functioning properly, and his energy level is low.

Although he is feverish, he is afraid of cold; he is thirsty, but he does not desire to drink; his pulse may be clear, but it lacks strength. Actually his is a yin sickness, commonly found in the advanced stage of a contagious disease when his body's natural defence has been worn down. Such is an example of a "solid yin disease manifested as empty yang symptoms."

On the other hand, a patient may appear to have yin symptoms. He does not sweat, his limbs are cold, he feels bodily pains, and he has "floating" pulse rate. However, his physiological functions are working well, and his energy level high. He does not need extra clothing, his body is warm, his urine yellowish, his faeces hard and smelly, and his pulse rate strong.

His case is "solid yang disease manifested as empty yin symptoms", often found in a strong, healthy person initially attacked by some contagious disease.

In his diagnosis, the physician needs to consider the following factors:

1. Location: whether the illness is "internal" or "external".
2. Body resistance: whether the illness is "empty" or "solid".
3. Behaviour of illness: whether the illness has the properties of "wind", "cold", "dryness", "dampness", "heat" or "fire".
4. Developmental stage: whether the illness is "superficial", "initial", "intermediate" or "advanced". The Chinese terms for these stages are "wei", "qi", "ying" and "xue". In physiological context, these terms have different meanings.

Four Diagnostic Methods

How does a Chinese physician discover whether a disease is external or internal, solid or empty, cold or hot, and initial or intermediate? The numerous techniques he can use to find this information are generalized into a system known as the "Four Diagnostic Methods", namely viewing, listening and smelling, asking, and feeling.

The following paragraphs give a general introduction to the clinical implication of the symptoms derived from the four diagnostic methods. Do not be discouraged if you find the information overwhelming: it is a summary of what Chinese medical students take many months to learn.

To avoid wordiness, terms like yin and yang deficiency are often used; readers who are unclear of their meaning may have to refer to the glossary or the relevant pages of this book for explanation.

Viewing

First, make an overall visual examination of the patient. View his general spirit, form and nature. If the patient's eyes sparkle, his face is bright, his movements unrestricted, and his voice clear, then his illness is likely to be yang, hot, external or solid. However, if his eyes are lacklustre, his face looks twisted, his movements unnatural, and his voice muffled, then his illness can be classified as yin, cold, internal or empty.

After the general viewing, we perform some localized visual examination. View the patient's skin, tongue, eyes, nose, and lips. Greenish skin indicates wind, cold and pain. Yellowish skin indicates dampness, heat or empty illness. Reddish skin indicates heat. Dark skin indicates cold. Whitish skin indicates that his natural body resistance has weakened.

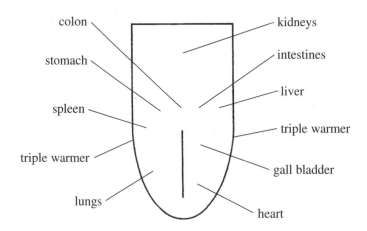

Fig 11.1 Internal Organs Manifested in Tongue

The conditions of various internal organs are expressed in the different parts of the tongue, as shown in Fig 11.1 above. A pinkish tongue suggests external illness, such as contagious diseases at the superficial or initial stage. A reddish tongue suggests hot or solid illnesses, such as contagious diseases that have developed to the intermediate stage.

A reddish tongue without fur, irrespective of whether the disease is contagious or not, indicates yin deficiency of the stomach or kidney systems, or deficiency of internal secretions. A whitish tongue suggests cold or apparent illnesses, such as anaemia and dysfunction of internal organs.

A purplish tongue suggests that hot illness has developed to the advanced stage. A light, shining purplish tongue suggests yang deficiency of the heart or kidney systems, often found in patients whose heart or lung functions have weakened. A hard tongue that has difficulty in movement indicates nervous or muscular dysfunction.

Eyes that are reddish, swollen or painful indicate the presence of wind and heat in the liver meridian. Dilated pupils suggest yin deficiency of the kidneys. Bulging eyes and swollen face suggest oedema (excessive retention of tissue fluid). Running nose with clear mucus indicates exogenous sickness due to wind and cold, whereas that with thick mucus indicate exogenous sickness due to wind and heat.

Pale lips indicate blood deficiency. Purplish green lips suggest blood stasis. Pale red lips suggest empty illnesses, often those caused by the dysfunction of the heart or lungs; whereas dark red lips suggest hot or solid illnesses. Sore lips indicate heat at the stomach and spleen; whereas crack lips indicate deficiency of body fluids.

Listening and Smelling

Listening involves listening to the patient's voice and breath. If his voice is loud and clear, the disease belongs to the solid type. If his voice is low and feeble, or he does not like to speak, his disease is empty and cold.

If the patient's breathing is fast and rough, his disease is hot. Fast, feeble breathing indicates that the disease is empty, especially when the patient looks weak. A patient who shows a preference of breathing in to breathing out, is likely to suffer from an empty illness; whereas the opposite situation indicates a solid illness.

If the patient's mouth emits foul smell, the illness is usually caused by heat of the stomach. If the phlegm is smelly, the illness is caused by heat of the lung, whereas odourless phlegm is caused by deficiency of lung yin.

Asking

We can obtain valuable information by asking about the patient's body warmth, sweating, excretion, appetite, and various bodily responses.

If the patient has a slight fever and is afraid of the cold, his illness is caused by the pathogenic agents of wind and cold. If the fever is high and he is thirsty, but only a little afraid of cold, the causes are wind and heat. Being afraid of cold is an indication that the sickness is at the superficial or initial stage.

When a patient no longer feels cold, but he is still constantly thirsty and the fever remains very high, this means that the illness has developed into the intermediate or advanced stage.

If the patient feels cold, but has no fever and his limbs are cold, the sickness is generally caused by yang deficiency with internal cold. If the patient has night sweating, and the centers of his palms are hot, then he generally suffers from yin deficiency with internal heat.

In diseases of the exogenous pathogenic nature, fever with sweating suggests the illnesses to be external and empty; without sweating suggests external and solid. Profuse sweating by a weak patient, although the weather is not warm, indicates yang deficiency. Night sweating indicates yin deficiency. Profuse sweating, severe fear of cold, cold limbs and hidden pulse rate indicate a serious, critical condition of yang-exhaustion.

If the patient's stool is hard and his abdomen full, the sickness is usually solid: whereas liquid stood and abdomen soft suggest empty illnesses. If the urine is yellowish or reddish, the disease is caused by heat; and if it is also short and painful, the hot disease is accompanied with dampness. Long, clear urine suggests a cold disease; and if it is frequent, the disease is caused by yang deficiency.

If the patient likes to take cold food, but often vomits, the sickness is caused by heat of the stomach. If he feels a full abdomen after food, the illness is caused by dysfunction of the stomach and spleen systems. If the patient feels comfortable after taking food, the sickness is usually empty: if he feels uncomfortable, it is generally solid.

If the mouth tastes bitter, the sickness is often caused by heat of the liver or gall bladder; if it tastes sweet, dampness and heat of the spleen; salty, heat of the kidneys; if it tastes flat, then heat of the stomach and bowel, or the illness is cold or empty.

Headaches, neck pains, feeling cold and fever often indicate external diseases. If the pain is at certain parts of the head or neck only, then the illness is often caused by internal wind or blood deficiency.

If the whole body and joints feel sour and painful, accompanied by fever, feeling of cold and headaches, the sickness is generally caused by exogenous wind and cold. If the numbness and pains are fairly fixed at certain parts, the sickness is caused by cold and dampness; whereas if the pain travels about in the body, it is caused by dampness and heat.

Chest pains, fever, with rust-colored phlegm indicates heat of the lung. Chest pains spreading to the left arm or back indicates problems of the heart or pericardium. Congested chest with shortness of breath suggests deficiency of energy.

Feeling

Feeling refers to feeling the pulse as well as feeling various parts of the body. Feeling the pulse is a major aspect of Chinese medicine. There is a common misconception that a skilful Chinese physician can tell the nature of a patient's illness just by feeling his pulse. This is not true, because the pulse, though very important, tells only part of the patient's conditions; it should be combined with other diagnostic techniques to obtain a more complete examination.

The pulse gives a good indication of the nature and volume of a person's energy flow. The pulse can be taken at many places, such as at the head, neck, arm-pit and legs. But generally it is taken at the wrist, where it is divided into three portions called "cun" (inch), "guan" (connection), and "chi" (foot). These portions on the left and the right wrists are related to different internal organs, Fig 11.2.

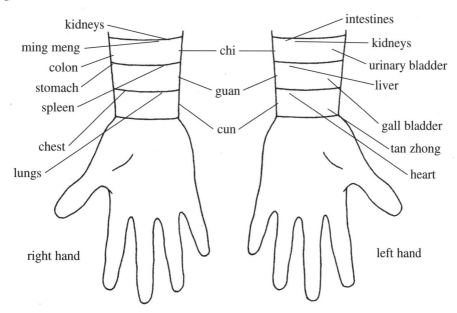

Fig 11.2 Internal Organs Reflected on Wrist Pulse

When we feel a pulse, we examine its frequency, rhythm, force, position and form. Great masters have classified the different pulses into 28 major types. Here we will study 6 typical pulse groups.

(a) Floating Pulse.
The pulse is clearly felt, as if floating at the skin surface. Its wavelength is wide, and its beat is strong. It indicates that the illness is external, and is generally found in contagious diseases at the superficial or initial stage.

(b) Submerged Pulse.
The pulse can only be felt when the fingers are pressed hard on the wrist. Its beat is slow, and its wave-length low. It indicates an internal illness.

(c) Slow Pulse.
The frequency is slow, less than 3 beats per breathing, or less than 60 times per minute. This pulse indicates cold illnesses where the nervous system is affected. It is often found in cardiovascular diseases.

(d) Frequent Pulse.
The frequency is fast, 6-7 times per breathing, or more than 100 times per minute. It indicates illnesses caused by heat, as found in contagious diseases.

(e) Empty Pulse.
The pulse can be felt at the surface, medial or deep level, but the beat is feeble. It indicates empty illnesses, where there is yang deficiency and energy deficiency. The body resistance and metabolic processes have weakened.

(f) Solid Pulse.
The pulse can be felt at the surface, medial and deep levels, and the beat is strong. It indicates solid illnesses. The patient's body resistance and metabolism processes are good, hence recovery is easier.

Other parts of the body also provide indications of the patient's conditions. Cold limbs generally show deficiency of yang energy, whereas heat at the centers of palms and soles suggests yin deficiency. Exogenous diseases are often indicated by warm palms; whereas cold, hard swelling indicates cold illnesses.

If you still wonder how do outward symptoms reveal internal conditions, like swollen eyes suggesting wind and heat at the liver, or reddish tongue indicating yin deficiency of the stomach, you have missed some fascinating information on man's internal cosmos and energy flow explained in Chapters 7, 8 and 9. This knowledge is not only essential to pathology and diagnosis, but also to therapeutics.

Basically, when we know how our body works, once we can correctly identify where our natural functions have gone wrong, it is not difficult to restore our natural functions.

In the next chapter we will learn how Chinese physicians classify the wide range of symptoms they have gathered, into convenient systems so as to restore their patients' health more effectively.

12

GETTING TO KNOW THE PATIENT BETTER

(Classifying Diseases According to Symptoms)

Sickness is not caused by evil spirits; it is caused by natural means.

Zhang Zhong Jing (150-219)

Classification of Illnesses

How does a Chinese physician understand his patient's illness so as to cure the patient after he has amassed a wide range of symptoms regarding his patient's condition?   Basing on the symptoms, he classifies the disease into various categories. The following are the main systems of his classification:

1. Six Syndromes.
2. Three Levels.
3. Four Stages.
4. Twelve Organ Systems.

These systems of classification are guidelines to enable the physician to know the patient's disease better. They are not compartmentalization of diseases. A physician could use one or more systems at the same time. The following description is only a brief introduction; Chinese physicians specializing in particular classifications can go deeply into each category in great details.

Six Syndromes

The Six Syndromes classification is the legacy of the great Han physician from the 2nd century, Zhang Zhong Jing, who resigned as a district governor to become a doctor. This gesture illustrating his genuine love for medicine and care for people was even more impressive when we know that in his time, a governor's life was comfortable and luxurious, whereas a doctor's was generally poor and often lonely.

His sacrifices, nevertheless, turned out to be a great blessing for the people, because this Six Syndromes classification devised by Zhang Zhong Jing to diagnose contagious diseases, saved thousands of lives during an epidemic in ancient China.

The terms used in this classification is the same as those for the primary meridians, namely taiyang (major yang), yangming (bright yang), shaoyang (minor yang), taiyin (major yin), jueyin (final yin), and shaoyin (minor yin), but their meanings are quite different. Here, they represent six typical conditions of the patient's reaction against diseases, particularly those caused by external factors.

The chief characteristics of taiyang (major yang) illnesses are "floating pulse, headache and being afraid of cold". It is usually found in infectious diseases at the superficial or initial stage.

Yangming (bright yang) illnesses shows symptoms like "body warmth, big pulse rate, and solid stomach system". ("Solid stomach system" refers to a stagnation of energy or sthenia-syndrome at the gastrointestinal tract due to heat-evil) Yangming syndrome indicates that infectious diseases have developed into the advance stage.

The stage between taiyang and yangming is shaoyang (minor yang), with characteristics like "bitter mouth, dry throat, and blur eyes". This syndrome shows that infectious diseases have reached the intermediate stage, but have not developed in the internal organs.

Taiyin (major yin) illnesses usually involves the spleen and the stomach, and its natures are cold and empty. (An "empty" disease refers to a disease where the body's physiological functions have been weakened, and the causes of the disease are not obvious.) The chief characteristics of taiyin illnesses include "full stomach, vomiting, stomach ache, and no desire for food".

On the other hand, the chief characteristics of jueyin (final yin) illnesses are "pain at the heart, hungry but with no desire to eat, and vomiting if eaten". This is an advanced stage of infectious diseases, where the body defence has been much weakened.

The main symptoms of shaoyin (minor yin) illnesses are "weak pulse, wanting to sleep, being afraid of the cold, cold limbs, and liquid faeces". This syndrome is indicative of energy deficiency of the heart and kidney systems, with cold and empty nature.

Hence, since the second century the Chinese already have had detailed knowledge concerning the nature and the developmental states of illnesses. This classification of illnesses according to six archetypical syndromes is particularly useful for contagious diseases.

Broadly speaking, diseases are divided into two main types according to the relationship between the potency of pathogenic agents, especially those of an infectious nature, and the efficiency of the patient's own defence system.

If it is obvious that pathogenic agents are mainly and actively responsible for causing the illness, the disease is classified as yang. On the other hand, if the chief causative factor is the weakening of the patient's own bodily systems, though exo-pathogens may also play a role in the illness, the disease is classified as yin.

Further, both yin and yang diseases are classified into three sub-types according to their developmental stages. Thus, yin diseases at the initial, intermediate and advanced stages are classified as taiyin, shaoyin and jueyin respectively. Yin diseases are those that occur because the patient's natural systems are too weak to contain pathogenic agents, irrespective of whether these agents have been inside the patient's body all this while or have just entered his body.

Yang diseases at the initial, intermediate and advanced stages are termed taiyang, shaoyang and yangming. Yang diseases are those that occur because of the potency of exogenous pathogens, even though the patient's natural systems may still be operating as usual.

It may be useful to remember that "tai" and "shao" which are prefixed to "yin" and "yang" in the above terminology, means "major" and "minor" respectively, suggesting the start and the continuation of the body's weakening or the pathogens' attack. "Jue" prefixed to "yin", and "ming" suffixed to "yang", means "final" and "bright", indicating that the body's defences has been drawn to its last stage, or the pathogens' attack is most intense.

This ingenious classification of diseases by one of China's greatest physicians, is both simple and effective. Western medical scientists, while maintaining their own mode of diagnosis and therapeutics, may draw some inspiration from such medical thinking.

Three Levels

Although the Six Syndromes system was developed in the ancient times by Zhang Zhong Jing, it is so useful against contagious diseases that it has been successfully employed by Chinese physicians until now.

Another historic development was made in the 17th century, two centuries before bacteriology was established in the west, when Wu You Xing (1582-1652) who braved possible fatal infection to study pestilent diseases, discovered that plagues, unlike other contagious diseases, are caused by "sinful energy" which consists of microscopic organisms that spread through the air. This led to the development of "wenyi" (virulent epidemic) diseases as a speciality from the other contagious diseases generally referred to as "shanghan" (cold and fever) diseases.

Later, Wu Ju Tong (1736-1820) synthesized past masters' invaluable knowledge on plagues which swept China previously, and devised the Three Levels classification for pestilent diseases. In Chinese, this Three Levels classification is called "san jiao classification". As "san jiao" is also the term for "triple warmer", it is easy for many people to mistake it as "triple warmer classification", again illustrating how easily Chinese medical thought can be misinterpreted by reading materials from honest writers who may lack the necessary linguistic or technical information, even though these writers may be eminently trained in their own fields. The Three Levels classification actually refers to the three distinctive developmental phases of virulent diseases.

At the first level when the disease first started, it is found at the lung meridian. Why must it be at the lung meridian, and not elsewhere? It is because the microbes that cause these virulent diseases are spread through the air, and breathed in by the patient into his lungs. Common symptoms include headaches, slight fear of cold, thirst, and cough. The patient's pulse becomes frequent; the "cun" (inch) region of the wrist indicates strong pulse, while the "chi" (foot) region indicates warmth. The patient feels warm after noon.

The second level is the intermediate stage of the virulent disease, when its manifestation is found in the spleen and the stomach meridians. If we recall our study of man's internal cosmos, we shall find that the lungs provide essential energy for the colon for its operation, and the colon is intimately connected to the spleen and stomach systems. Hence, if attacking microbes are not checked at the lungs, they spread to the spleen and stomach via the meridian network.

The patient is feverish but he is not afraid of cold. Common symptoms include reddened face, rough respiration, yellowish fur on tongue, and solid faeces. The patient's condition worsens in the afternoon, such as feeling muddled in his thinking, body heavy, no desire for food, wanting to vomit, whitish fur on his tongue, and difficult urination.

As the illness develops into the third level, it is manifested in the kidney and the liver meridians. Our study of man's internal cosmos explains that the stomach and the spleen are responsible for the production and regulation of nutrient essence, which in turn forms the basic ingredients of blood. The kidneys and the liver are the principal organs for the storage and regulation of essence and blood respectively. Hence, as the virulent disease develops into the advance stage, its microbes spread to the kidneys and the liver.

Some typical symptoms of the advance stage of virulent diseases are that the patient's face becomes red, his body warm, his lips crack, his throat sore, and his hearing difficult. The patient often feels depressed and dejected.

How is it that virulent diseases can affect a person's mental performance or emotions? Again the Chinese knowledge of man's internal cosmos provides a logical answer. Kidney energy is directly responsible for the production of "sui" or marrow, which flows to the brain and affects its performance.

In Chinese medical philosophy, emotions are controlled by the heart, not by the brain, and as the heart is also the chief organ for blood circulation, its function in emotional control is thus affected by "contaminated" blood. The heart, as the "emperor organ", is affected in various ways by all types of illnesses.

With this understanding from Chinese medicine, we should be more tolerant to people who become "unreasonably" emotional when they are sick. Indeed, if after brain surgery or psychotherapy, neurologists and psychiatrists still find nothing clinically wrong with their patients, they may derive some unexpected result if they care to investigate the premise that their patient's problem may be patho-physiological instead of neurological or psychiatric.

The three developmental stages of virulent diseases roughly correspond to the three levels of the triple warmer. At the start, the disease is found at the lung level or top warmer; it is at the stomach level or middle warmer during the intermediate stage; and at the kidney level or bottom warmer in the final stage.

It is tempting to ask whether Europe would be more able to handle her epidemics that spared neither rich nor poor in the 19th century if western doctors knew about such knowledge of the Chinese masters who successfully contained epidemics in the east. While we cannot turn back history, we can learn from it. Qigong therapy, a major branch of Chinese medicine still little known in the west, and which will be discussed in later chapters, is an excellent curative and preventive measure against cardiovascular diseases, the top killer in the west today.

Four Stages

Another system of disease classification is called the Four Stages, devised by the great physician of the Qing Dynasty, Ye Tian Shi (1667-1746), who, despite being born into a generation of Chinese physicians, learnt from 17 other physicians at a time when he was already an acknowledged master. The demonstration by this great master of his willingness and courage to learn from others amidst a traditionally conservative society, may inspire us to do likewise in modern times.

The Four Stages described four typical developmental stages of pestilent diseases, namely "wei", "qi", "ying" and "xue", which may be translated as the superficial, initial, intermediate and advanced stage. In physiological context, the four terms refer to "defence", "energy", "nutrient", and "blood" respectively. Such apparent confusion, which does not cause any problems to the initiated, is one of the reasons why western scholars can sometimes misinterpret Chinese medical writings, especially when they know the Chinese language or medical system inadequately. They may, for example, report these stages as "defence stage", "energy stage", "nutrient stage" and "blood stage", which will, albeit the good intentions of the authors, further confuse western readers. Yet, in some situations, which will be explained later, translations of such terms in their physiological context may be more appropriate!

This apparent confusion will be cleared when we understand the relationship between the developmental stages of the disease and the physiological response of the patient. At the wei or superficial stage, it is the defence energy (known as wei qi) of the patient that is most active in fighting the disease.

When microbes have succeeded in passing through the body defence and entered the qi or initial stage of their development, they spread to other parts of the body along the energy (qi) flow of the meridian system. If this is not checked, the disease develops into the ying or intermediate stage where the level of the patient's nutrient energy (ying qi) is affected, resulting in the general weakening of his natural systems.

At the xue or advanced stage, microbes attack internal organs and tissues, spread by blood (xue) circulation. Ye Tian Shi summed up this pathological development of pestilent diseases in his famous, concise statement, "pestilent-evils come from the air, enter the lungs, and settle at the pericardium".

How does a physician know which developmental stage the disease is in? There are typical symptoms, and the following is a brief description.

At the "wei fen" or superficial stage of pestilence diseases, common symptoms are fever, mild chilliness, floating and rapid pulse, little or no sweating, headaches, body pains, cough, blocked nose, white fur on tongue, and tastelessness.

When the virulent epidemic disease progresses to the "qi fen" or initial stage, common symptoms include high fever without chilliness, profuse sweating, thirst with desire for cold drink, congested chest or stomach, wanting to vomit, solid faeces, yellowish and dry fur on tongue, smooth and rapid pulse, or large and bouncing pulse.

If the pestilent disease breaks through the outer defence of the body and reaches the "ying fen" or intermediate stage, common symptoms are restlessness, predominant fever at night, sleeplessness, dry lips and mouth but no desire for drink, skin rashes, crimson tongue, delirium, and small and rapid pulse.

At the "xue fen" or advanced stage, the virulent epidemic disease has entered the interior. Symptoms include high fever predominant at night, delirium, convulsion, crimson tongue, skin eruption, bleeding, black faeces, and small and rapid pulse. Usually only two or three symptoms may appear, but they show that the sickness is very serious.

A remarkable contribution by Ye Tian Shi was his explanation that pestilent diseases are different from other contagious diseases in nature, behavior, causes and treatment. This distinction helped to save countless lives.

In Chinese, pestilent diseases are called "wen yi" (virulent epidemic), whereas other contagious diseases are referred to as "shang han" (cold and fever). Ye Tian Shi also pointed out that virulent epidemic diseases may be dormant for some time. Hence when they surface, the first symptoms may already be at the "ying" (intermediate) stage; as they progress to the outside of the body, "wei" (superficial) and "qi" (initial) symptoms appears later!

This feature may apply to other kinds of sickness besides pestilent diseases. So, a patient suddenly relieved of grave symptoms like high fever, delirium, and weak and rapid pulse, may not necessarily be a good sign if he also sweats profusely, feels congestion in his chest or abdomen, and has yellowish, dry fur on his tongue.

Although his syndromes change from the "ying" stage to the "qi" stage, his illness is actually worsening. This explains why some patients "suddenly" die though they appear to be recovering. Doctors who understand this principle will surely be in a better position to save lives. Indeed many lives were saved by physicians who applied this classification of diseases when pestilence swept China in the 17th and 18th centuries, when people referred to pestilent diseases as "evils from the sky".

This classification, like other classifications of diseases, helps the physician to plan his therapeutic program. Obviously, the physician should attack the disease at its appropriate level; attacking it elsewhere is not only wasteful but may also be injurious to the patient. For example, administrating cold herbs (antibiotics) to kill microbes is suitable at the wei and qi, or superficial and initial, stages; but doing so at the ying and xue, or intermediate and advanced stages may further weaken the patient.

Ye Tian Shi gave the following advice: "At the wei stage, apply sweating technique; only when the disease has reached the qi stage, should the physician clear qi; at the ying stage, warm and circulate energy; when the disease has entered the xue stage, cool blood and disperse stagnation."

This means that the physician could use antibiotic herbs at the superficial stage and dispel the microbes through sweating; at the initial stage, antibiotic herbs can clear the microbes in the meridians; at the intermediate stage, the physician should improve the patient's metabolic processes and energy flow; at the advanced stage, cold herbs (antibiotics) are not suitable, but the physician can eliminate microbes by using cool herbs (with milder antibiotic effect), while making sure that "blood stagnation", which occurs as a result of the cooling effect, must be taken care of.

During a tuberculosis epidemic, Ye Tian Shi, whom the people called "doctor from heaven", cured countless of patients not by prescribing antibiotic herbs but by improving their metabolic processes so that their own body systems can overcome the dreaded disease.

Anyone who thinks that Chinese medicine is unscientific because of his inadequate understanding or because he had read misleading or inaccurate information, should reconsider his opinion after reading such profound knowledge with regards to the cause, development and treatment of pestilent diseases.

In view of the resurgence in western societies of tuberculosis and other infectious diseases that have become resistant to antibiotic treatment, western experts could derive some useful ideas from Chinese medical thinking.

Classification According to Internal Organs

The fourth category of disease classification depends on the patient's physiological response to the disease, enabling the physician to understand where and what is wrong with the patient. He determines which organ or meridian systems are diseased, and which pathogenic factors are responsible. It does not matter whether he starts with the "where" or the "what" factors; the conclusion is similar.

For example, by examining the patient's nose, face, pulse and numerous other features of the four diagnostic techniques, the physician may conclude that the disease is located at the lungs, and symptoms like yellowish phlegm, thirst, back pains and a strong pulse rate indicate that the pathogenetic cause is fire. The disease, therefore, is described as excess fire at the lungs.

This classification is very popular, as it enables the physician to treat the cause and site of illness directly. In this case, the main therapeutic principle is to dispel fire at the lungs, and it can be realized in many ways to be explained in later chapters. The example here is simplified for readers' easy understanding; real cases are often more complex, but the underlying principles are the same.

The internal organs and their meridians involved are the heart, small intestine, liver, gall bladder, spleen, stomach, lung, colon, kidney, urinary bladder, pericardium, and triple warmer. They are examined against pathogenetic factors like cold, heat, empty, solid, yin and yang deficiency.

It must be pointed out again that pathological terms like "cold" and "heat" should be interpreted symbolically, not literally; this apparent "strangeness" is as much the result of linguistic and cultural discrepancies, as of different medical thinking.

The following is only a brief description of the symptoms and other features that Chinese physicians employ for their classification. Not all disease types are shown.

In Chinese medical philosophy, diseases of the heart system concerns the circulatory and the nervous systems. Symptoms of illness due to "cold" at the heart include pain at the heart, cold limbs, and slow pulse. Dry and painful tongue, and feeling of oppression in the chest indicate diseases caused by "heart-fire". Illnesses resulting from "yin-deficiency of the heart" is indicated by being easily frightened, loss of memory, and sleeplessness.

Diseases at the small intestine can usually be divided into the "empty, cold" type or the "solid, hot" type. "Empty, cold" illness of the small intestine is indicated by clear urine, purging, stomach pains, weak pulse and whitish fur on tongue; whereas "solid, hot" illness is reflected by reddish urine, swollen abdomen, pain at waist and spine, sore tongue, and yellowish fur on tongue. "Empty" and "solid" here refer to the weakening of physiological functions, and the potency of pathogenic agents respectively.

The common pathogenetic causes of liver diseases are cold, heat, empty or solid conditions. Cold illnesses of the liver system show the following symptoms: spasms, pain at the genitals, slow and sunken pulse, and smooth and greenish fur on tongue. Pain at the ribs, swollen and reddish eyes, sleeplessness, reddish tongue, and frequent pulse show hot illness of the liver. Sound in the ear, blur eyesight, lacklustre nails, weak pulse, and pale tongue without fur indicate illnesses caused by deficient liver energy. Pain at the ear, crimson tongue, yellowish fur on tongue, strong pulse, and being easily prone to anger show that the illness is due to excessive liver energy.

Hence, if your ears are painful but your ear specialist finds nothing wrong with them, you should start examining your liver system.

Disease at the liver systems often affect the gall bladder system; therefore there are many similarities between the two. Headaches, vomiting, flatulence, sleeplessness, and weak pulse are common symptoms of energy deficiency of the gall bladder. Excessive gall bladder energy is indicated by bitter taste in the mouth, chill alternating with fever, blur eyesight, hard of hearing, and rapid pulse.

"Dampness" is a very common pathogenetic cause of the spleen system. Insufficient yang resulting from "dampness" and "cold" are manifested as abdominal pains, purging, inability to digest food, slow and sunken pulse. Spleen illness due to "dampness" and "heat" are yellowish fur on tongue, short yellowish urine, solid and rapid pulse, and excessive body fluid. Generally, sweet taste in the mouth is indicative of spleen system problem.

The spleen system and the stomach system are closely related; hence illnesses at one system often affects the other system. Symptoms of stomach illnesses caused by yang deficiency are abdominal pains, tastelessness, wanting to vomit, cold limbs, slow and sunken pulse. Excessive fire in the stomach is indicated by great thirst, hunger, smelly breath, and bleeding gum.

Illnesses of the lung system is often manifested in the nose, throat and skin. When "cold" and "wind" attack the lungs, the symptoms are blocked nose, cough, thin and whitish phlegm, whitish fur on tongue, and floating and smooth pulse.

If the lungs are attacked by "fire", symptoms are reddish face, yellowish phlegm, phlegm with blood, thirst, chest and back pains, whitish spots on throat, yellowish fur on tongue, and a strong pulse. Lung illnesses are due to deficiency of yang energy and is indicated by shortness of breath, pale face, cold limbs, frequent urine, cough, dry skin, hair dropping, weak and empty pulse.

Symptoms like liquid faeces, clear and long urine, abdominal pains, whitish fur on tongue, and weak pulse indicate cold diseases of the colon. Solid faeces, short urine, pain at the anus, yellowish fur, and frequent pulse show that the colon illness belongs to the hot type.

Diseases of the kidneys are often manifested in the eyes, ears and genitals, and are more often "empty" rather than "solid" in nature. Nocturnal emission, tinnitus, lumbago, dizziness, blur eyesight, red tongue without fur, weak and rapid pulse indicate yin deficiency of the kidney system. Its yang deficiency is shown by symptoms like premature ejaculation, impotency, flaccidity of lower limbs, and chilliness at the waist and legs.

Women who fail to bear children despite trying hard, and despite being repeatedly told by gynaecologists that they are clinically normal, may have amazing result after consulting Chinese physicians regarding their kidney system.

Sickness concerning the urinary bladder system is often reflected in the urine. Clear, frequent urine shows cold urinary bladder disease, whereas short, painful urine shows the disease is of the hot nature. Uncontrollable urination indicates empty illness; congested, painful urination indicates solid illness. However, although the diseases may be at the urinary bladder system, they are frequently related to the lung and the kidney systems.

In this classification of diseases according to the organ systems, the pericardium and the triple warmer are not mentioned because diseases of the pericardium system are similar to those of the heart system, and since the triple warmer contains all the other internal organs, its diseases are included in these organs.

This classification concerns not only physical but also psychological diseases, as the Chinese have always regarded the soma and the psyche as one unity. Perhaps western doctors and psychiatrists may derive some insight from the Chinese concept that emotional disorders are related to physiological ailments.

A useful approach to this classification is to apply the Eight Principles of cold, hot, empty, solid, internal, external, yin and yang to the organ systems. For example, once we know that the patient's problem lie in his liver system, we can then determine whether the disease is cold or hot, empty or solid, internal or external, yin or yang.

Alternatively, having established that the patient's condition is yang, hot, solid and external, we find out which organ system the disease is located at.

Chinese physicians classify diseases not for academic pleasure, but for practical usefulness.

It is therefore a gross mistake to suggest, as some misinformed writers do, that the Chinese are in the habit of classifying factors or processes in medicine and other fields according to philosophical concepts for no better reasons than following convention, such as grouping syndromes into six classes, and not five, seven or any other number because the Yi Jing (I Ching) mentions six divisions of yin-yang, or classifying disease development into three levels so as to conform to the Confucian concept of the three levels of heaven, earth and man.

One writer even mentioned that to complete the pairing of yin-yang organs, the Chinese invented the triple warmer concept to match the pericardium!

Let's Diagnose a Patient

Of the four systems of disease classification discussed in this chapter, the Six Syndromes classification is mainly used for contagious diseases; the Three Levels classification and the Four Stages classification for virulent, epidemic diseases; and the organ system classification for all groups of diseases.

It must be remembered that disease classification is only a convenient tool; it must never be taken as rigid compartmentalization. Whatever system or systems the physician uses, he must always treat the patient as a whole person, not merely attend to his disease nor diseased parts only.

Lets say you are a Chinese physician; see if you could employ what you have just read to diagnose an imaginary patient. It must be emphasized that this is meant for fun. In real life, diagnosing and treating a patient is a serious affair. Thus no one should attempt a diagnosis, unless he has been properly trained by qualified instructors.

Mr Sickman consults you, and as a responsible physician you give him a thorough examination, applying all your four diagnostic methods of viewing, listening, asking and feeling.

You notice that although he is anxious and hesitant, his physical movements are unrestricted and his voice clear. You also notice that his skin is slightly yellowish, and his lips sore. You ask him to open his mouth, and you notice his tongue is pinkish. His breathing is fast and rough, and he has a slight fever.

To your questions, he says that he feels cold, does not sweat, and his urine is yellowish, short and painful. You ask him if he has taken any food lately, and he replies that he does not like food as it makes him uncomfortable, but his mouth tastes sweet! He complains of headaches, purging and abdominal pains. He has had this sickness since the previous night.

You feel his pulse at his wrist, and find it strong and floating at the surface. Its frequency is fast, more than a hundred times a minute. His palms are warm too.

In accordance with Chinese medical philosophy, we do not ask what his disease is, but ask what is wrong with the patient. From the diagnosis we know that he is affected by external causes of "dampness" and "heat", and his disease is at the superficial stage.

His sore lips and yellowish urine indicate heat at the stomach and spleen; and his lack of sweating suggests that the illness is external and solid. His short and painful urine confirms that the hot disease is accompanied with dampness, and his feeling uncomfortable after food confirms it is solid.

His purging and abdominal pains, as well as sweet taste at the mouth further indicate dampness and heat of the stomach and spleen systems. His headaches, warm palms and floating and frequent pulse suggest that the illness is external, contagious and at the superficial or initial stage.

With this rich information, we are ready to classify the patient's symptoms into convenient groups for better understanding. Using the Six Syndromes system, we can say the patient's illness belongs to the "tai-yang" (major yang) type. Nevertheless, it also has some features of a "taiyin" (major yin) illness. Although this disease is infectious (or "shanghan" disease), it is not virulent and epidemic (or "wenyi" disease); so the Three Levels and Four Stages systems are not so suitable.

However, if we want to attempt a classification, we can say that it belongs to the First Level, and to the Superficial Stage of diseases.

Using the organ system of classification is the most appropriate in this case. The disease can be described as hot, solid, external, yang disease of the spleen and stomach systems caused by dampness and heat. Indeed, such is the traditional way of naming diseases in Chinese medicine, which incidentally is not verbose in the Chinese language. Chinese physicians do not give a particular name for a disease as in western medical practice; they refer to the disease by the pathogenetic conditions of the patient.

However, mainly for the convenience of comparison with western medicine, modern Chinese physicians sometimes use the Chinese translations of western medical terms to describe diseases. The closest modern term for the above example is diarrhoea.

But notice what a vast difference of information is contained between the western and the Chinese traditional term. This difference also influences the therapeutic approaches between the west and the Chinese.

The western approach is thematic; western doctors will consider their job well done when the patient's diarrhoea is cured.

The Chinese approach is holistic; Chinese physicians are satisfied only when the patient's health is restored, including eliminating all his patho-genetic symptoms like yellowish skin, sore lips, short and painful urine, and floating and frequent pulse rate. How Chinese physicians accomplish this, will be explained in subsequent chapters.

TREATING THE PATIENT, NOT THE ILLNESS

(The Principles of Chinese Therapeutics)

By concentrating on smaller and smaller fragments of the body, modern medicine perhaps loses sight of the patient as a whole human being, and by reducing health to mechanical functioning it is no longer able to deal with the phenomenon of healing.

Prince Charles,
speaking to the British Medical Association in 1982

Curing the Patient as a Whole Person

Regarding the human being as one united entity, not just a composition of various parts, is an essential principle in Chinese medicine. In his therapeutics, the Chinese physician, therefore, seeks to cure the patient as a whole person, and not merely attempts to cure the disease or the affected parts only.

Man is made up of complex, but united and coordinated, organs and systems. These organs and systems are interrelated and interdependent. The respiratory system, for example, depends on the circulatory system for the supply of food and energy, which in turn are derived from the digestive system. The digestive system also has to depend on the circulatory, respiratory and other systems for its maintenance and functioning.

This inter-connectedness of our body is even better appreciated when we understand its intricate meridian systems, which links not only outwardly unconnected organs like the eyes and the liver, but also every part of our body. All our internal organs — lung, liver, kidneys, etc — are connected to the external organs —skin, eyes, ears.

The external organs keep man aware of his surroundings, thus helping him to maintain the harmony between himself and his environment. Environment is ever changing, as in the change of the surrounding air and micro-organisms as well as climatic conditions, geographical localities and emotional influences.

If the environmental changes are too drastic or sudden, man may not be able to accommodate himself to these changes. Once the balance between man and his environment, or between his internal and external systems is disturbed, sickness may occur.

As man's organs and systems are interrelated by various meridians, injury to or sickness at any one part will affect other parts, resulting in loss of harmony and occurrence of the disease.

For example, as expressed in the saying "liver diseases affect the spleen system", when the liver is diseased, the sickness frequently causes the disruption of the spleen system, resulting in the loss of appetite and general health.

Thus it is utmost important for the physician to treat the patient as a whole person: not merely attend to his head when he complain of headaches, or to his stomach when he complain of stomach pains.

Prescribing Therapeutics According to Illness

The principle of "Prescribing therapeutics according to illness" dictates that the physician must first find out the cause and nature of the illness, only then he prescribes the appropriate therapeutics for the patient. The importance and necessity of this principle are obvious, but in practice it is astonishing how many doctors fail to observe this principle adequately, as the number of unsuccessful treatment of simple ailments explicitly suggests.

If the cause and nature of an illness are correctly determined, then the illness — perhaps with only a few exceptions — can be easily and readily cured by using the appropriate therapeutics.

Hence, diagnosis is extremely important: if the illness is correctly diagnosed, recovery will be a matter of course. In his diagnosis, as we have seen in previous chapters, the physician considers the location, potency in relation to the body's resistance, behavior, and developmental stage of the illness. He examines the external (six evils) as well as the internal causes (seven emotions). He uses the four diagnostic methods, and is guided by the eight principles. He then employs one or more ways to classify the illness so as to understand it better.

The Battle Between Goodness and Evil

Chinese physicians figuratively refer to our health in relation to illness as a battle between goodness and evil. "Goodness" and "evil" here have no religious or metaphysical connotation. They refer to two relative situations in health and illness.

Goodness refers to "good qi", the life force or vital energy that is responsible for the maintenance of living. It includes the healthy functioning of bodily organs and systems, the natural resistance against internal and external disease-causative agents, and the natural ability and tendency to recuperate and rebuild.

Evil refers to "evil qi", that is the illness, including all the causative agents that cause the illness, as well as the symptoms and manifestations brought about by these agents. Health or sickness is a continuous process of the battle between goodness and evil. The incidence of illness, its development and manifestations are times when evil is victorious. When goodness triumphs, as when a person is charged with good qi, illnesses can never occur.

This figurative description of the battle between goodness and evil may strike some readers as primitive or simplistic; but actually it represents in its most concise form, a profound medical truth learnt from observation and study through the ages. If we can understand its significance and master its application, we can not only cure illnesses, but more positively, prevent diseases and promote longevity.

Hence, all therapeutic methods can be summarized into two fundamental principles of "Restoring Goodness" and "Eliminating Evil". Restoring goodness refers to using medicine, nutrition, exercise and other means to restore the vital energy of the body, strengthening the body, and enhancing its defence systems, curative and self-generative abilities, so as to overcome pathogenic agents and restore health.

Eliminating evil refers to employing various therapeutic methods, such as herbal medicine, acupuncture, massage, qigong therapy, etc., to eliminate evil qi, removing pathogenic agents or their effects, restrict or terminate their development, so that illness is eliminated.

Restoring goodness and eliminating evil are interrelated. But for convenience, we can classify therapeutics into the following approaches:

1. Restoring goodness only.
   This is used when the patient is actually weak, and external pathogenic agents are not present. This applies particularly to patients suffering from organic diseases.

2. Eliminating evil only.
   This is used when external pathogenic agents are present, but the patient is fit and healthy. This applies particularly to contagious diseases.

3. Restoring goodness cum eliminating evil.
   The patient is weak and pathogenic agents are present, but the patient's weakness is more notable.

4. Eliminating evil cum restoring goodness.
   The patient is weak and pathogenic agents are present, but the pathogenic agents are more urgent.

5. Restoring goodness then eliminating evil.
   Both physical weakness and pathogenic agents are present, but eliminating evil first may further weaken the patient. For example. prescribing antibiotics may drastically enfeeble an infirm patient.

6. Eliminating evil then restoring goodness.
   Both physical weakness and pathogenic agents are present, but restoring goodness first may increase the severity of the illness. For example, enhancing the energy level of a person suffering from internal blockage, may actually cause him more injury.

Whatsoever the therapeutic methods or approaches are, the ultimate factor is restoring goodness. This clearly contrasts with the western emphasis on eliminating evil. In Chinese medical philosophy, the patient's good qi (vital energy) is the basic factor in overcoming evil (sickness). Moreover all therapeutic means (herbal medicine, acupuncture, etc.) depends on the patient's qi for their working.

Obviously, our modern doctors can draw much benefit from the above philosophy. For example, the prevailing philosophical impetus behind medical researches for degenerative diseases, the most pressing medical problem of the 20th century, is finding ways to eliminate diseases, that is "eliminating evil", rather than to restore the patient's physiological functions, that is "restoring goodness".

And when the organic illness requires surgical operation, the question is more often whether the patient can afford to pay for the surgery, that is "eliminating evil", than whether the patient can recover without resorting to surgery, as many of my qigong students have accomplished, that is "restoring goodness".

The Concept of Branch-Root

The concept of Branch-Root refers to the secondary and primary aspects in a relationship. It is frequently used in Chinese medicine, and is manifested in many ways.

In the relationship between health and sickness (goodness and evil), a person's natural resistance against disease is considered primary (root), and disease causative agents are secondary (branch). Hence, in therapeutics, restoring the patient's general vital energy always takes precedence over merely curing particular diseases.

In diagnosis and therapeutics, the cause of illness is primary, whereas the symptoms are secondary. Hence, the physician should not just judge by the outward symptoms of a disease, but attempt to find out its cause. He should not merely cure the symptoms, but treat the cause of the illness.

Regarding the development of an illness, old illness or illness that was contracted earlier is primary; new illness or illness that was contracted later, is considered secondary. Illness that is internal is primary, whereas an external illness is secondary. Regarding the cause of illness, internal causes are primary and external causes are secondary.

The usual therapeutic approach is first cure the primary, then cure the secondary. For example, a patient suffering from deficiency of heart energy may experience pain in the arm. If we just eliminate the pain at the arm, but is not aware of the heart problem, we fall into the not uncommon practice of "treating the symptoms not the cause". This explains why a great many patients suffering from chronic diseases never permanently recover from their ailments.

The concept of branch-root will help us to guard against this mistake. Differentiating between primary cause and secondary symptom, we treat the cause by enhancing his heart energy; his symptoms, the pains in the arm, will automatically disappear.

Nevertheless, in our zest to treat the cause, we must not neglect the symptoms. We may explain to the patient the actual cause of his illness, but to him his symptoms from which he suffers from, are real, and perhaps more meaningful than his heart-energy deficiency which he probably does not experience immediately. And if we do not relieve him of his pain in the arm, he may soon lose faith in our healing, though we are actually doing good work with his energy deficiency.

Moreover, by relieving him of the symptoms, like opening the meridians along the arm, we can also speed up the enhancing of his heart energy.

Sometimes, however, the symptoms may become more urgent than the cause of the disease. In this case, we have to treat the symptoms first. For example, liver dysfunction can bring about excessive fluid at the abdomen. The liver dysfunction is the primary cause, and the excessive abdominal fluid is the secondary symptom. But if the accumulation of fluid has become so severe that the abdomen is bloated, and excretion and breathing difficult, we have to treat the symptom first, using purging to flush out the excessive fluid.

The Eight Techniques

The following are eight fundamental therapeutic techniques employed in internal medicine.

1. Sweating (Diaphoresis).
   Sweating is useful for external diseases such as fever and cold, pyogenic infection, and excessive fluid (oedema). Some common herbs that induce sweating are ma hwang (Herba Ephedrae), kwei chi (Ramulus Cinnamomi), fang feng (Radix Ledebou-riellae), po he (Herba Menthae), ji hua (Flos Chrysanthemi) and chai hu (Radis Bupleuri).

2. Induced Vomiting (Emesis).
   Induced vomiting is used to dispel poisonous food that has not yet been

absorbed into the body. Materia medica that can induce emesis are kwa ti (Pedicellus Melo), li lu (Veratrum Nigrum) and chang san (Radis Dichroae).

3. Purgation
Purgation is used for diseases that are internal, real and hot, especially at the spleen and stomach systems, such as difficulty of excretion, bloated abdomen, excessive fluid, blood and chi stasis. Some purgative materia medica are ta hwang (Rhizoma Rhei), mang sheow (Natrii Sulfas), fu tze (Radis Aconiti Praeparata), kan jiang (Rhizoma Zingiberis), fo ma ren (Fructus Cannabis), yuan hua (Flos Genkwa), and da ji (Radis Euphobiae Pekinensis).

4. Reconciliation.
Reconciliation refers to the regulation of functional relationships between yin and yang and between organs. Unlike in other techniques where certain herbs are used for sweating, others for purging, etc., in this technique there are no particular material medica for reconciliation.

The physician has to find out what causes the imbalance in the patient, and choose the appropriate materia medica to overcome the imbalance.

However, sao Chai Hu Tang (Radix Bupleuri Decoction) and Xiao Yao San (Xiaoyao Powder) are two popular prescriptions for achieving reconciliation.

5. Warming.
The warming technique is used to eliminate cold diseases and to enhance yang energy. It serves three main functions: dispelling coldness at the middle level, cleansing blocked meridians, and strengthening physiological functions.

Relevant materia medica include fu tze (Radis Aconiti Praeparata), kan jiang (Rhizoma Zingiberis), yi kwei (Cortex Cinnamomi), sao huai xiang (Fructus Foeniculi), and hua jiau (Pericarpium Zanthoxyli).

6. Heat-Clearing.
This technique employs cooling materia medica to clear away heat and fire. It kills bacteria, dissolves phlegm and reduces fever. This technique is frequently used to treat contagious diseases at the intermediate and advanced stages.

Popular materia medica for heat-clearing include hwang lean (Rhizoma Coptidis), hwang chin (Radis Scutellariae), jin yin hwa (Flos Lonicerae), lung tan chao (Radis Gentianae), and xi jiao (Cornu Rhinoceri).

7. Dispelling.
This technique is used to dispel blockages caused by energy and blood stasis, fluid, dampness, food and other materials. Its usage is very wide, and includes removing wind, removing dampness, regulating qi, regulating blood, digesting and absorbing food, dispelling phlegm and excessive fluid, dispelling stones, and reducing abscess and inflammation.

Some relevant materia medica are chuan kung (Rhizoma Ligustici Chuanxiong), fu qin (Poria), muk tung (Caulis Akebiae), muk xiang (Radis Aucklandiae), hung hwa (Flos Carthami), san cha (Fructus Crataegi), chuan pei mu (Bulbus Fritillariae Cirhosae), hwang po (Cortex Phellodendri), and tao ren (Semen Persicae).

8. Invigoration
The invigoration technique enhances the patient's physiological functions, natural resistance and self-recuperative and self-regenerative abilities. It is also used to rebuild the patient's health after curing him of his illness. There are five major areas of invigoration: qi, blood, yin, yang and internal organs.

Relevant materia medica include tang shun (Codonopsis Pilosula), hwang chi (Radis Astragali seu Hedysari), dang gui (Radis Angelicae Sinensis), he sau wu (Radis Poligoni Multiflori), pa ji (Radis Morindae Officinalis), and ti hwang (Radis Rehmanniae).

Various Therapeutic Methods in Chinese Medicine

It is a common misconception to think that Chinese medicine mainly consists of taking herbal decoctions. Herbal medicine is only one aspect of Chinese medicine. Chinese medicine is very rich in therapeutic approaches; the major ones are as follows.

1. Herbal Medicine
This involves the taking of medical decoctions brewed from prescriptions of herbs, minerals, animal and other matters. The medical prescriptions can also be in other forms, like bolus, pills, powder and tincture. The Chinese have an incredibly wide range of material medica.

The Great Herbal Pharmacopeia of Li Shih Chen, for example, lists 1892 different types of materia medica and over 10,000 medical prescriptions.

2. External Medicine

This refers to other types of therapies besides taking of oral medicine. In its wide sense it includes acupuncture, massage therapy and traumatology; in its restricted meaning, it comprises the use of ointments, plasters, vaporization, scraping-therapy, heat-therapy, cupping therapy and surgery.

It is a common mistake to think that Chinese medicine is weak in surgery. In fact, the Chinese were successfully performing major operations long before the west knew about anaesthetics.

3. Traumatology.

This includes various types of therapeutics for external as well as internal injuries caused by incision, contusion, dislocation, fracture and violent means. Colloquially, it is known as "die da", (pronounced as "thiet ta") meaning "therapy for injuries sustained from falling and from being hit" and is closely linked to the practice of kungfu. The traumatology therapist deals mainly with bruises and sprains, orthopaedics, visceral damage and internal injuries.

The Chinese, especially great kungfu masters, set very high standards in the field of traumatology.

4. Acupuncture and Moxibustion.

Not too long ago many people would laugh when told that illnesses could be cured by inserting needles into the patient's body; but now acupuncture has been accepted beyond doubt to be an efficient and self-contained therapy system.

The basic principle is that every part of the body is connected by a comprehensive network of channels and collaterals, and by manipulating the energy flow at these meridians, health can be restored.

Where acupuncture is not appropriate, moxibustion is used. Moxibustion is the application of moxa wool or rolls on the affected parts at the patient's skin, and it is based on the principles of acupuncture.

5. Massage Therapy.
   Massage therapy is based on the same principles as acupuncture; but the therapist's hands instead of needles are used to harmonize energy flow in the patient.

   It may surprise many uninitiated to find out that, like acupuncture, massage therapy is self-contained; there are many major massage techniques to produce different effects on different tissues, muscles, vital points and meridians. Thirty of these major techniques are described in the chapter on Massage Therapy in this book.

   Massage therapy together with acupuncture and herbal medicine were the three earliest of the various Chinese therapies to be awarded the professors' chairs at the Imperial University of Medicine (the world's first medical school) during the Tang Dynasty.

6. Health Exercises.
   Health exercises include physiotherapy, qigong exercises and martial arts. Therefore their preventive function is as important as their curative purpose. A crucial difference between Chinese and western health exercises is that the Chinese emphasize not just bones and muscles, but also internal organs and systems.

   The Chinese were probably the earliest people to use health exercises in medicine. Early records show that prehistoric men in China employed dances and physiotherapy to cure diseases like rheumatism and arthritis.

   Great medical classics also describe the importance and techniques of health exercises. Some famous examples are Hua Tuo's Five-Animal Play, Shaolin Eighteen Lohan Hands, Taijiquan (Tai Chi Chuan) and the Eight Pieces of Embroidery.

8. Qigong Therapy.
   Traditionally, qigong therapy refers to the use of qigong exercises to cure illnesses. In its modern narrow context, it refers to the therapeutic approach whereby the therapist channels qi to the patient; but in its wide meaning, it is an umbrella term covering all therapeutic methods that utilize the harmonizing of qi flow as the basic principle to restore health.

Hence, it includes relevant methods like massage therapy, acupressure and physiotherapy. As the fundamental principle of Chinese medical philosophy (as well as all other medical philosophies known to man, except conventional western philosophy) assumes that the harmonious flow of vital energy is essential to health, qigong therapy is perhaps the most natural of all therapies.

Chinese medicine is, therefore, an exceedingly wide and exciting discipline. This is not surprising if we remember that it is mankind's longest continuous medical system and has been used by the world's largest population. The different therapeutic approaches mentioned above represents the many and varied ways the Chinese have successfully used to combat illnesses since millennia. We shall examine them in some detail in subsequent chapters.

GINSENG, CINNAMON BARK AND REINDEER'S HORN

(Chinese Pharmacology and Herbalism)

For creatures your size I offer,
a free choice of habitat,
so settle yourself in the zone
that suits you best.
In the pools of my pores,
or the tropical forests
of arm-pit and crotch,
in the desert of my forearm,
or the cool woods of my scalp,
Build colonies: I will supply
adequate warmth and moisture,
the sebum and lipids you need,
on condition you never do annoy me
with your presence
but behave as good guests should,
not rising into acne or athlete's foot
or a boil.

W. H. Auden

Military Strategy and Poetry

Can you guess why Chinese physicians often read poetry? It is not because they are particularly poetic — though some are; but because it is part of their work if they practice internal medicine.

Internal medicine is probably the most popular of the various branches of Chinese medicine, to such an extent that many people erroneously believe that Chinese medicine is only internal medicine. Because herbs form most of the materia medica of Chinese internal medicine, it is often called herbal medicine or herbalism, though the rich Chinese pharmacology also include minerals and animal matter. Conventionally, the term "herbs" includes all types of materia medica.

Chinese physicians of old had a saying that "using medicine is like using an army." When a physician helps a patient to fight a battle against an illness, the physician, like a general, must first collect all relevant information — pathogenetic symptoms; next he must plan an effective strategy — working out a therapeutic program; then he manoeuvres his resources for the operation — applying materia medica against the disease. These three procedures — diagnosis, strategy and medication — are the essential steps of Chinese herbal medicine.

Chinese medication is traditionally in the form of herbal decoctions. A mixture of appropriate herbs is placed in an earthen pot mixed with three bowls of water. The mixture is brewed over a small fire until about eight-tenths of the decoction is left, and the decoction is drunk while lukewarm. The residue is discarded. (To save money, the residue may be brewed again for another similar decoction, then discarded.)

Readers who are used to the pill and syrup mixture of western medicine and who think that Chinese medicinal decoction is old fashioned, would be surprised to learn that pills, syrup mixture and other forms of western medication were used in ancient China. Decoctions, tincture, pills, pellets and powder were mentioned in Nei Jing 2000 years ago.

In his famous "Treatises of Epidemic Colds and Fevers", written in about A.D. 210, Zhang Zhong Jing gave directions for washing, soaking, fumigating and applying ear and nose drops, nasal and oral administration, ointment and suppositories. His alum pill for treating leukorrhea was probably the first gynaecological suppository in the world.

Later, but still much earlier than in western medicine, during the Song Dynasty (960-1279) when the government set up imperial dispensaries to maintain high standards in pharmacy, medicinal tablets and syrups were common and patent medicine was popular.

Why then is the traditional decoction, with its obvious inconvenience when compared to the pill, syrup or tincture, still the most popular form of Chinese medication? This is because the medicinal recipe, instead of patent medicine, provides the greatest range for the physician to select his herbs for the specific needs of individual patients.

He can prescribe a different medicinal recipe each time a patient consults him. When the herbs have been prescribed by his physician, brewing it into a decoction is the easiest way for the patient.

There are over three thousand types of materia medica in Chinese medicine. While modern physicians may prescribe their own recipes according to the needs of their patients, famous physicians in the past have left behind a legacy of a rich collection of medicinal recipes for common syndromes. These established medicinal recipes run to thousands and are commonly employed by today's physicians as bases for their prescriptions.

For example, a Chinese physician diagnoses that his patient suffers from "cold of the lungs with a slight fever, coughing with yellowish phlegm, short of breath and sore throat, and the disease is found to be external at the initial stage." The great ancient physician, Zhang Zhong Jing, has bequeathed a medicinal recipe for illnesses with this kind of syndromes and this recipe is poetically called "Little Green Dragon Decoction".

The modern physician often prescribes this "Little Green Dragon"; he may add or subtract a herb or two and will decide on the amount of each of the herbs in this recipe according to the specific needs of his patient. If you wonder why a modern physician still uses this medicinal recipe which was first prescribed in ancient times, the answer is that it has been found to be effective throughout the ages.

How does a physician remember thousands of medicinal recipes? How could he even remember the three thousand odd types of materia medica? In practice, he will be sufficiently equipped if he can keep in his mind or notebook a few hundred herbs and recipes.

Moreover, past masters have made the task easier for him by recording such information in the form of songs or verses which work on the principle of mnemonics. The "Little Green Dragon", for example, could survive nearly twenty centuries because of the following poem!

> Miraculous cure little green dragon has
> External cold, cough, congestion at chest
> Xi xin, ban xia, gan and wei
> Jiang, gui, ma huang, shao the best

Those not familiar with the Chinese language and Chinese medicine may find the above verse nonsensical, but it concisely contains the necessary information regarding the syndrome and the main materia medica to be used.

This medicinal recipe is effective against illnesses with symptoms of cold and fever, cough with plenty of phlegm, cold at lungs, and congestion at chest. The herbs necessary for this mixture, as represented by the Chinese words in the verse, are respectively Herba Asari, Rhizoma Pinelliae, Radix Glycyrrhizae, Fructus Schisandrae, Rhizoma Ephedrae, Romulus Cinnamomi, Herba Ephedrae, and Radix Paeoniae.

While the English terms may be tongue twisters, the Chinese names are poetic and meaningful. Xi xin, for example, means "small suffering", ban xia "midsummer", gan cao (represented by gan above) "sweet grass", and wu wei zi (wei above) "fruit of five tastes".

Not only are the major medicinal recipes and materia medica recorded in verses, but other important medical knowledge, such as meridians, acupuncture points and therapeutic principles, are also recorded in rhyming verses to make it easier for physicians to remember.

If you like poetry, you will get an extra bonus when you study Chinese medicine in the Chinese language.

Basic Principles of Chinese Pharmacology

To help physicians in their prescription, Chinese masters have classified the properties of material medica into four energies, five tastes and twelve meridian systems.

The nature and functions of materia medica are generalized into four energies, namely cold, heat, warmth and coolness. Cold materia medica refer to those that have properties of eliminating heat and fire and neutralizing poison. (If you wonder what "eliminating heat and fire" means, you have missed some important information in previous chapters on Chinese pathology and diagnosis. The terms "heat" and "fire" are figurative.)

Western antibiotics belong to this class of herbs in Chinese pharmacology. Examples of cold herbs include bai tou ong (Radix Pulsatillae) and huang lian (Rhizoma Coptitis).

Hot materia medica refer to those herbs that expel cold, enhance yang and strengthen the immune system. Examples include rou gui (Cortex Cinnamomi) and fu zi (Radix Aconiti Praeparata).

Warm and cool materia medica are moderate versions of hot and cold medicine. Examples of warm herbs are hong hua (Flos Carthami) and du zhong (Cortex Eucommiae); and of cool herbs are xi cao (Radix Rubiae) and niu huang (Calculus Bovis).

There is also a fifth group of herbs that are neither hot nor cold, warm nor cool and are therefore termed "neutral". Some examples include pei lan (Herba Eupatorii) and jin ying zi (Fructus Rosae Laevigatae).

Besides the four energies, Chinese materia medica are classified into five tastes, namely acrid, sweet, bitter, sour and salty.

Acrid materia medica have properties of dispelling external evil, inducing diaphoresis (sweating), regulating vital energy, and waking the patient from unconsciousness. Examples of acrid herbs are ma huang (Herba Ephedrae) and mu xiang (Radix Aucklandiae).

Sweet herbs have properties of reconciliating the physiological functions of the spleen and stomach systems and invigorating vital energy and blood. Examples of such herbs are kan cao (Radix Glycyrrhizae) and tang shen (Radix Codonopsis Pilosulae).

Bitter herbs can eliminate heat, quench fire, dry dampness and cleanse blockage. Examples of materia medica with bitter taste include da huang (Radix et Rhizoma Rhei) and mo yao (Rasina Commiphorae Myrrhae).

Sour materia medica can implement astringent therapy, consolidate functions and resources, promote body fluid and relieve cough. Examples of sour herbs are wu wei zi (Fructus Schisandrae) and wu mei (Fructus Mune).

Materia medica with a salty taste have properties of mositurizing dryness, softening hardness, facilitating excretion and clearing blockage. Examples are lu jiao jiao (Colla Cornus Cevis) and mang xiao (Natrii Sulfas).

The classification of materia medica into meridian systems indicates which meridians (please see Chapters 8 and 9) the energies of the herbs will flow. These refer to the twelve primary meridians of the lung, colon, stomach, spleen, heart, small intestine, urinary bladder, kidney, pericardium, triple warmer, gall bladder and liver.

Because the intricate meridian network links every part of the body together, the prescribed medication while being focused at a particular meridian system, can also reach other parts of the body.

Chinese medical prescriptions, therefore, are not merely prescribing herb A for disease X, or herb B for disease Y. For a particular disease, the physician has a wide range of therapeutic herbs.

His choice will depend on factors such as the developmental stage of the disease, the meridian system where the battle is likely to take place, as well as the physiological and psychological conditions of the patient, as shown by indicators such as his pulse rate, facial and other bodily appearances and his reactions to the disease-causing agents.

The physician may prescribe between two to twenty or more kinds of materia medica for each mixture. As the patient's conditions change during the prognosis, the physician will modify his prescription accordingly.

The physician, like a general in a battle, has to evaluate the holistic situation of the patient, who resembles the battle ground in this analogy, and map out a comprehensive strategy to fight the disease.

Unlike narrow-minded generals, he would not simply inject a foreign infantry to fight the invaders, nor drop a few bombs to destroy the areas where his enemy has established himself, for he is concerned that such measures even if successful would harm his own territory, which is the patient.

The physician's preference is to strengthen the territorial army to fight the invaders, or to mobilize the local citizens to rebuild the damaged parts. Hence, employing antibiotics or surgery is usually his last resort.

If he ever has to use them, the physician has to make sure that after the defeat of the enemy, the patient's own army (which is his vital energy and blood systems) and his own citizens (his cells) are adequately rehabilitated to carry on their normal functions. The Chinese physician considers his job done not when the disease-causing agents have been eliminated, but when the patient has been restored to health.

Hence, after antibiotics or surgery have successfully accomplished their purpose, a competent physician always follows up with a program of strengthening and nourishment, which are considered an integral part of the treatment.

Yin-Yang and Five Elemental Processes

The principles of yin-yang and five elemental processes apply to the nature and behavior of the Chinese materia medica. Naturally, herbs that are cold and cool are regarded as yin, whereas those that are hot and warm are yang.

Concerning the yin-yang of the five tastes, herbs that are salty, sour and bitter are regarded as yin, and those which are acrid, sweet and taste flat are yang.

Herbs have affinity with particular meridians. Those that have affinity with meridians linked to the yin storage organs — heart, liver, spleen, lung, kidney and pericardium — are known as yin herbs. Yang herbs on the other hand, are closely connected to meridians that are linked to the yang transformation organs. And yang transformation organs are small intestine, gall bladder, stomach, colon, urinary bladder and triple warmer.

From their long years of observation and study, Chinese masters in the past discovered that in their operation, the different nature, taste and behavior of the materia medica correspond to archetypical processes. These masters generalized them into the five elemental processes.

Cold herbs are symbolized as water, cool as wind, hot as fire, warm as metal, and neutral herbs as earth. Concerning the five tastes, acrid herbs are symbolized as metal, salty as water, sour as wood, bitter as fire, sweet as earth.

Herbs classified by meridian systems follow the elemental processes of their respective organs: lung and colon as metal, kidney and urinary bladder as water, liver and gall bladder as wood, heart and small intestine as fire, spleen and stomach as earth.

As the pericardium relates to the heart, herbs that have affinity with the pericardium meridian are symbolized as fire. As the triple warmer actually comprises all other organs, herbs that have affinity with the triple warmer meridian are represented by the respective organ systems that their effects are focussed at. The table in Fig 14.1 will make these relationships clearer.

Elemental Processes	Metal	Water	Wood	Fire	Earth
Nature	Warm	Cold	Cool	Hot	Neutral
Tastes	Acrid	Salty	Sour	Bitter	Sweet
Organs and Meridians	Lungs Colon	Kidneys Urinary Bladder	Liver Gall Bladder	Heart Pericardium Small Intestines	Spleen Stomach

Fig 14.1 Five Elemental Processes in Chinese Herbs

This classification is made not because Chinese physicians merely wish to correspond the herbs to the concepts of yin-yang and the five elemental processes for speculative discussion, as some misinformed writers imply, but because it serves some very useful practical purposes which will become clear as the book unfolds.

It must be emphasized that the terms "metal", "water", etc are symbolic and they refer not to the basic ingredients that make up the universe, but to archetypes of all processes. For example, when Chinese physicians say that "cold herbs belong to water" or "acrid herbs belong to metal", they do mean that cold herbs are mainly made from the element water, nor acrid herbs from the element metal.

What they meant was herbs that are classified as cold, have the properties of the water process, like quenching fire, which is a symbolic expression for eliminating pathogenic micro-organisms; and that herbs which are classified as acrid, have the properties of the metal process, like the reverberating sounds of a metal bell, which figuratively describes induced sweating as a therapeutic process.

A scholar once mentioned that because the Chinese had devised a classification of five elements (a common mistaken translation for the five elemental processes), they tried to force everything into this classification, including the tastes of their medicine and the emotions of their patients. It is obvious that even a brief description like the paragraph above illustrates that this scholar's opinion is wrong.

Yin-yang and the five elemental processes are used to describe Chinese materia medica because this enables Chinese physicians to express many medical ideas concisely. These concepts also provide them with a philosophical framework for many medical operations. For example, after a physician has diagnosed his patient's illness as yin (revealed by symptoms like pale face, weak pulse, clear urine and general debility), to restore harmony, he would prescribe yang herbs.

When faced with a wide choice of herbs, his task is made half easier if he only refers to his pharmacopoeia and discards all those that are labelled "yin".

If the physician wants to strengthen the patient's spleen and stomach systems, for here is where he has found his patient's weakness lies, he would choose herbs that taste sweet because sweet herbs, possessing the earth process, will nourish the spleen and stomach.

So far the application of the yin-yang and the five elemental processes principles is quite simple: using yang herbs to balance yin illnesses and using earth herbs to nourish earth organs. But let us say there is a small complication. Although the source of the patient's weakness lies in his spleen and stomach, these organs are too weak to absorb nourishment. What should the physician do? The inter-creativity principle of the five elemental processes may suggest an answer.

Using the principle of "fire creates earth", which means increasing the patient's fire can indirectly improve his earth, the physician prescribes herbs with fire behavior to strengthen the patient's heart and small intestine systems.

When these organs are strong, there will be sufficient fire to create earth, meaning that his spleen and stomach will improve and he will be able to take nourishment on the road to recovery.

If you think the physician uses this method just because the five elemental processes concept stipulates that the heart and intestine correspond to fire and the spleen and stomach correspond to earth, and the inter-creativity concept stipulates that fire creates earth — if you think the physician does so just because the theory says so — you are, like the scholar above, presuming that the Chinese put their cart before their horse.

Unlike the ancient Greeks who put forward their theories to speculate on the universe, the ancient Chinese did the reverse: they studied the universe first, then put forward theories to explain what actually happened. The theories of the Chinese, therefore, are explanations, not speculations.

And if you ask how does a Chinese physician know that sweet herbs can invigorate energy at the stomach, or that one can improve stomach functions through the heart system, it is like asking a western doctor how does he know antibiotics like erythromycin and tetra-cycline can kill infectious pathogens, or that infusion of insulin can alleviate the sufferings of a diabetic.

The doctor may answer that he learnt it at medical school and that although he has not personally conducted experiments to confirm the validity of his medical authorities, this knowledge has been proven correct in practice.

Similarly, the physician may say that he learnt this from past masters, who probably discovered it through years of study and observation and although he himself has not conducted scientific tests on it, he can trust the masters because their discoveries have been proven correct in practice.

One notable difference, however, is that while the western practice has been carried on for decades, that of the Chinese has been carried on for centuries. Hence an understanding of the yin-yang and five elemental processes principles enable the Chinese physician to unlock and apply invaluable knowledge masters have accumulated over the ages.

Seven Modes of Medical Prescriptions

Chinese herbs are usually prescribed in suitable combinations rather than on its own. There are seven modes of medical prescription in Chinese herbal medicine, figuratively called the "Seven Emotions of Materia Medica". These seven emotions are different from the seven emotions describing the seven internal causes of disease.

These seven modes refer to seven ways of combining materia medica in Chinese medicinal recipes, namely "Single Way", "Mutual Combination", "Mutual Enforcement", "Mutual Restraint", "Mutual Inhibition", "Mutual Rebellion" and "Mutual Destruction".

When there is only one kind of materia medica in a recipe, it is called the "single way". The famous ren sheng (Radix Ginseng) steamed alone in water, known as "Single Ginseng Decoction", excellent for invigorating vital energy, is a classic example.

When two kinds of materia medica with similar properties are used together in a medicinal recipe to reinforce each other, this mode of prescription is known as "mutual promotion". An example is the "Little Pinelliae Decoction", comprising of ban xia (Rhizoma Pinelliae) and sheng jiang (Rhizoma Zingiberis Recens), which is an effective recipe to stop vomiting.

If we use other kinds of herbs to enhance the effect of the main herb or herbs, this mode is known as "mutual enforcement". An example is using huang lian (Rhizoma Coptidis) and huang ling (Radix Scutellariae) to enhance da huang (Radix et Rhizoma Rhei) in the "Purging Stomach Fire Decoction" to relieve fire (micro-organic attack) at the stomach system.

When two kinds of materia medica are employed together and both retrain the properties of each other, or one restrains the properties of the other, the mode is called "mutual restraint". For example, ban xia is toxic (similar to western antibiotics) and may be harmful to the patient if in excess; but if a few slices of ginger (Rhizoma Zingiberis Recens), are added, the toxicity is controlled.

When two kinds of materia medica cancel each others' properties, or when one cancels the properties of the other, the mode is known as "mutual inhibition". Ginger (Rhizoma Zingiberis Recens) has the properties of dispelling cold and inducing warmth; but if huang lian (Rhizoma Coptidis), which has the properties of detoxification and clearing heat, is added, it will inhibit the effects of ginger. Thus, this mode of "mutual inhibition" is generally avoided in medicinal prescription and physicians are aided by the "Song of Nineteen Inhibitions". Nevertheless, it is useful for neutralizing herbs taken in by mistake.

If two kinds of herbs result in drastic side effects when used together, the mode is known as "mutual rebellion". For example, both ban xia (Rhizoma Pinelliae) and chuan xiong (Rhizoma Ligustici Chuan-xiong) are acrid and warm. When they are used together, they will increase the toxicity of ban xia, causing harmful side effects.

Past masters have bequeathed the "Song of Eighteen Rebellions" to help physicians avoid combinations of certain herbs.

On the other hand, two different herbs that may be toxic when used separately, may cancel each others' toxicity when used together, or one harmless herb may destroy the toxicity of the another. Such a mode is called "mutual destruction". For example, ba dou (Fructus Crotonis) is toxic and is an effective antibiotic if used appropriately.

However, a patient will have its antibiotic effects destroyed or greatly reduced if he unwittingly eats a bowl of green bean gruel, because green bean (Semen Phaseoli Radiatus) destroys the toxicity of ba dou.

Brief Glimpses of Chinese Pharmacology

A Chinese physician is required to know a wide range of materia medica, which are classified into convenient groups for his easy reference, such as regulating vital energy, strengthening blood, stabilizing emotions, clearing heat, facilitating fluidity, purging and sweating, poisons and external application.

The materia medica are divided into three main classes: herbs that promote invigoration like ginseng and reindeer's horn belong to the first class, those that restore psychological and physiological functions belong to the second class, while those which the west would call antibiotics and which the Chinese label as poisons belong to the third class.

The following are brief examples of the basic information usually included in a Chinese pharmacological list. Because of space constraint, only an example of each class is given below. Readers who wish to find out more about Chinese medicinal herbs need to refer to a good pharmacopoeia.

Ren Sheng (Radix Ginseng), literally meaning "Human Root".

> Sweet's the taste of this wonderful herb
> Invigorating you with health sublime
> Quenching thirst and generating fluid
> Nourishing and defending you at all time

> Background:
>   Plant belonging to ginseng family. Root used for medicine. Found in
>   Northeast China and Korea.

> Nature:
>   Warm. Sweet, slightly bitter. Flow in spleen and lung meridians.

> Application:
>   Excellent for invigorating primordial energy. Relieve coma and asthenia.
>   Benefit blood and generate fluid. Improve appetite and strengthens the
>   body. Suitable for: asthenia, insomnia, anorexia, yang deficiency, sexual
>   impotency, sudden loss of energy, breathlessness, diabetes, swollen
>   limbs, coldness of body and purging.

Combination:

Alone as "Single Ginseng Decoction" for invigoration. With fu zi (Radix Aconiti Praeparata) as "Ginseng Aconiti Decoction" for loss of blood and vital energy. With fu qin (Poria), bau shu (Rhizoma Atractylodis Macrocephalae) and gan cao (Radix Glycyrrhizae) as "Four Gentlemen Decoction" for general weakness after prolonged illness.

Amount:

5 to 15 gm.

Caution:

Not suitable for those with cold and fever, "solid" illnesses and internal injuries. Inhibited by wu ling zi (Faeces Trogopterorum); and destroyed by li lu (Veratrum Nigrum).

Yuan Zhi (Polygala tenuifolia wild), literally meaning "Far-Sighted Ambition".

Warmth is the nature of yuan zhi
Good remedy for fright and anxiety
Dispels worry and clears your phlegm
Cures sores and improves your memory

Background:

Plant; bark and root used for medicine. Found in Henan and Shanxi Provinces.

Nature:

Warm, bitter. Flow in the heart and kidney meridians.

Application:

Stabilizes emotions. Cleanse blockage between heart and kidney meridians. Disperse worry and clear phlegm. Suitable for relieving fright, loss of memory, insomnia, cough, phlegm and sores.

Combination:

With fu qin (Poria), bo zi ren (Semen Biotae), mai dong (Radix Ophiopogonis), tian dong (Radix Asparagi), ren sheng (Radix Ginseng), dan sheng (Radix Salviae Miltiorrhizae), yuan sheng (Radix Scrophulariae), wu wei zi (Fructus Schisandrae), di huang (Radix Rehmanniae), jie geng (Radix Playticodi), suan zao ren (Semen Ziziphi

Spinosae) dang gui (Radix Angelicae Sinesis) as "Heavenly King Invigorating Bolus" to cure excessive worry, deficiency of "heart-blood", poor memory and various mental discomforts. After being heated and soaked in wine, it is used as external application for sores.

Amount and Treatment:
3 to 15 gm. Used raw, or treated with honey or heat.

Caution:
Not suitable for those with deficiency of heart energy and kidney energy; and not to be used by those with "real fire" (microscopic pathogens) and those who vomit blood.

Huang Lian (Rhizoma Coptidis), literally meaning "Yellow Lotus".

Bitter and cold Yellow Lotus may be
Congestion at heart and abdomen it'll dispel
Heat and poison it'll disperse with glee
Making gastrointestinal system strong and well

Background:
Plant of the Coptidis family. Root used as medicine. Found in Sichuan, Yunnan, Guizhou, Hubei, Anwei and Lingxia.

Nature:
Cold and bitter. Flows in the heart, liver, spleen, stomach, gall bladder and colon meridians.

Application:
Cooling blood and dispelling fire. Dry dampness and clear heat. Clear congestion and neutralize poison. Quench thirst and remove worry. Suitable for "hot purging" (purging due to micro-pathogenic attack), vomiting caused by contaminated food and evil heat (external pathogens), painful or swollen eyes, oral ulcers, nose bleeding and various sores.

Combination:
With mu xiang (Radix Aucklandiae) as "Fragrant Lotus Bolus" for diarrhoea and profuse reddish and whitish viscid vaginal discharge. With wu zhu yu (Fructus Euodiae) as "Left Gold Pill" to relieve

vomiting. With huang ling (Radix Scutellariae), shan zhi (Radix Pittospori) and huang bai (Cortex Phellodendri) as "Yellow Lotus Detoxification Decoction" to cure various sores, rashes and other skin diseases.

Amount and Treatment:
5 to 15 gm. Used raw or fried.

Caution:
Not suitable for illnesses not caused by real fire (infectious diseases) and those deficient in stomach or spleen energy.

Having a sound knowledge of the numerous herbs and their properties is of course an essential part of the Chinese physician's practice. But he goes beyond this. He does not merely prescribe a certain herb for a certain complaint; he prescribes a range of herbs to correct his patient's pathogenetic conditions and restore him to health. For example, when a patient complains of gas in the stomach, vomiting and cough with plenty of phlegm, he does not say, "Look, yours is a complicated case. Let's tackle it one thing at a time. Take this for your stomach gas, this to stop your vomiting, this for your cough, and this to clear your phlegm."

Instead, he evaluates his patient's pathogenetic conditions holistically, considers some strategies and tactics, then prescribes an appropriate medicinal recipe, which in this case could be the "Fragrant Six Gentlemen Decoction". We shall read about this in the next chapter.

15

PLANNING AND FIGHTING THE BATTLE

(Strategies and Tactics in Chinese Herbal Medicine)

Like any other names in science, cancer is just a shortened way
of saying something that cannot be simply defined. ... Cancer is a
disease of organization, not a disease of cells.
                    Dr D.W.Smithers, a world cancer specialist.

Medicinal Recipe as Unit of Medication

There are at least three things a general must do if he is to fight a battle well: know the enemy, plan a strategy and use his men efficiently. Similarly a herbalist must do three things to fight illnesses; know the disease, plan a therapeutic program and use herbs effectively.

Diagnosing the disease has been dealt with in previous chapters. Here we will learn how to plan healing strategies and use herbs. After knowing the properties of individual herbs, the physician combines them in a suitable manner to get the best effects. The principles of mutual promotion, mutual enforcement and mutual restraint, as explained in the previous chapter, are used to increase the efficiency of medicinal recipes. He would guard against mutual inhibition, mutual rebellion and mutual destruction as these modes of prescription would reduce the intended effects. Sometimes he may use only one herb in the single way mode.

In Chinese, this prescription of medication is known as "fang ji", which means applying principles and techniques to combine appropriate materia medica for restoring the patient's health.

The term indicates that it is not just a matter of knowing which herbs can cure what diseases and applying the appropriate herbs when the disease is diagnosed. Although such a procedure is practiced by some healers and may produce some startling cures, it is comparatively amateurish.

A competent physician understands not only pharmacological principles (as explained in the previous chapter), but also the structure of a medicinal recipe and the strategies and tactics of its application.

Unlike in western medicine where individual drugs constitute the basic units of oral medication, in Chinese medicine the basic unit is the medicinal recipe, not the individual herbs which make up the recipe. This difference is significant on at least three counts.

If western medical scientists find certain herbs hold promise of possible cures for some difficult diseases, studying the essence of the herbs or even the whole herb in isolation may not be sufficient to yield positive results, because these herbs operate in combination with other herbs in a medicinal recipe.

Secondly, Chinese herbal medication, including those with antibiotic properties, does not have the common side-effects of western drugs, because these side-effects have been neutralized or inhibited by other herbs in the same recipe.

Thirdly, medicinal recipes comprising many herbs operating harmoniously, enable the Chinese physician to treat the patient holistically, instead of the specific disease.

Structure of a Medicinal recipe

The various kinds of materia medica in a medicinal recipe may be classified into four types according to their functions in the recipe. These four types are jun, chen, zuo and shi, which are figuratively translated as monarch, minister, deputy and ambassador.

Monarch herbs are the primary medicine against the disease. Minister herbs are those that enhance the effect of monarch herbs. Deputy herbs help to relieve secondary symptoms, or restrain any drastic action of the primary or other herbs so that there are no unfavorable side-effects. Ambassador herbs act as guides to lead other herbs or act as a catalyst.

Obviously, monarch herbs are the most important. They are regarded as "zheng yao" or main medicine. All the others are "fu yao" or supplementary medicine. However, one should not be mistaken to think that supplementary medicine is unimportant; not only it greatly increases the effectiveness of main medicine, it also removes the unfavorable side-effects for which western drugs have been notoriously known.

It is not necessary that all the four groups of medicine are present in a prescription. In the examples given in the previous chapter, in the "Single Ginseng Decoction", ginseng being the only herb, is naturally the monarch herb.

In the "Little Pinelliae Decoction", both ban xia (Rhizoma Pinelliae) and sheng jiang (Rhizoma Zingiberis Recens), are monarch herbs as they are of equal importance as the primary medicine.

But in the "Purging Stomach Fire Decoction", da huang (Radix et Rhizoma Rhei) is the monarch, while huang lian (Rhizoma Copti-dis) and huang ling (Radix Scutellariae), which are employed to enhance the primary medicine, are the ministers.

Ban xia (Rhizoma Pinelliae) being toxic is an effective antibiotic. A few slices of ginger (Rhizoma Zingiberis Recens), are often added to a medicinal recipe where ban xia acts as the monarch. The ginger, which restrains the toxicity of ban xia, is the deputy herb.

In such a prescription, gan cao (Radix Glycyrr-hizae) is also often added to coordinate the various herbs, and it is called the ambassador medicine.

Let us try to use these four groups of herbs in a medicinal recipe. In Chapter 12 we diagnosed our imaginary patient to be suffering from a hot, solid, external, yang disease of the spleen and stomach systems caused by dampness and heat.

The principal target of our treatment, therefore, is to dispel dampness and heat at the stomach and spleen systems. As this disease is "solid", that is caused by "real fire" (pathogenic micro-organisms), huang lian (Rhizoma Coptidis) and da huang (Radix et Rhizoma Rhei) are effective remedies, as these herbs flow in the stomach and spleen meridians, dry dampness, clear heat and dispel fire. Hence, they are employed as monarch herbs.

To enhance the effects of the monarch herbs, we add huang ling (Radix Scutellariae) and mu tong (Caulis Akebiae) which will dry dampness, clear heat and dispel fire at the related lung, colon, intestine and urinary bladder meridians. They are, therefore, ministers.

It is worthy to note that all these monarch and minister herbs are "cold" and "bitter", which are figurative terms meaning that they possess pharmacological properties to fight "hot", "solid" and "external" diseases.

To speed up the relief of the patient's headaches and to dispel "external evil", we may add fang feng (Radix Ledebouriellae), which is thus an deputy herb. To coordinate the actions of all the herbs, we add gan cao ((Radix Glycyrrhizae), the ambassador herb.

Hence, with this concept of monarch, minister, deputy and ambassador, the Chinese physician is able to increase the effectiveness of his medical prescription. Some western books on Chinese medicine mention that Chinese medical philosophers superimpose political concepts into medicine. Such misleading information can easily make Chinese medical philosophy appear ludicrous.

In the above example, it is obvious that terms like "monarch" and "minister" have no political connotations. Should there be any debate regarding the suitability of these terms, it is a linguistic, not a political or medical question.

The Chinese physician treats a patient as a living organization, in which the disease has interrupted its systematic operation and this classification of materia medica into different kinds according to their therapeutic functions in their respective medicinal recipes, helps the physician achieve his purpose better.

If he merely prescribes herbs according to the disease without considering other factors, he may not achieve the optimum effects, because the same herbs and disease may behave differently in different situations and environments in the organization of the patient's body.

In a battle, for comparison, if a general merely sends his solders to fight the enemy without considering factors like weather, terrain and psychological settings, he may be described as having an army, but not having any tactics and strategies.

Similarly, the Chinese regard a physician who only knows which herbs cure which disease as "you yao wu fang", meaning "although there is medication, there are no techniques and principles".

Seven Strategies in Prescribing Medicine

The analogy between employing medicine to cure illnesses and employing an army to repel an enemy is both apt and illuminating. The enemy need not necessarily be foreign invaders (infectious diseases); it may be a case of civil war (cancer), breakdown of essential functions (organic illnesses), or disorganization of the country's intellectual activities (psychiatric disorders).

In all cases the battle field is in our own territory. This means that whatever damage that has been inflicted in the fighting, even when the battle is won, has to be borne by our own citizens (body cells). So, even if we have big guns and bombers, we have to use them with great care.

Obviously, the tactics and strategies used to fight a platoon of enemy commandos operating in a crowded area, are different from those used to fight an enemy battalion in an open field.

Similarly, a Chinese physician uses different categories of medical prescriptions to fight different kinds of diseases. There are literally thousands of established prescriptions, but masters have classified them into archetypes for the physician's convenience. This classification is known as "Seven Strategies and Twelve Tactics".

The Seven Strategies refer to seven major principles of medical prescription to meet different categories of illnesses. These strategies are "large", "little", "gradual", "urgent", "single", "multiple" and "combined".

If the disease is potent and widespread, or has a wide range of complications, the physician uses a "large prescription" with a large number, high dosage and/ or great potency of herbs. The "Large Green Dragon Decoction" and the "Large Bupleuri Decoction", both for infectious diseases at the intermediate stage, are two examples.

If the sickness is minor, it is not necessary to use elaborate medication. As soon as the sickness is alleviated, medication should stop so as not to affect the patient's natural state of vital energy. Such a strategy is known as a "little prescription". The "Little Ban Xia Decoction" and the "Little Purgative Decoction" are examples.

Illness that is chronic and asthenic requires a "gradual prescription" where medication spreading over a period of time can strengthen and nourish the patient. Those who suffer from frequent back pains due to inadequate blood, or those whose lung system has been weakened through grief will respectively find the gradual prescription of "Four-Substance Decoction" and "Zhi Gan Cao (Radix Glycyrrhizae Praeparata) Decoction" useful.

If the illness is serious or acute, an "urgent prescription", in which the medication may be drastic or potent, is necessary. For example, when a patient's disease is of the yangming syndrome, where an infectious disease has developed to an advanced stage, when his pulse is sunken and solid, his abdomen swollen, his bowel stagnant and the patient in coma, an "urgent prescription", like the "Potent Purgative Decoction", has to be used.

A "single prescription" is used when the illness is straight-forward. The term "single" as used here does not mean that only one herb is prescribed, or the patient needs to take the medication only once.

It means that since the patient does not show complications, the medical prescription has only a single purpose directly targeted at the cause of the patient's illness. For example, when a patient is attacked by pathogenic micro-organisms, with symptoms of fever and sore throat, the physician's "single prescription" is to expel the "poison" with a simple medication like "Hong Huang (Realgar) Antibiotic Pill".

On the other hand, if the causes of the illness are complex, different types of monarch herbs have to be prescribed, constituting a "multiple prescription". For example, a patient, because of excessive anxiety that has injured his spleen system, suffers from anorexia (loss of appetite) and asthenia (loss of strength).

His kidney system is also weak and he has frequent nocturnal seminal emission. He feels pain all over his body as his vital energy is sluggish.

A physician may use "Angelicae Sinensis Invigorating Spleen Decoction" as the base to strength his spleen system and add as main herbs, shan zhu yu (Fructus Corni), shu di (Rhizoma Rehmanniae Praeparatae) and du zhong (Cortex Eucommiae) to improve his kidney systems and relieve him of his seminal emission, as well as add ren sheng (Radix Ginseng) and huang qi (Radix Astragali seu Hedysari) to promote his energy flow.

A "combined prescription" is one where two or more recipes are mixed together to form one recipe, or are prescribed to the patient alternately. For example, half the dosage of "Four Gentlemen Decoction", which is effective for promoting vital energy and half the dosage of "Four-Substance Decoction", which is effective for promoting blood, are combined into one dose for a chronically weak patient. Or the two decoctions can be prescribed to the patient in turns.

These strategies reveal that the Chinese have had an advanced philosophy of medical prescription. They represent the development of Chinese thought on medication over many centuries. Besides these "Seven Strategies", Chinese physicians also employed "Twelve Tactics".

Twelve Tactics to Restore Health

The "Twelve Tactics" refer to twelve general methods of restoring health. They are based on the principles of yin-yang and five elemental processes and illustrate that the onus in Chinese medicine is to restore the natural functions of the patient, rather than defining and curing diseases. For example, if the vital energy in the body has become too warm, which is symbolized by yang, the remedy is to cool it, symbolized by yin.

If the normal reproduction of certain body cells is inhibited, symbolized as stagnation of the wood process, the remedy is to nourish the relevant parts of the body with vital energy, which is a water process, to restore the natural cell production.

As early as the 6th century, a great physician, Xu Zhi Cai (492-572), crystallized the approaches of past masters into ten tactics. Later physicians added another two tactics. These twelve tactics are explained below. Do not be surprised to read about terms such as "real, hot evils" and "windy, cold diseases"; if you are puzzled by such figurative terms, please refer to Chapter 12 which is on Chinese Pathology.

1. "Dispersion dispels Congestion" (Xuan Ke Qu Yong). Prescription with a dispersing effect can dispel the congestion-syndrome. Congestion may be caused by "real evils", which correspond to exogenous pathogens like gems and bacteria, or "apparent evils", like weakening of physiological functions. The "Dispersing Toxic Substances Decoction" is an example of a medicinal recipe for dispersing "real" congestion.

2. "Cleansing dispels Retention" (Tong Ke Qu Zhi). Prescription with a cleansing effect can dispel the retention-syndrome. Retention of body fluid, for example, may cause abdominal flatulence. The "Wu Ling San" (Powder of Five Herbs including Poria) is effective for cleansing this retention.

3. "Invigoration removes Debility" (Bu Ke Qu Ruo). Prescription with invigorating effects can remove the debility-syndrome. Debility is the underlying cause of diseases. There are four main kinds of invigoration, that of yin, yang, blood and energy. The "Lu Wei Yuan" (Bolus of Six Herbs) is an example of a medicinal recipe for invigorating yin.

4. "Purgation removes Closure" (Xie Ke Qu Bi). Here "closure" refers to blockage due to "real evils", corresponding to pathogenic micro-organisms, which may be "hot" or "cold". Prescription with a purgative effects can remove this closure-syndrome. An example of purgative prescription is "Purgative Decoction" for removing "real, hot evil".

5. "Light dispel Real" (Qing Ke Qu Shi). "Light" here refers to herbs that induce sweating or diaphoresis; "real" refers to pathogenic micro-organisms at the superficial or initial stages. In other words, this tactic

involves the use of diaphoretic herbs against infectious diseases at the early stages. Depending on the typical behavior of the pathogenic micro-organisms, Chinese physicians describe them as "hot evil" or "cold evil" and the term "wind" is often used to describe the patient's condition if the disease location tends to change rapidly. The "Ma Huang (Herba Ephedrae) Decoction" is an example of diaphoretic prescription against "windy and cold" infectious diseases.

6. "Heaviness stabilizes Fright" (Zhong Ke Zhen Qie). "Heaviness" here refers to herbs with stabilizing or calming effects; "fright" refers to negative emotions as well as mental disorders like shock, insomnia and amnesia. Chinese medicine is quite rich in herbs dealing with emotional and mental ailments, with the advantage that Chinese prescriptions do not have the common negative effects of western sedative drugs because the side-effects if any are neutralized or inhibited by "deputy" herbs in the medicinal recipes. The "Cinnabaris Tranquilizing Pill" is an example of a stabilizing prescription.

7. "Lubrication removes Coagulation" (Hua Ke Qu Zhou). "Coagulation" here refers to any mass that stagnates in the body, but it does not have the virulence of "real evils" (pathogenic micro-organisms). Prescriptions with a lubricating effects can remove or flush out the coagulation, such as the "Dong Kui Zi (Semen Malvae Verticillatae) Lubrication Decoction" for curing urinary stones.

8. "Astringency overcomes Collapse" (Se Ke Qu Tuo). Astringent measures are those that can cause contraction and stop discharges. "Collapse" refers to the loss of essence and body fluid as in involuntary bowel movement, nocturnal emission and night sweating, due to collapse of yin, yang, blood or energy, i.e. collapse of essential body functions. The "Golden Lock Bolus for Keeping Kidney Essence", for example, can overcome nocturnal seminal emission.

9. "Drying overcomes Dampness" (Zao Ke Qu Shi). Dampness is one of the exogenous pathogenic causes, resulting in disorders like edema, dysuria, diarrhoea, cough and dyspnea. Prescription with a drying effect can overcome these disorders, such as the "Bolus of Double Wonders" to relieve diarrhoea.

10. "Moisturizing overcomes Dryness" (Shi Ke Qu Zao). Dryness refers to the deficiency of "blood" and other body fluids. Dryness of the

lungs is one of the symptoms of tuberculosis, which the Chinese refer to as weakness of the lungs. The "Heat-Clearing and Lung Nourishing Decoction" is an example of a "moisturizing prescription".

11. "Cold expels Heat" (Han Neng Qu Re). Prescription with the cold-effect can overcome the heat-syndrome. Medicinal recipes that clear heat, dispel fire and generate body fluids are "cold prescriptions" and many of them correspond to what are called antibiotics in western medicine. The "White Tiger Clear-Heat Decoction" and the "Yellow Lotus Antibiotic Decoction" are examples.

12. "Heat expels Cold" (Re Neng Qu Han). Prescriptions with the heat-effect can overcome the cold-syndrome. Medicinal recipes that can increase yang energy (physiological functions) as well as yin defence (blood and immune systems) belong to warm or hot prescriptions. The "Four Herbs Restoring Yang Decoction" is an example of a hot prescription to expel internal cold and the "Gui Ji (Ramulus Cinnamomi) Decoction" to expel external cold.

Examples of Famous Medicinal recipes

A medicinal recipe, the basic unit of Chinese oral medication, is a mixture, not a compound. This means that the amount of each ingredient, as well as the ingredients themselves may vary. Indeed, Chinese physicians often vary the amount as well as adding and subtracting a few ingredients according to the particular needs of the patient, while maintaining the general nature and dosage of the recipe. Naturally, children and those who are weak will be given a lighter dosage.

Chinese physicians, like generals planning each battle, prescribe a different medicinal recipe for every patient, basing on a thorough diagnosis and a careful consideration of the various strategies and tactics they can use.

Nevertheless, great physicians in the past have left behind a legacy of effective medicinal recipes with detailed explanations of their principles and modern physicians of course make full use of this accumulated wisdom.

Three famous examples of established medicinal recipes are given below. The amount listed for each ingredient is only a suggestion. Those who wish to pursue this topic further may refer to a good Chinese pharmacopoeia.

Ma Huang Decoction

In the ma huang decoction use gui ji
Xing ren, gan cao four herbs join in glee
Infectious disease, fever, headache and cold
Dispersed with profuse sweating they'll be

Ingredients:

Ma huang (Herba Ephedrae)	15 gm
Gui ji (Ramulus Cinnamomi)	10 gm
Xing ren (Semen Armeniacae Amarum)	15 gm
Zhi gan cao (Radix Glycyrrhizae Praeparata)	5 gm

Suitability:

Infectious diseases with fever, fear of cold, headaches, bodily pains, floating pulse, no sweat and short of breath.

Preparation:

Brew the mixture with three bowls of water in an earthen pot over a small fire until about eight-tenth of a bowl of the decoction is left. Drink the decoction while lukewarm.

Fragrant Bolus of Su He

Su He fragrance comprises eight kinds
She an mu ding tan chen fu combine
Xi jiao bing pian and bai shu
Covered with ju sha nourish the mind

Ingredients:

50 gm each of the following.
Su he xiang (Resina Liquidambaris Orientalis)
She xiang (Moschus)
An xi xiang (Benzoinum)
Mu xiang (Radix Aucklandiae)
Ding xiang (Flos Syzygii Aromatici)
Tan xiang (Lignum Santali)
Chen xiang (Lignum Aquilariae Resinatum)
Xiang fu (Rhizoma Cyperi)
Xi jiao (Cornu Rhinoceri)
Bing pian (Borneolum Syntheticum)
Bai shu (Rhizoma Atractylodis Macrocephalae)

Suitability:
Clear "wind" (mental disorders), stabilizes emotions and revive unconsciousness.

Preparation:
Grind into powder and make into bolus about 2 cm in diameter. Cover with a coating of zhu sha (Cinnabaris) and encase each bolus in a round shell of wax. Take one bolus each night washed down with ginger soup.

Four Gentlemen Decoction

Four Gentlemen Decoction makes you strong
Sheng, shu, ling, cao flow along
Ban xia, chen pi six gentlemen be
Cure yang deficiency and increase energy
Ban xia away Wondrous Powder achieved
Mu xiang, sha ren stomach cold relieved

Ingredients:
Ren sheng (Radix Ginseng)	5 gm
Bai shu (Rhizoma Atractylodis Macrocephalae	10 gm
Fu qin (Poria)	15 gm
Zhi gan cao (Radix Glycyrrhizae Praeparata)	5 gm

Suitability:
Remedy for energy deficiency, debility of stomach and spleen systems and shortness of breath.

Variation:
Add 5 gm of chen pi (Pericarpium Citri Retriculatae) to basic recipe to form "Five Herbs Wondrous Powder" for deficiency and stagnation of energy in children, hot deficiency of spleen and stomach, oral ulcers, vomiting, cold limbs and eyes exposed while sleeping.

Add 10 gm of ban xia (Rhizoma Pinelliae Praeparatae) and 8 gm of chen pi (Pericarpium Citri Retriculatae) to basic recipe to form "Six Gentlemen Decoction" for curing dysfunction of spleen and stomach, chest congestion, abdominal flatulence and cough with plenty of phlegm.

Add 5 gm of mu xiang (Radix Aucklandiae) and 3 gm of sha ren (Fructus Amomi) to Six Gentlemen Decoction to form "Fragrant Six Gentlemen

Decoction) for curing energy stagnation in the middle warmer, chest congestion, vomiting and purging, abdominal pains and rumbling sounds in the gastrointestinal tract.

Preparation:
Brew the mixture of herbs in three bowls of water until about eight-tenth of the decoction is left. Drink the decoction while lukewarm.

Hopeful Possibilities

The different medical philosophy between Chinese and western medicine is quite obvious. While the western approach is reductionist and mechanical, reducing disease to its smallest possible unit, the Chinese approach is holistic and organic, regarding disease in relation to the totality of the patient.

Indeed the Chinese physician does not treat the disease; he treats the patient as a whole person. His approach, therefore, is not so much the elimination of the disease, but the restoration of health.

This difference of approach is more than just a matter of perspective; it affects the whole range of medical principles and practices from pathology and diagnosis to pharmacology and therapeutics.

Hence, the Chinese have never really bothered to quantify diseases nor define them into specific types. Their knowledge of diseases in western scientific terms, such as the types of specific bacteria and viruses that cause infections, or the types of enzymes necessary for certain metabolic processes, is exceedingly poor.

On the other hand, Chinese physicians exhibit a profound interest and understanding in their patient as a person. They observe, albeit intuitively without the aid of measuring instruments and sophisticated technology, the minute changes the patient undergoes when he is unwell and they classify his disease not according to the agents that cause it, but according to the patient's pathogenetic conditions in reaction to the disease.

Hence, in their treatment, Chinese physicians emphasize not on removing the disease-causing agents, but on correcting the patient's pathogenetic conditions. For example, when treating a patient suffering from an infectious disease, their onus is not on defining the pathogenic micro-organisms and killing them, but on defining the patient's pathogenetic conditions, which in this case may be described as external heat at a particular organ system and correcting the deviated conditions.

Because the Chinese and the west look at illnesses from different angles, it is irrelevant to find the exact corresponding Chinese terms for diseases named in English. For example, a disease known in western medicine as peptic ulcer may be interpreted in Chinese medicine, depending on the patient's pathogenetic reaction, as stomach pains due to deficiency of stomach energy, or stomach pains due to "empty-cold" in the stomach.

There are, nevertheless, equivalent Chinese names for diseases known by western terms. Peptic ulcer, for instance, is called "wei kui yang", which literally means "stomach ulcer". But such names, though they are widely used in modern Chinese for convenience, are Chinese translations of western terms — strictly speaking, not Chinese medical terms themselves.

In fact the traditional Chinese terms are more exact. While western doctors are quite uncertain of the cause of peptic ulcers, the Chinese know that it is caused by deficiency of stomach energy or empty-cold in the stomach.

So, while western doctors prescribe drugs to neutralize the gastric acids that erode the stomach wall, or cut away the stomach sore in a surgical operation — both of which are actually treating the symptoms and new ulcers may appear as soon as the drugs are stopped, or some time after the operation; Chinese physicians treat the cause by invigorating stomach energy or dispelling empty-cold in the stomach.

The Chinese approach is holistic; it does not isolate the disease as if it will always behave the same way irrespective of its environment inside the patient's body, but treats it in relation to the patient as a living organization.

In this connection, we can hopefully ask whether this holistic approach to restoring the patient's health — rather than the reductionist approach of focusing on the specific disease — may provide answers to Dr Smithers' search for a cancer cure after his conviction that cancer is a disease of organization, as quoted at the beginning of this chapter.

We can also hopefully ask whether a shift of attitude from a reductionist, mechanical approach to a holistic, organic one may provide answers to cures for AIDS and other so-called incurable diseases.

Chinese physicians openly and proudly tell their patients to seek western medical treatment whenever they realize that western treatment is better or speedier. Hospitals in China use western medical instruments and methods extensively. They always do so in a spirit of competency, confidence and professionalism; they never ever have any tincture of inferiority complex nor being threatened that referring their patients to a medical system other than their own may imply any inadequacy on their part.

Of course no one suggests that western doctors discard the methods they have been trained in in favor of the Chinese system, even if they were to find the Chinese system superior.

But wouldn't it be sensible, once western doctors and medical scientists have the courage to transcend provincial prejudice or arrogance, to adapt some of the successful principles and practices from other healing systems into their own in their noble endeavor to find cures for as-yet-incurable diseases in western medicine, especially when these so-called incurable diseases have been cured in other systems? The material provided in this chapter offers some possibilities.

More to come in subsequent chapters.

16

A CUP, A COIN AND A SLAB OF STONE
(Chinese External Medicine)

Certainly an empirical medicine that has survived thousands of years of civilization has something to offer the West.

Richard Hyatt.

External Medicine for Internal Illness

If you think that Chinese external medicine is merely for external injuries, you will be in for a surprise. It covers a wide range of therapeutic approaches and provides rich material for thought, not only for medical researchers, but also for sport instructors who may adopt some handy Chinese methods to treat their injured athletes on the spot and enterprising producers who may develop some Chinese ideas into health gadgets to make fortunes.

Chinese external medicine refers to other types of therapies besides taking of oral medicine. This include acupuncture, massage therapy and traumatology, but in its restricted sense, it comprises the use of ointments, plasters, cupping, scraping-therapy, heat-therapy, surgery and some extraordinary techniques. Actually the Chinese were very advanced in surgery, successfully performing major surgical operations many centuries ahead of the west.

Acupuncture, massage therapy and traumatology are regarded as independent branches of Chinese medicine and will be explained in detail in separate chapters. Surgery is not explained here because I am not competent to do so, although it actually constitutes the major part of external medicine.

External therapies are so called in the Chinese medical system not because they are meant for external injury, but because they are applied externally. Nevertheless, they can be used to treat external ailments as well as internal sicknesses, both topically as well as for the whole body.

Instead of taking appropriate herbs into the stomach from where our energy flow and blood circulation transport the medication to the diseased parts as in internal medicine, in external medicine the medication is diffused through the skin at suitable points into the body to be transported by our meridian systems to where it is needed.

Its principles and applications are more profound and extensive than those of western intravenous medication.

Serious Injury from Internal Force

I personally benefited from an aspect of Chinese external medicine in the form of a medicinal plaster, which was very effective though it would look primitive to some people. Long ago during a sparring session with my senior in my Shaolin Kungfu training, I managed to grasp both his arms as he executed a double punch. As I was to learn later, it was his trick; with a skilful manoeuvre, he unexpectedly released my grip and gave me a lighting punch within a few inches onto my chest.

I took no notice of this apparently gentle tap. But a few days later, I felt cold and feverish and began to cough. My eyes became blood-shot and there was slight pain at my chest, though there was not the slightest sign of injury on the outside. I knew it was not an ordinary illness, for since I started practicing Shaolin Kungfu and qigong, I was always healthy.

When my master, Sifu Ho Fatt Nam, who is an accomplished Chinese physician and traumatology specialist, examined me, he said it was a serious internal injury, caused by energy blockage at my tan-zhong energy field (located in the middle of the chest above the heart). This internal injury was unwittingly caused by the internal force of my senior through his punch, though he had no intention to hurt me.

Had I not experienced it myself, I would not have believe that such an innocent-looking punch with apparently no visible force, could cause any internal damage.

My master opened some energy points on my chest. Then he applied a medicinal paste in the form of a plaster. I also drank some medical decoction to cleanse the energy blockage and practiced some qigong therapy exercises. The medicinal plaster was changed every alternate day. During the change of plaster, I could see a dark purplish patch on my chest, which my master explained was "dead blood" drawn out from the injury by the medicinal paste. I recovered in about two weeks.

Besides verifying that the incredible destructive effects of a kungfu master's internal force is real, this experience also provides us with another useful lesson. Had I consulted a conventional doctor, he would not be able to cure me.

He would say there is nothing wrong with my chest (just as years later some of my patients were told the same thing by their conventional doctors) because energy-blockage, the real cause of the internal injury, is absent in the western medical vocabulary.

The conventional doctor might prescribe medication for my blood-shot eyes, cough, cold and fever, but the real cause of the disease would escape his notice. A person with such serious internal injuries uncured would die within a few months, with hardly anybody knowing the reason!

External Application

Medicinal plaster is one of the many techniques of external application of medication. External application, known as "fu yao" in Chinese, is an important aspect of Chinese external medicine.

An appropriate medicinal recipe of herbs is ground into powder and is usually treated with honey or rice wine. The essence of the medicine, its heat, or its coldness is diffused through the skin into the patient's body, where his meridian system transmits the therapeutic effects into internal organs and other parts of the body for restoring the patient's health. Sometimes flour, earth and other material may be used as a base to mix the medicinal powder.

The common places of application are the patient's palms, soles, back, chest and certain energy points on the arms and legs. The medicinal mixture may be prepared in vaseline, an ingredient that the Chinese have learnt from the west and applied as ointment. The following are some examples of external application, with their therapeutic principles briefly explained.

Knead some flour into a small ball. Warm it and apply it to the sole of the patient. Change the warm flour every two hours. Appropriate herbs in powder form may be added to the flour.

This treatment is useful for sprains or spasms of the leg, sores on the legs, excessive urination due kidney weakness and nose bleeding (for which there are many causes, like abnormal rushing up of lung-heat forcing blood out of the vessels, hyperactivity of liver-fire, attack of stomach-heat, deficiency of lung-yin or kidney-yin, attack of wind on the head such as caused by over-drinking).

It is not difficult to see that the heat diffused into the leg through the sole would facilitate energy flow with therapeutic effects for its sprains, spasms or sores. But how does it work for excessive urination and nose bleeding? The important yongquan energy point is found at the sole and it leads along the kidney meridian to the urinary bladder and kidneys.

Heat transmitted along this meridian can activate the kidney energy, thereby alleviating excessive urination. As the kidney meridian is also linked to the lungs and liver, increased activity at the kidney meridian helps to palliate rising lung-heat and liver-fire, thus relieving nose bleeding.

Appropriate herbs in powder form are mixed with yellow or red earth, which needs to be washed previously. The mixture is applied to the patient's chest and useful for relieving high fever, cough and internal injuries in the chest. It can be fastened by either bandage or plaster.

The therapeutic principle is that the cold-effect from the earth and appropriate medicine is diffused into the chest and spread by the defence-energy in the triple warmer to lower body temperature, cool the lungs thus soothing cough and clear the heat of the chest injury. This method should not be used in winter, because the intense cold absorbed by the earth mixture may be harmful.

Prepare a mixture of herbs that are effective for activating blood flow, loosening muscles and cleansing meridians. Grind them into powder, heat the mixture and make it into a stick. Apply the heated stick of medicine on the cheng shan energy point at the back-middle of the calf.

This is a useful treatment against sprains and spasms, involuntary urination and the "numbness-syndrome" (characterized by numbness, arthralgia and dyskinesia) at the leg. A viable idea for a creative manufacturer is to put the medicine in concentrated form in an elongated container, to be carried about conveniently by sportsmen like a large sized pen, which they can use to treat themselves effectively against common sports injuries.

Cheng shan is an important energy point along the urinary bladder meridian which controls much of the muscle system of the body. Hence this technique is effective for relieving sprains, spasms and the "numbness-syndrome" at the leg. Involuntary urination can be remedied when the urinary bladder energy is improved.

Another traditional method is to apply a paste of leaves on the navel. Leaves from medicinal plants with properties of clearing heat and neutralizing toxins (a Chinese term for antibiotics) are the best; but any leaves or vegetables can be used. The leaves are pounded into a paste and secured to the navel with plasters or bandages. Change the paste after half a day, or when it becomes dry.

This technique is useful for relieving high fever, abdominal pains due to stomach heat and infantile convulsions (caused by hyperactivity of heat and wind evils, or by impairment of stomach and spleen and upward attack of apparent yang due to liver dysfunction).

At the navel is located the shenque energy point (meaning "gate of the human spirit") which leads directly into the abdomen. Hence the cold-effect of the leaves can be diffused into the stomach, spleen and liver to clear heat. This cold-effect is also spread by the defence-energy of the body to reduce fever.

Prepare appropriate herbs, grind into powder and mix with vaseline. Apply to the middle of the patient's back as ointment a few times a day. This technique is useful for relieving asthma, coughing, cold and fever (caused by wind-cold and by wind-heat) and wounds. The herbs must suit the type of illness.

There are a few energy points at the back of the body. In the middle is lingtai (meaning "spiritual platform"), which leads to the chest. Appropriate medication applied here, therefore, can relieve asthma, cough, cold and fever. For wounds, the ointment is applied directly on them.

Cold compression is an external medical technique. Wet a towel in cold water and apply it over the dazhui energy point (at the back just below the neck). Repeat after a few minutes. This technique is useful against sunstroke, nose bleeding and common cold due to wind-heat. It is not suitable if there are sores or wounds at the dazhui area.

The dazhui energy point lies along the du or governing meridian and has access to the head and face. The cold-effect of the cold compression is diffused to the head to relieve nose bleeding and "heaty" common cold and spread by the du meridian over the body to palliate sunstroke.

On the other hand, warm or hot compression is used for other types of illnesses. Wet a towel in warm or hot water, and apply it over the patient's forehead. Ensure that it is not too hot or it might hurt the patient. It is useful for relieving headaches due to cold and fever, feeling of severe cold and unconsciousness.

The therapist may continue to add warm or hot water gradually to the towel so that the heat is diffused into the patient's head. The heat-effect of the towel placed at the forehead "opens" meridians at the head, promoting better energy flow and stimulate the senses, thus relieving headaches and unconsciousness.

Heat Therapies

There is an interesting group of external therapies known as "yun tang", which literally means "ironing with heat". It is actually a group of heat therapies. It may take many forms and is economical but effective, including for some serious diseases. However, it is not suitable for hot diseases and where there is bleeding.

Fry some salt in a pan, then wrap it in some dry, clean cloth. Roll the packet of heated salt over the patient's palms, soles, back or abdomen to let the heat diffuse in. Salt has properties of clearing blockages.

This method is a good relieve for sprains and spasms, purging and vomiting and sicknesses due to cold-dampness retained in the abdomen, as the heat from the salt packet stimulates better energy flow, clear cold and dry dampness.

Enterprising manufactures could make a fortune from this method: the salt packet, if it can be heated conveniently at will, should have a wide market as it is a handy treatment for some common medical complaints.

Some vinegar and xiang fu (Rhizoma Cyperi) in powder form can be added to the fried salt, to be mixed and wrapped in a packet. Xiang fu, which is acrid in taste and flows to the liver and triple warmer meridians, has properties of regulating energy flow, stopping pain and dispersing congestion. Vinegar has properties of overcoming collapse and stopping discharge.

When the heated packet is ironed over diseased parts, it helps to relieve cold limbs, body pains due to retention of cold and dampness, abdominal flatulence, internal haemorrhage, fever and infantile convulsion.

Fry some salt until hot, then add slices of garlic leaves and continue frying for about two minutes. (Do not fry for too long or else the therapeutic properties of garlic may be lost.) Garlic can activate energy flow, induce sweating and dispel cold.

Wrap the mixture in a piece of dry, clean cloth. It is suitable for cold and fever due to wind and cold, shortness of breath with plenty of phlegm and hemiplegia, or paralysis of one side of the body. Hemiplegia is caused by deficiency of yang energy and defence energy leading to disorder of vital energy flow, or by the attack of evils simultaneously. This cheap, unsophisticated method can relieve hemiplegia by dispelling cold, cleansing blockages and promoting vital energy flow.

Even eggs can be used as a therapeutic agent. Boil an egg; make sure that there are no cracks on the shell. While it is hot, roll the egg swiftly over the patient's abdomen, limbs or other parts of the body. This is useful for relieving cold and fever, cold-dampness in the abdomen, cold limbs and purging due to collapse-syndrome.

As all these ailments are due to cold evil and dampness evil, the heat from the egg help to remove them. The egg must not be eaten after use.

A slab of stone, iron, chinaware and other suitable material may be used for hot compression. After heating the material, wrap it in a piece of clean cloth. Some ginger or garlic may be added to the slab. Heat from the slab diffuses into the disease parts of the body to dispel cold-evil and is effective against abdominal pains due to cold and dampness, fear of cold, frostbite and chilblain due to sever cold weather.

This method is also useful for reverting an unfavorable prognosis caused by deficiency of the body energy and hyperactivity of the pathogenic agent.

Prepare a mixture of herbs with properties for cleansing meridians, activating energy and blood flow, dispelling cold and eliminating toxins. Fry the mixture in a pan, then place the mixture on the diseased parts. The essence and heat of the herbs diffuse into the body with the above mentioned effects.

This technique is suitable for relieving arthritis and rheumatic pains, numbness and debility of limbs and itching of skin.

Medication through Orifices

One special group of Chinese external therapeutic methods is medication through the orifices. In Chinese medical philosophy, the orifices are directly connected to their respective internal organs by meridians. They are, therefore, entrances to man's internal cosmos.

The Chinese physician not only can have a good idea of the condition of the internal organs by examining their orifices, he also can administer medication to the internal organs through these orifices.

How are they connected? The eyes are connected to the liver; the nose to the lungs; the mouth to the stomach; the tongue to the heart; and the ears as well as the external sex organs and the anus are connected to the kidneys. If the orifices are healthy and strong, they act as effective defence to prevent diseases attacking their respective internal organs.

Grind the following herbs into powder: 2 gm each of xiong huang (Realgar), bin pian (Borneolum Syntheticum), zhu sha (Cinnabaris), she xiang (Moschus) and 4 gm of yan xiao (Sal Nitri). Using the tip of a clean, pointed brush, dot a bit of the powder onto a corner of the patient's eye once or twice a day. Close the eyes for some time after dotting the medication. As the eyes lead to the liver, the essence of the medicine can be transmitted to the internal organ.

It is suitable against food poisoning, sunstroke, epidemic evil and scarlet fever, as the herbal mixture has antibiotic effects, clear heat and dispel fire. It is also effective as a preventive measure to be applied once a week.

Grind 6 gm of zao jiao (Spina Gleditsiae) and 1 gm of bing pian (Borneolum Syntheti-cum) and blow some of the powder into the patient's nose. Let him sneeze. As the nose leaks to the lung systems and the medicine has properties of clearing heat and eliminating toxins, it is suitable for relieving cold and fever, blocked nose, tight jaws and diseases caused by epidemic evils.

Place appropriate herbal mixture, like shi chang pu (Rhizoma Acori Graminei), ai ye (Folium Artemissiae Argyi), da suan (Bulbus Allii), in a container and pour boiling water over it. Let the steam and fragrance of the medicine flow into the patient's nose. This treatment, to be carried out twice a day, is effective against cold and fever, running nose, dry nose and insomnia. Add boiling water or herbal mixture when the steam has become inadequate.

Grind appropriate herbs and sprinkle the powder over gauze or cotton wool. Fold the medicated gauze or cotton wool into tubes and tuck one or two tubes into one or both of the patient's nostrils. This is useful for curing or preventing contagious or virulent-epidemic diseases, as these microscopic pathogens usually enter through the nose and attack the lung system. Suitable herbs include those that clear heat, dispel fire and cleanse pulmonary blockages. Enterprising manufacturers may make a fortune producing such preventive gadgets during an epidemic.

Alternatively, such medicated gauze or cotton wool can be push into the ears. Be careful not to push too far in. This method is suitable for ailments like hard of hearing, noises in the ear, migraine and various ear complaints. The correct herbs appropriate to the ailments must be used.

Instead of using gauze or cotton wool, the medicinal powder may be blown into the ears. It is suitable for relieving pains in the ears, noises in the ears and secretion from the ears. If there is secretion, dry it with some cotton wool before blowing in the medication.

Use a feather, which must be aseptic, to tickle a patient's throat inside his mouth to make him vomit. This is a simple, mechanical method to relieve food poisoning, foreign matter stuck in the throat and thick phlegm along the esophagus.

Medication may be pushed in through the anus. Grind the appropriate herbs, make the powder into a tiny tube and coat it with oil. This method is suitable for diseases like purging, constipation, piles, worms in the alimentary canal and prolapse of the rectum.

Some Extraordinary Chinese Methods

Some of the external therapies described here are quite extraordinary. Although some uninformed people may regard them as primitive or unscientific, there are actually sound medical principles to explain their working. And the fact that they have been practiced for a long time can attest to their usefulness.

Cupping, which was a main therapeutic method in Europe for many centuries, is still used by some Chinese because it is simple, economical and effective. The inside of a cup, bowl or glass is heated by burning inside it a ball of cotton wool soak in alcohol. Then the vessel is inverted over the diseased parts of the patient's body, who is usually lying down.

An alternative method is to fasten a candle firmly to a coin, place the candle with the coin as a base on the targeted part of the patient's body. Light the candle, then place the vessel over it.

In either case, the partial vacuum in the vessel causes evil qi or energy, in a gaseous form, being sucked out of the patient's body.

The common sites where the cupping vessel is placed and the ailments it can relieve are as follows: on navel for abdominal pains due to cold and dampness, abdominal flatulence, purging and involuntary urination amongst children; on chest for chest pains, cough, chest congestion and disorder due to rising stomach energy; on mid-abdomen for constipation, worms in alimentary canal, vomiting and mid-abdominal pains; on middle back for cough due to heat or cold, shortness of breath, cold and fever; on lower back for lumbago, constipation, purging, numbness and dyskinesia of lower limbs, sprains and pains; on limbs for arthritis, rheumatism, internal haemorrhage, sprains and muscular pains.

Looking at this list, it is no wonder that cupping was a principal therapeutic in the past.

I had a personal experience to verify the effectiveness of cupping. When I was a child, I once had a severe abdominal pain in the middle of night. My mother applied cupping on my navel. The process took less than half an hour and the relief was immediate! Had she rushed me to the hospital, the treatment would be more complicated.

Another interesting but simple method is scraping. Let the patient lie face-down without his shirt. Use a copper coin or a porcelain table spoon to scrape the patient's back firmly in one direction from below the neck to his waist. Some water or oil may be applied to facilitate the movement and a piece of towel or cloth may first be place at the patient's back to soften friction, especially for children.

Other places that may be scraped are the arms, the thighs and the neck. Scraping improves energy flow and the nervous system in the body. It is useful against ailments such as dizziness, nervousness, unconsciousness, high fever, infantile convulsion, vomiting and sunstroke.

Two related methods that would strike many people as odd are pinching and nibbling. In pinching, the healer bends his second and middle fingers at the knuckles and rapidly pinches his patient until his skin is red. This can promote energy and blood circulation and is effective for relieving infantile convulsions, unconsciousness and vomiting due to cold and dampness.

In nibbling, the healer slowly nibbles at the patient's body, particularly his chest, abdomen, palms and soles, until the patient's skin becomes red. Like pinching, nibbling promotes energy and blood circulation and is useful for infantile convulsion, difficult bowel movement and urination, abdominal pains and flatulence. Pinching and nibbling are usually used on children.

If you practice Chinese external medicine, you may have a chance to hit your patient with a whip, yet get paid for it! Of course Chinese physicians are not sadists and this whip is not an ordinary whip.

It is called a medicinal whip, obtained by dipping some soft branches, like those of the morus and willow trees, into medicated wine and is used to hit the patient's diseased parts.

The medicine from the medicated wind diffuses into the patient and is useful against arthritis, rheumatism, infantile polio-myelitis and paralysis of limbs.

Selected herbs should have properties of clearing wind, stopping pains, cleansing meridians and activating blood and energy flow. Soak a mixture of suitable herbs in rice wine for about three weeks before use.

A common treatment for children, though it can also be used on adults, is the wearing of a "fragrant bag". Appropriate herbs, especially those with fragrant smells, for the particular diseases are seasoned with rice wine and gently heated over a fire.

If fragrant smelling herbs are not in the list, then some are added principally for their fragrance. The mixture is packed into a bag to be worn by the patient all the time. The essence of the medicine diffuses into the patient's body. It is effective for virulent-epidemic sicknesses, infectious diseases, febrile rashes on the skin and smelly sweat.

Alternatively, the herbal mixture can be packed into a pillow for the patient to sleep on. Add some fragrant material if the mixture does not contain fragrant herbs. The essence of the medicine diffuses into the patient's head and it is suitable for diseases like stiff neck due to coldness, headaches, dizziness and insomnia.

An extraordinary therapy for serious illnesses is called fire treatment. Place a lighted wick burning with organic oil on various energy points and as soon as a soft explosion is heard, swiftly withdraw the fire. This will stimulate his nervous system and energy flow and is effective for relieving headaches due to cold and fever and for tetanus and epilepsy! After treatment, apply some ointment on the patient's heated parts.

A more common method is the medicinal bath. Appropriate herbs are brewed and then poured into a tub. As the patient takes a bath in the warm medicinal water, the essence of medication diffuses into his body. This is an effective therapy for rheumatism, febrile rashes, dry skin and various skin diseases. He must take care that the medicinal water does not get into his ears, eyes and navel and should apply some talcum powder over his body after the bath.

Instead of water, steam can be used. Prepare a mixture of herbs according to the targeted illness. Brew the mixture and then pour the steaming concoction into a container on which the patient sits. Sit for about thirty minutes and let the essence of the medicine vaporize into the buttocks. This method, known as sitting therapy, is suitable for constipation, difficult urination, pro-lapse of rectum, itchiness and pains at external sex organs and hernia.

Vaporization is a popular therapy against numerous diseases. Prepare a mixture of suitable herbs for the targeted disease. Slowly brew the herbs until the concoction is steaming, in an enclosure or small closed room with the patient, so that the medicinal essence in the form of vapour diffuses into him.

The patient should also gently breathe in the vapour. This technique is effective for diseases like scabies, measles and rheumatism. Vaporization therapy can also be used for treatment at a localized area. In this case, place the diseased part over the steaming concoction.

Medicine without Medicine

It is amazing how rich and varied the Chinese external therapies are. But this becomes no longer a surprise if we remember they represent some of the healing methods of the world's largest population for more than 20 centuries.

Many of these therapies do not need medicine and if you have understood the Chinese philosophy on pathology and therapeutics, you can see that they follow sound medical principles of relieving illnesses by removing its cause. For example, if the cause of the illness is wind, cold or dampness, or energy blockage, the physician removes the disease-causing "evil" or clear blockages, sometimes by ingenious means without using any materia medica.

These external therapies are simple, economical and effective and have efficiently served many rural people, who do not have ready access to modern hospitals and expensive medicine. Some, ironically are doubtful of their effectiveness because they are unsophisticated.

Nevertheless, even if you are rich and scientific, you do not carry modern medical technology with you wherever you go. So knowledge of such methods may prove to be very useful if one day you or your friends have only a cup, a coin or a slab of stone and a pressing illness.

INJURIES FROM FALLS AND HITS
(Introduction to Chinese Traumatology)

The art of medicine consists of amusing the patient while nature cures the disease.

Voltaire.

Traumatology and Chinese Kungfu

Traumatology, or "shang ke", is a special aspect of Chinese medicine, probably unique in the world, a speciality for the treatment of injuries caused by incision, contusion, dislocation, fracture and violent blows resulting in internal damage. It is closely related to Chinese martial arts.

In Chinese culture, a person's cultivation can be classified into two main divisions: "wen" or the arts of the scholar and "wu" or the arts of the warrior. In classical China, the emperor's high officials were divided into "wen guan", scholarly ministers, and "wu jiang", army generals. A person who is trained in both the scholarly and martial disciplines, known as "wen wu shuang quan", is much admired.

The development of traumatology in classical China was closely related to the martial cultivation. Kungfu masters were usually traumatologists as kungfu training and fighting often resulted in injuries that required traumatological treatments. The famous Shaolin Monastery, regarded by many as the pinnacle of kungfu, was well known for its traumatology. Traumatological injuries are often caused by falls or hits. Hence this unique aspect of Chinese medicine is also known as "die da", which in romanized Chinese is pronounced as "th'iet ta" in English spelling and which means "falls and hits".

Traditionally, the normal way to learn traumatology or "die da" was to follow a traumatologist, who was usually a kungfu master. The onus was on practical treatment, with little theory learning. Hence, as time went by, many traumatologists who were excellent in their practice, were not familiar with medical theory. Indeed, traumatology virtually operated outside the main stream of Chinese medicine proper.

The situation is accentuated by the practice that people generally differentiate an injury (shang) from a disease (bing): thus, a traumatologist treat patients with injuries, whereas a physician treats patients with diseases.

Even now, most Chinese physicians have scant knowledge of and little skill in traumatology, because even if they studied traumatology in their training, few would specialize in it, as patients who need traumatological treatment almost always consult kungfu masters instead of Chinese physicians.

This odd situation is rather unfortunate because Chinese traumatology is actually very advanced and has much to offer the world, but if its practitioners are not in the main stream of Chinese medicine, its role and contribution in medical circles will certainly be affected.

In this connection, I am lucky, because two of my four kungfu masters, Sifu Ho Fatt Nam and Sifu Choe Hoong Choy who taught me Shaolin Kungfu and Wing Chun Kungfu respectively, were Chinese physicians who specialized in traumatology.

My first kungfu master, Sifu Lai Chin Wah, who taught me Shaolin Kungfu too, was a traditional traumatologist, though he was not trained in Chinese medicine proper; while my other kungfu master, Sifu Chee Kim Toong, who taught me Wuzu Kungfu, was a Chinese physician but he did not specialize in traumatology.

The situation of traumatology now in Chinese medicine is promising. Returning from an international conference on Chinese medicine in China recently, Sifu Ho told me that traumatologists now enjoy very high esteem amongst medical practitioners in China, higher than acupuncturists, herbalists and other specialists, but second only to surgeons.

It is interesting to note the changing prestige of these specialists in Chinese medicine. During the Zhou Dynasty more than 20 centuries ago, the official ranking was as follows: herbalists, acupuncturists, surgeons (including traumatologists and massage therapists) and dieticians.

Classifications of Traumatology

For convenience, Chinese traumatology is divided into two main groups, namely external injuries and internal injuries. External injuries refer to injuries of skin, muscles and bones; whereas internal injuries refer to those of vital energy, blood and internal organs. These divisions and their sub-divisions are meant for easy study; in practice there is much over-lapping of classification.

Injuries to the skin and flesh are of two kinds. If the skin is torn, the injury is termed incision or cut; if the skin is intact but the injury has gone beyond into the flesh, it is termed contusion or bruise.

The injury may be simple, like a wound caused by a blade or pointed object, or a blood clot in the flesh; or complex, like the skin and flesh being injured by vehement impact damaging bones and blood vessels, or internal haemorrhage affecting energy flow and blood flow to internal organs.

The Chinese regard the skin as a wall protecting the interior: any break may result in external evil entering, or internal essence escaping. Hence, even for a simple cut, it is necessary to prevent infection and to stop the bleeding.

Injuries to muscles and tendons are amongst the most common in traumatology, especially amongst adults. The Chinese have many figurative terms to describe such injuries, such as muscles and tendons being discontinued, twisted, slanted, displaced, overturned, loosened, softened, strengthened and locked. These injuries can also be classified according to whether they are caused by spiral, turning force, or by direct, impact force; and according to whether the muscles and tendons are severed or not severed. Simple injuries of muscles and tendons affect bodily movements, while complex injuries may interrupt energy flow and injure internal organs.

While many people would consider a bone fracture a serious injury, which would need a few months to heal, in medical convention, bone injuries are classified as external injuries, compared to internal ailments like a viral attack on body cells or defective tissues in an organic disorder. Injuries to bones are first classified as minor or major.

Minor bone injuries affect only the bone surface without any serious damage. Major bone injuries involve joint dislocations and fractures. Dislocations may be partial or total; and may be forward, backward, upward or downward. Fractures are of three kinds, namely the bones being cracked, broken into two or more parts and smashed into many pieces.

Simple bone injuries do not present complications and treatment is often topical; but complex bone injuries, like when a fracture has pierced an internal organ or a spinal dislocation has affected the nervous system, demand great skills and knowledge.

Internal injuries in traumatology are of three main kinds: injuries to vital energy, injuries to blood and injuries to internal organs. The term "internal" is used here relative to external injuries of muscles, bones and skin.

Traumatology, as a branch of surgery, belongs to external medicine, where the healer normally deals with discernible body parts, compared to internal medicine where oral medication is taken into the body for operation at the cellular level. These terms are meant for convenience; irrespective of whether he practices internal or external medicine, the Chinese physician always treats the patient as a whole person.

Injury of vital energy is an area where the west may learn a lot from the Chinese. Because energy flow is not visible and its concept is absent in western medical philosophy, western doctors are generally not familiar with this type of injury.

Actually in Chinese medical philosophy, all illnesses are caused by the interruption of harmonious energy flow; in traumatology, the term "injury of vital energy" is particularly used to refer to the blockage or stagnation of energy flow caused by an external force, such as a forceful blow or a heavy fall, where the impact is so powerful that its force is transmitted into the body causing energy blockage or stagnation.

Because harmonious energy flow is essential for health, such an injury may have serious repercussions, like affecting the functions of various organs, disrupting the feed-back system and causing nervous disorders.

In advanced Shaolin Kungfu, there is an incredible art known as "dan xue", or dotting energy points, where an expert using internal force can interrupt the energy flow of his opponent by striking his energy points with a finger, causing serious delayed injuries which the opponent may not know!

Reversely, by opening certain energy points and transmitting vital energy into a patient, a Shaolin master can cure injuries and illnesses! We shall read more about these curing techniques in later chapters on acupuncture, massage therapy and qigong therapy.

Injury of vital energy often leads to injury of blood and vice versa. A Chinese medical principle states that "qi is the commander of blood", meaning that energy flow paves the way for blood circulation. Hence, energy blockage or stagnation unfavorably affects blood circulation.

A Chinese medical saying explains that "injury of vital energy causes pain; injury of blood causes swelling." Blood injury may also result in internal haemorrhage, where "disorderly" blood is forced out of its vessels and clots inside the body; or in haemorrhage disorder, where such "disorderly" blood is forced out of the body abnormally like vomiting blood, passing out blood in faeces or urine and blood gushing out through the nose, eyes or ears.

Injury of internal organs can be direct or indirect. Direct injury is caused by agents such as powerful blows, heavy falls, forceful pressure, penetrating weapons and fractured bones, where the agents physically damage the organs.

Injury can also be indirect, such as the result of energy blockage or blood disorder, where the function rather than the structure of the internal organs is injured. Injury may also be cause by negative emotions, such as excessive anxiety injuring the spleen and excessive grief injuring the lungs.

Wrong or deviated training in martial arts or qigong may cause internal injury of organs. For example, an uninformed student jabbing his fingers into granules in prolonged training without prior preparation may injure his heart or eyes, because meridians link the finger tips to the heart and eyes; prolonged forced breathing in qigong practice injures the lungs, because air sacs and lung muscles that have not been properly exercised for a long time are not given sufficient time to adjust to the new energy level of the forced breathing.

Hence, a knowledge of traumatology is important for martial art training, especially for instructors. Because in my kungfu training, traumatological medication, like medicated wine, injury-cleansing bolus, pills for activating energy flow and remedial qigong exercises, was always ready, I was quite shocked when I first learnt that many martial art students merely jumped about to loosen their muscles and improve blood circulation as means to lessen their injuries sustained in contact sparring.

Such injuries in sparring as well as in vigourous training, if untreated, may lead to serious health problems. This may explain why many sportsmen, despite their regular training which is supposed to make them fit and healthy, often have organic disorders; and some even collapse for no apparent reasons.

Principles of Traumatological Treatment

The saying that "the doctor does the dressing; God does the healing" is particularly apt for western treatment of traumatological injuries. In Chinese traumatology, however, the traumatologist does much to help God in his healing. And the traumatologist is guided by the following three principles:

1. Balance between local and holistic treatment.
2. Attention to both external and internal injury.
3. Coordination between static and dynamic approaches.

Let us take a simple fracture of the ulna as an example. Treating the ulna topically is only part of the trumatologist's job. He must remember that treating this injury locally will have repercussions over the whole body; so he takes appropriate measures to look after his patient holistically.

Chinese medical philosophy explains that "damage to a limb is an external injury, but it will cause internal injury of vital energy and blood, affecting the patient's nutrient energy and defence energy and consequently his internal organs may be disorientated."

Hence, besides the local treatment of the ulna, the traumatologist ensures that the patient's energy flow and blood circulation are back to normal, all parts of his body continues to receive their share of nutrients, the defence system maintains its vigilance against exogenous pathogens and all organs continue their perfect coordination.

In this way, not only the patient does not allow external as well as internal pathogenic causes to take advantage of his injury, his recovery will also be fast. This is the balance of local and holistic treatment.

A fractured ulna will cause blood flowing out of its vessels and since the skin is not broken, the disorderly blood will clot internally. This mass of internal blood clot not only affects a proper rejoining of the fractured ulna, it also affects the transportation of nutrients to and the removal of dead cells from the injured site. Hence appropriate medication should be applied locally as well as taken orally to remove the blood clot and to enhance energy and blood flow.

Moreover, the traumatologist should prescribe suitable mixtures of herbs to strengthen the patient's liver and kidneys, the organs that are mainly responsible for producing and regulating blood and bone respectively. The traumatologist, therefore, pays attention to the external methods of bone setting and external medication, as well as the internal methods of promoting energy and blood flow and strengthening the relevant internal organs.

When the fractured bone is properly set, it is important to keep it in place so that it will grow and unite into one piece again. While many western orthopaedists permit a margin of displacement if the function of a fractured bone is restored, the Chinese traumatologist considers the appearance of the bone as important as its function. I still remember the fantastic skills of my master.

Twenty years ago in the 1970s when a patient with a fractured leg often leave the hospital with the injured leg slightly shorter, my master treated a patient, who had one leg broken at seven parts because of a motor accident, so skilfully that nobody could notice it when he recovered!

While the orthopaedist prefers to cast a fractured limb in plaster of Paris, which often serves the patient better as a convenience for his visitors to sign their autographs than for immobilizing his limb, because he can still easily move his muscles which may affect his bone, the Chinese traumatologist usually uses splints and bandages to fasten a patient's fractured ulna.

Unlike the western method where the wrist is also immobilized, the Chinese traumatologist makes sure that the upper and the lower joints of a fractured bone — in this case, the elbow and the wrist — are free. (At the initial stage, however, some traumatologists also immobilize the wrist.) This, of course, is to allow movement of the elbow and wrist — in line with the principle of coordinating static and dynamic approaches. The Chinese onus is that only the fractured part is immobilized; other parts of the same limb are encouraged to move.

Why do the Chinese encourage such movements? So as to maintain, as much as sensibly feasible, the normal activities of the limb, such as movements of its muscles and flow of blood and mental impulses along it, while the fractured part heals. Will these movements affect the alignment of the set bone? They may. The alignment may still be affected even if the arm is cast in a plaster; that is why many patients' arms are slightly shorter after the plasters are removed. But while the orthopaedist hopes for the best as he removes the plaster after, say, three months; the traumatologists works for the best every alternate day, as he removes the splints and bandages to examine the prognosis. If he finds the slightest misalignment, he corrects it immediately.

In other words, unlike the western orthopaedist who sets a fracture only once and sees its result three months later, the Chinese traumatologist examines the healing fracture every alternate day and resets it as many times as needed.

The recovery is at least two times faster, because besides the various other medications, the patient's fractured arm is restore to normal conditions as much and as fast as possible. He is spared the torment of suffering from itchiness in the arm while being able to scratch only the outside of the plaster.

He is also spared the ordeal of seeing his arm shrivelled and rigid when the plaster is finally removed and he does not have to exercise his arm for another month or so to bring it back to life because he can exercise it while the fracture heals.

Internal Methods of Traumatology

Chinese traumatological treatments can bring speedy recovery because the traumatologist treats injuries from many angles. For convenience, treatment may be classified into internal and external methods, which are applicable to both internal and external injuries. Internal methods are subdivided into beginning, middle and concluding stages.

These methods and stages are useful guidelines, not rigid rules. Although the internal methods are mentioned first in the description below, both the internal and the external methods are employed at the same time.

Almost all traumatological injuries involve injury of blood. Therefore, at the initial stage, it is important to treat blood injury, which is usually internal haemorrhage or blood disorder.

There are three main techniques, namely "eliminating internal haemorrhage by draining", "dispelling internal haemorrhage by activating vital energy" and "clearing heat and cooling blood". Chinese medical terms, here and elsewhere, should be interpreted figuratively.

Cleansing internal haemorrhage is very important, failing which the production of new blood and its harmonious flow are affected. When "injured blood" is retained in the body, an effective remedy is to eliminate it by draining. "Tou Ren (Semen Perisae) Decoction" and "Da Cheng (Great Success) Decoction" are two examples of medicinal recipes that drain internal haemorrhage by purging.

In Chinese medicinal recipe, naming a decoction by a particular herb, unless it is a single-herb decoction, means that that herb is the main, but not the only, ingredient in the decoction. In the "Tou Ren Decoction", for example, five herbs are used, of which tou ren is the main ingredient.

When internal haemorrhage causes swelling or qi stagnation, an effective way to overcome this situation is to dispel the injured blood by activating energy flow. This technique is also a useful, though slower, substitute for "eliminating internal haemorrhage by draining" if the patient's conditions — like old age, general weakness, pregnancy and blood deficiency — do not favor the more drastic method of the latter.

Two examples of medicinal recipes for activating energy are "Generating Blood and Stopping Pain Decoction" and "Harmonizing Energy and Generating Blood Decoction".

The third technique, clearing heat and cooling blood, is useful for blood disorder as well as for gun-shot injuries and blood infection. Blood disorder refers to pathogenetic conditions where blood flows disorderly outside the blood vessels but still inside the body and may gush out abnormally through any of the orifices.

Two examples of such medicinal recipes are "Xi Jiao Di Huang (Cornu Rhinoceri and Radix Rehmanniae) Decoction" and "Cleansing Heart Decoction". The traumatologist, however, must take care that the medication should not be over-cold, which would result in the stagnation of blood and energy flow.

If the patient is weak, the traumatologist must also nourish energy, as injury of blood often brings about injury of energy.

Harmony at the Middle Stage

When the treatment at the beginning stage has accomplished its purpose, the traumatologist moves to the middle stage. The criterion for transition depends on the patient's prognosis, not on the number of medication he has taken, nor the number of days of treatment, though generally this takes place somewhere between the third and tenth medication and between the fifth and the twentieth day of treatment.

The guiding principle at the middle stage is "harmony", that is, reconciling or restoring the natural functions or abilities of the patient. The follow three techniques are often employed at this stage: "harmonizing nutrients and stopping pain", "joining bones, muscles and tendons" and "loosening muscles and cleansing meridians".

The three earlier techniques at the beginning stage are concerned with "eliminating evil", that is, attacking the pathogenetic causes of internal blood clot and blood disorder. When these pathogenetic causes have been eliminated, or when they are not yet totally eliminated but further attack on them may harm the patient, the technique of "harmonizing nutrients and stopping pain" is beneficially applied.

This harmonizing technique is concerned with "restoring good", that is, enhancing the natural self-curative and self-regenerative abilities of the patient. Examples of such medicinal recipes are "Eliminating Pain and Harmonizing Blood Decoction" and "Harmonizing Nutrients and Activating Energy Powder".

The technique of "joining bones, muscles and tendons" is applied at the middle stage when a fracture is properly set, muscles and tendons are well aligned and swelling has subsided. In conjunction with "harmonizing nutrients and stopping pain", the principal objectives of this technique are to clear away dead cells, increase blood circulation and energy flow, promote bone production and enhance muscles and tendon functions.

Useful medicinal recipes include "Decoction for the Rejoining of New Injuries" and "Pills for the Rejoining of Muscles and Tendons".

The technique of "loosening muscles and cleansing meridians" is an effective remedy at the middle stage for pathogenetic conditions like energy and blood stagnation, residue of blood clot still remaining at the site of the injury, stiffness of muscles and joints and rheumatic pains.

Useful medicinal recipes include "Loosening Muscles Cleansing Meridians Bolus" and "Loosening Muscles Activating Blood Decoction".

Nourishment at the Concluding Stage

After restoring the patient's natural functions, or when the restoring process has been placed on a sound basis, the traumatologist may move to the concluding stage of treatment. This transition may occur about two weeks in the case of internal injury of vital energy, or about two months in the case of fractures.

The main principle in this concluding stage is nourishment and four effective techniques to achieve this objective include "invigorating energy and nurturing blood", "nourishing spleen and stomach", "nourishing liver and kidneys" and "warming and clearing meridians".

Anyone suffering from internal or external injuries, being confined to bed for some time and lacking regular exercise, is bound to be deficient in vital energy and blood. The logical step, therefore, is to improve his energy and blood levels so that he may not succumb to other diseases and that he can soon return to normal life.

Two excellent medicinal recipes for this purpose are "Eight Precious Herbs Decoction" and "Ten Herbs Holistic Great Invigoration Bolus".

A recuperating patient usually has lost his appetite during his illness. He is, therefore, deprived of getting nutrients from good food. Even if he forces himself to take good food, his body may not be ready to accept it. (This, if fact, is the reason why he has no appetite and swallowing or injecting multivitamins at this stage may do more harm than good.)

As the stomach is mainly responsible for transforming food into nutrient energy and the spleen for storing and regulating this energy to all parts of the body, it is sensible to "nourish his spleen and stomach" to restore their normal functions which had been affected by the illness.

Useful medicinal recipes for this purpose include "Ginseng Poria Atractylodis Powder" and "Strengthening Spleen Nurturing Stomach Decoction".

In Chinese medical philosophy, "the liver is responsible for muscles" and "the kidney is responsible for bones". Moreover, the liver stores and regulates blood circulation, while the kidney affects the vitality of the whole body.

Hence, "nourishing liver and kidneys" is a significant technique at the concluding stage of traumatological treatment, especially when the patient suffers from a fracture or an injury to the muscles.

Effective medicinal recipes are "Generating Blood and Nourishing Marrow Decoction" and "Purple Gold Pill".

If a patient takes a long time to recover, exogenous pathogenic causes of wind, cold and dampness may have entered his body; or his energy flow and blood circulation may have stagnated. "Warming and clearing meridians" is an effective technique to overcome these problems.

Examples of such recipes are "Ma Gui (Herba Ephedrae and Ramulus Cinnamomi) Warming Meridians Decoction" and "Activating Meridians Pills".

All the therapeutic techniques described above are termed internal methods, because they involve taking medication into the stomach to be transformed into appropriate medicinal energies and transported to the site of injury at the cellular level.

They are applicable not only to internal but also to external injuries and not only in traumatology, but also in all other branches of Chinese medicine. It is obvious that anyone who regards as primitive or unscientific, any medical system with such profound philosophy, clearly has no knowledge of its theory and practice even at the elementary level.

All the methods described above, the internal methods, are only one part of Chinese traumatological treatment. The other part which are the external methods, are explained in the next chapter.

TREATING AN INJURY FROM DIFFERENT ANGLES

(Various Methods of Chinese Traumatological Treatment)

In modern medicine, the basic sciences have made great progress, but the therapeutics remain rather poor. In Kanpo medicine (Chinese traditional medicine in Japan), the reverse is true.

Yasuo Otsuka.

Holistic Treatment of the Patient

In Chinese traumatology, as in all other branches of Chinese medicine, a good traumatologist does not just treat the injury; he treats the patient as a whole person. For example, when treating a simple external injury like a dislocation of a shoulder joint or a simple internal injury of a blood clot inside the body, the Chinese traumatologist ensures not only that the dislocation is set right (which takes only a few minutes), or the blood clot is cleared (which western doctors often ignore), but also that all other functions of the patient are operating normally.

Otherwise, there may be after-effects. For instance, if the dead blood cells in either case are not flushed out of the body, years after the injury has been "cured" the patient may feel pains at the shoulder whenever the weather turns humid, or the residue of the "dead blood", while not manifesting directly or immediately as an illness, may affect the intricate workings of the body in such ways that complications may result indirectly.

It may seem far-fetched, but it is worthwhile to investigate or at least speculate, whether such insidious complications caused by "dead blood" and other interruptions to normal body functions may not be some of the contributing factors why some people fail to react effectively against some infectious microbes or even to AIDS or cancer.

When treating an injury, the traumatologist draws upon a rich repertoire of therapeutic principles and methods. For example, when treating a fracture, he does not merely set the bones right and let God do the healing; he assists God in numerous ways like promoting better energy and blood flow to clear away dead cells as well as generate faster replacement of needed tissues, continuously checking that the bone and muscles are in correct alignment, enhancing the internal organs that are actively involved in the recuperating work like the spleen, stomach, liver and kidneys and strengthening the patient holistically so that both endogenous and exogenous pathogenic agents have no chance to exploit the situation.

His therapeutics can be conveniently divided into internal and external methods. Internal methods have been discussed in the previous chapter; in this chapter we will examine the external methods.

External Methods of Traumatology

External methods may be classified into three groups: external application of medicine, manipulative skills and physiotherapy. These external methods are used for both internal injuries as well as external injuries and are used simultaneously with internal methods.

The five main techniques of external application of medication, which is a very common method in traumatology, are "stuck on medication", "rubbed on medication", "steam medication", "water medication" and "ironing medication". Sometimes the traumatologist also uses the numerous techniques of external medicine described in Chapter 16.

Suitable herbs are made into a paste, plaster or powder, and stuck onto the site of the injury by means of bandages or adhesive tapes. Such stuck on medication is used to reduce swelling, stop pain, promote energy flow and blood circulation, generate joining of fractured bones and severed muscles, clear cold and dampness and harmonize physiological functions.

For relieving rheumatic pains and for detoxification, medicinal plasters are often used; while medicinal powder is used on cuts and wounds to stop bleeding, prevent infections, generate growth, dispel cold and clear meridians.

Rubbed on medication may be in the form of medicinal wine, oil, powder and ointment. Medicinal wines are very popularly used in kungfu schools. Appropriate herbs, which have properties of clearing internal blood clots and activating blood circulation, are soaked in white rice wine for about two months and the medicinal wine is rubbed onto the injured parts.

Being effective for relieving sprains, bruises, muscle fatigue and internal blood clot, it can be a handy form of medication for sportsmen. Medicinal wine is also usually applied to the injured parts to facilitate setting of dislocations and fractures. Medicinal oil is sometimes used, but medicinal powder and ointment are not as common.

Steam medication is prepared by boiling some appropriate herbs and placing the injured parts over the vapour. This technique is useful for clearing internal blood clot in new injuries, as well as relieving rheumatic pains from old injuries.

In water medication, appropriate herbs are brewed slowly and then the concoction is allowed to become lukewarm. The warm concoction is used to bath the injury. The concoction is boiled again and can be reused for a few times.

In Shaolin Kungfu training, students often wash their arms and hands in these concoctions before and after hard force training like hitting sandbags, striking poles and jabbing their palms into granules. In this way, their arms and hands will not become rough nor deformed.

In ironing medication, an appropriate mixture of herbs is treated with wine and heated. It is then wrapped in a piece of dry, clean cloth and is used to roll over the patient's injured parts as if ironing some clothing. The essence of the medicine and heat diffuse into the patient's body.

Eight Techniques of Manipulation

Manipulative skills are extremely important in Chinese traumatology. Its essential role is obvious in dislocations and fractures, but it is also significant in other injuries.

No matter how effective is the internal and external medication, if a dislocation or a fracture is not well set, the patient cannot heal properly. Personally I go to the extent of considering it "sinful" for a traumatologist to set a fracture poorly, because when it heals, the patient will carry this "deformity" for life.

I remember that when treating a patient with a limb that was shorter or out of alignment because it had been badly set by a previous practitioner, my master, Sifu Ho Fatt Nam, sometimes broke the limb again to reset it. "If a healer is not confident or competent enough to treat his patient well, he must refer that patient to another healer. There should never be any feeling of shame nor inadequacy," he advised me, "for we must only practice according to our ability."

Since the Tang Dynasty when massage therapy became a speciality in Chinese medicine more than 10 centuries ago, the art of manipulative techniques for correcting dislocations and fractures have been developed continuously. It is, therefore, not difficult to imagine how rich Chinese manipulative techniques are. In traumatology the myriad methods are generalized into eight main techniques, known as Eight Manipulative Techniques for Correcting Bones. They are mo, jie, duan, ti, an, mo, tui and na, which means palpating, setting, replacing, lifting, pressing, stroking, pushing and gripping.

Each of these principal techniques, which are further classified into finer techniques, constitute a major part of the traumatologist's training. They are briefly described below.

Palpating refers to feeling the bones. Setting means joining two or more pieces of a fractured bone together. Replacing refers to placing one end of a fractured bone correctly to its other end, or placing a dislocated joint back to its proper location. Lifting refers to using the hands to raise a bone, joint or muscle, or using an aid like a rope to pull the patient as a means of traction.

Pressing means pressing and releasing the fingers or palms on the patient's energy points or meridians to activate energy and blood flow. Stroking is moving the fingers or palms to and fro along the patient's meridians or other parts of his body to activate energy and blood flow. Pushing refers to pushing a bone back to its proper position, or pushing the flow of energy or blood through a blockage. Gripping means holding the patient's skin, flesh, muscles or tendons and performing various movements to facilitate healing.

As in any art, the important thing is not merely knowing the techniques, but how to apply them skilfully. Chinese masters have devised some ingenuous ways for traumatology students to improve their skills. These training methods include throwing and grasping small sandbags, exercising with weights and pulleys, gripping one's own or a partner's specific energy points, muscles and bones swiftly and accurately and internal force training.

A medical saying advises that the physician should be so skilful in his application that "in setting a dislocation or fracture, the patient is not even aware of the manipulative movements, but as soon as he feels some pain, the dislocation or fracture is already set properly."

To help the traumatologist execute these techniques skilfully, Chinese masters have advocated certain principles, such as "Thorough understanding of the patient's conditions", "Planing of exact procedure before actual treatment", "Readiness of all tools and medicine before commencing treatment", "The right amount of strength applied during manipulation", "Ease and gracefulness in manipulative movement" and "One-pointed mind during treatment".

Through the years, various effective methods for setting dislocations and fractures have been developed for the convenience of the traumatologist. The diagrams below show some examples of these established methods, with poetic names, taken from Shaolin traumatology.

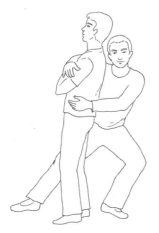

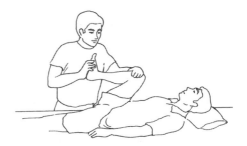

Fig 18.1 Across the Plain into the Cave
(for dislocation of a spinal vertebra)

Fig 18.2 Playing with the Unicorn
(for dislocation of the femur)

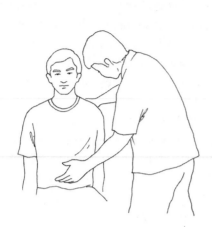

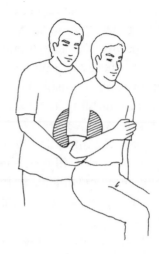

Fig 18.3 Strumming the Lute
(for fracture of a rib)

Fig 18.4 Treasure under the Arm-Pit
(for fracture of a collar bone)

Physiotherapy in Traumatology

Physiotherapy, which itself is a major branch of Chinese medicine, is often employed in traumatological treatments. The concept and practice of physiotherapy is wider in the Chinese medical system than that in the western and many physiotherapy exercises prescribed by Chinese traumatologists may appear unorthodox to a western physiotherapist. These exercises can be conveniently classified into three types, namely for topical treatment, for holistic treatment and those practiced with the help of tools.

Physiotherapy exercises for topical treatment are meant to loosen relevant muscles and tendons, facilitate joint movements, as well as promote better energy and blood flow to the injured area. Unlike in western medicine where physiotherapy is usually applied after the traumatological injury has healed, so as to restore muscular and joint movements, in Chinese medicine it is also employed in the beginning and the middle stages as a remedial process itself.

For example, a patient with a fractured arm may be asked to grip and release his fist regularly as a means to enliven his muscles and tendons as well as to promote energy and blood flow to and from his fractured arm to speed up his recovery.

Like exercises for topical treatment, those for holistic treatment can be applied at the beginning, the middle or the concluding stages of the injury. For example, a patient with internal injury of vital energy, may be taught physiotherapy exercises that stimulate energy flow as a main technique to cure his internal injury right at the beginning stage. Or the exercises may be taught at the middle stage to supplement treatment of appropriate medicinal decoction.

They may also be taught at the concluding stage to harmonize energy flow and balance energy levels, a procedure that is very helpful to a patient whose energy is often depleted and unbalanced due to his injury.

Besides common tools like weights, rollers and poles, the Chinese also use some extraordinary yet simple means to help the patient restore his physiological functions at the start of, during as well as after his recovery. A patient who has weakened his muscles at the elbow may be asked to straighten his arm, then bend his elbow to touch his shoulder with his fingers. He may be asked to repeat this exercise fifty times per session, ten sessions per day. Later he would have to hold some object, like a stone, in his hand and gradually increase the weight of the object as he progresses.

A more unusual exercise is to ask a patient whose fingers have become stiff due to injuries, to pick up peas using different fingers from one side of a table to another, then use the fingers on the other hand to transfer the peas to their original side.

The following diagrams illustrate two physiotherapy exercises taken from "Eighteen Lohan Hands", which are qigong exercises that originated from Bodhidharma at the Shaolin Monastery.

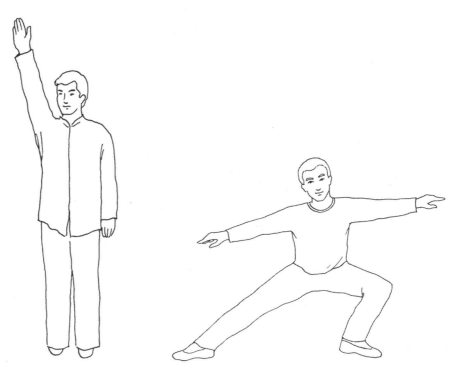

Fig 18.5 Big Windmill   Fig 18.6 Dancing Crane

Repertoire of the Traumatologist

To have a comprehensive picture of the traumatologist's art, the following table summarizes his various techniques described in this and the precious chapters.

(A) Internal Methods.

    1. Beginning Stage:
        (a) Eliminating internal haemorrhage by draining.
        (b) Dispelling internal haemorrhage by activating vital energy.
        (c) Clearing heat and cooling blood.
    2. Middle Stage:
        (a) Harmonizing nutrients and stopping pain.
        (b) Joining bones, muscles and tendons.
        (c) Loosening muscles and cleansing meridians.
    3. Concluding Stage:
        (a) Invigorating energy and nurturing blood.
        (b) Nourishing spleen and stomach.
        (c) Nourishing liver and kidneys.
        (d) Warming and clearing meridians.

(B) External Methods.

    1. External Application of Medicine:
        (a) Stuck on medication.
        (b) Rubbed on medication.
        (c) Steam medication.
        (d) Water medication.
        (e) Ironing medication.

    2. Eight Manipulative Techniques:
        (a) Mo — Palpating.
        (b) Jie — Setting.
        (c) Duan — Replacing.
        (d) Ti — Lifting.
        (e) An — Pressing.
        (f) Mo — Stroking.
        (g) Tui — Pushing.
        (h) Na — Gripping.

3. Physiotherapy Exercises:
    (a) For topical treatment.
    (b) For holistic treatment.
    (c) Practiced with tools.

Examples of Medicinal Recipes

The following are some examples of established medicinal recipes frequently used in Chinese traumatology. The amount of each ingredient is decided by the traumatologist depending on the needs of the patient. The first two examples are meant for internal use, as in internal medicine and the next two are for external applications.

Tou Ren Decoction

Suitability:
  Blood retention in the body, thoracic and abdominal pains, and feverish and agitated conditions.

Ingredients:
  tou ren (Semen Perisae), da huang (Radix et Rhizoma Rhei), mang xiao (Natrii Sulfas), gui zhi (Ramulus Cinnamomi), gan cao (Radix Glycyrr-hizae).

Application:
  Brew for internal consumption.

Activating Meridians Pills

Suitability:
  Clearing internal blood clots, dispersing blood stagnation, dispelling cold in blood circulation, cleansing meridians.

Ingredients:
  tian nan xing (Rhizoma Arisaematis), chuan wu (Radix Aconiti), cao wu (Radix Aconiti Kusnezoffii), di long (Lumbricus), ru xiang (Resina Pistacia), mo yao (Resina Commiphorae Myrrhae).

Application:
  Grind into powder, treat with wine, and make into pills for internal consumption.

Powder for Reducing Swelling

Suitability:
Reduce swelling, stop pain and clear blood clot.

Ingredients:
Huang bo (Cortex Phellodendri), cang shu (Rhizoma Atractylodis), da huang (Radix et Rhizoma Rhei), jiang huang (Rhizoma Curcumae Longae), chen pi (Cortex Citri), xiang fu (Rhizoma Cyperi), hong hua (Flos Carthami) and gan cao (Radix Glycyrr-hizae).

Application:
Grind into powder, mix with wine or honey for external application.

Medicinal Wine for Activating Blood Flow

Suitability:
Activate blood flow, cleanse meridians, clear internal blood clots, loosen muscles and tendons, relieve bruises, sprains and muscular fatigue.

Ingredients:
Ru xiang (Resina Pistacia), mo yao (Resina Commiphorae Myrrhae), hong hua (Flos Carthami), xue jie (Resina Draconis), chuan bei mu (Bulbus Fritillariae Cirhosae), mu xiang (Radix Auckland-iae), hou pu (Cortex Magnoliae Officinalis), chuan wu (Radix Aconiti), cao wu (Radix Aconiti Kusnezoffii), bai zhi (Radix Angelicae Dahuricae), xiang fu (Rhizoma Cyperi), zi ren tong (Pyritum), mu gua (Fructus Chaenomelis), dang gui (Radix Angelicae Sinensis), du huo (Radix Angelicae Pubescentis), xu duan (Radix Dipsaci), hu gu (Os Tigris) and chuan xiong (Rhizoma Ligustici Chuanxiong).

Application:
Soak in white rice wine for external application.

Treating a Traumatological Patient

Let us say you are a traumatologist. Using the four diagnostic methods of viewing, listening and smelling, asking and feeling, you discover your patient has two broken ribs and a fractured shin, but there are no cuts nor wounds.

Luckily his fractured ribs did not damage his heart nor lungs; otherwise, you will have to refer him to a surgeon. From certain signs, like his eyes, breathing and color of his nails, you know that his injuries are not life threatening. But his vital energy is not flowing smoothly and there are internal blood clots at his chest.

Setting the fractured ribs is comparatively easy; if you spread apart the fractured ends properly, they will readily spring back in place. You must feel with your fingers that the ribs and the muscles are in correct alignment. Apply an appropriate medicinal paste on the injured ribs to stop pain, reduce swelling and promote blood circulation; and fasten the stuck-on medication with bandages which will also keep the set ribs in proper alignment.

If the injured shin is swollen, you should not attempt to set the fracture yet. It is important to assure the patient that it is perfectly all right to leave the fractured bone untreated for a few days; in his case, it is definitely better to let the swelling subside first. Apply some stuck-on medicinal paste to reduce pain and swelling and to promote energy and blood flow. Immobilize his injured leg firmly with splints so that he cannot move his fractured bones.

However if the swelling has not developed, you should set the fractured shin immediately. If you have a trained assistant, let him hold the injured leg firmly just below the knee; otherwise, fasten it with ropes and bandages so that the upper part of the fractured shin will not move when you pull the lower part.

Apply some medicinal wine with anaesthetic properties on the injured part. Massage his leg muscles to loosen them. If you are familiar with energy points, press on the relevant points at the thigh and knee to make his lower leg numb. With your fingers, feel the alignment of the shin and muscles. Ask the patient to relax and while holding the lower part of the fractured shin, manipulate it with some preliminary movements.

Then, strongly but gracefully, tract the two ends of the fractured shin apart — against the natural pull of his leg muscles — and with the feel of your fingers and the sight of his foot and leg in line, carefully release your traction so that the two fractured ends come together exactly. You could hear a gentle sound of the two ends joining if they lock into each other properly.

This is the most crucial moment of the bone setting process, representing the climax of the traumatologist's manipulative skills. If this joining is not done properly, there will be some deformity when the bone heals.

Loosen his energy points, especially those you pressed earlier, to promote energy and blood flow. Apply some external medication on the site of injury to reduce swelling, stop pain and promote blood circulation. Then fasten the shin with bandages and splints to immobilize it. You may tie the foot of his injured leg to a weight on pulley to maintain traction, countering the natural pull of his leg muscles.

Every night for about five nights, the patient should be given internal medication to drain away his internal haemorrhage. The Tou Ren Decoction, which will clear the blood clot in his chest and promote energy flow, besides flushing away dead cells at the fractured ribs and shin, is a suitable prescription.

You have to see your patient at least once every two days. Examine his eyes, complexion, breathing, pulse and other features and ask about his appetite, bowel, his reaction to the medication and other pathogenetic conditions. It is quite likely that he will complain of pain and internal movement at the chest, as if some force is cleansing him inside. Tell him that this is an expected reaction as the Tou Ren Decoction clears his internal injury.

Each time you see him, remove the stuck-on medication at his ribs and shin and ensure that the set bones are in order. If there are any misalignments, you must manipulate the bones and muscles to correct it. When everything is in order, apply new medicinal paste to the injuries and fasten them firmly. You also have to apply medicinal powder on his body to prevent sores developing due to lying on bed for a long time.

After about five nightly doses of the Tou Ren Decoction to drain internal haemorrhage, the patient's internal blood clot at the chest will be much relieved. This can be indicated by his facial complexion, pulse and breathing and the patient will say that he no longer feels any pain in his chest.

Then change the decoction to "Harmonizing Energy and Generating Blood Decoction" to activate energy flow.

In about ten days, his internal injuries will be cured and his fractured bones would have started to grow together. You can now remove the weight on his foot. The patient is now onto the middle stage of the treatment. Change the stuck-on medication to herbs with properties of promoting energy and blood flow and generating bone growth.

For internal medication, change to herbs that harmonize physiological functions, like "Harmonizing Nutrients and Activating Energy Powder".

After another ten days, when you find that the newly joined bones are quite strong, introduce some gentle physiotherapy exercises for him to practice while still lying in bed. For example, he can spread open his arms as he breathes in gently and close them again as he breathes out. But should he feel any pain at his ribs, he should stop the exercises. He wrinkles his toes and move his ankle, but without moving his shin, as many times as he can every day. He has to exercise both legs, one leg at a time.

For internal medication he takes "Decoction for the Rejoining of New Injuries" for about five days, then "Pills for the Rejoining Muscles and Tendons" for the following five days. Now you see him once about every five days, instead of every alternate day.

About two months after the first day of treatment, you may proceed to the concluding stage. By now his bones have grown together quite strongly. But all this while you continue to examine his ribs and shin, check their alignment, apply appropriate external medication and immobilize them. Now you can remove the splints, but continue to bandage his shin, together with the stuck-on medicinal paste which facilitates blood and bone growth.

Tie the foot of his injured leg so that the free end of the rope, going through a pulley, drops just in front of the patient. By pulling the rope, he can bend his knee. He exercises his leg in this way as often as he can, but it must be at least a total of 500 times a day. He must exercise the other leg, without the aid of a pulley, as often as he can too. Also prescribe other physiotherapy exercises for other parts of his body.

His ribs should be recovered by now. Instead of stuck-on paste, apply rub-on medicinal oil on his chest to promote energy and blood flow. Continue to apply stuck-on medicinal paste, with properties to strengthen bones, on his shin for another ten days, after which stop bandaging the shin and apply medicinal wine on both the injured and the free leg to promote energy and blood flow. For internal medication, take herbs that invigorate energy and nurture blood, like "Eight Precious Herbs Decoction".

When the legs are quite strong, about three months since his first treatment, ask him to stand at the edge of the bed. Make sure that he stands on both legs. He probably needs a lot of prodding and encouragement. With his hands on the bed for support, ask him to bend his knees and squat. Practice this exercise everyday as often as he comfortably can.

After a few days, ask him to walk round his bed, at first only once, but gradually increase the number of times. A few days later the patient will walk away from the sick-bed, back to normal life.

Throughout the period of treatment, you must be ready to change or modify your medication according to the conditions of the patient. For example, if you find his appetite poor, you may add "deputy" herbs that enhance his spleen and stomach; or if he becomes infected, you should add herbs with antibiotic properties to "cool" his blood.

The difference between how western and Chinese medicine treat traumatological injury is glaring. With the great advantage of modern high technology, western medicine is in a favorable position to improve the art and science of treating injuries for all humanity if western medical scientists are ready to adopt some of the useful principles and methods of Chinese traumatology.

It is also interesting to note how ingenuously the Chinese overcome their lack of scientific instrumentation in traumatology as well as other branches of Chinese medicine. Acupuncture is a striking example. Without x-ray, radioactive tracers, kidney-dialysis, laser beams, computerized topography and not even drugs, the Chinese use only needles to cure all types of diseases! We will look at this extraordinary branch of Chinese medicine in the next chapter.

19

THE MAGICAL NEEDLE OF CHINESE MEDICINE

(Introduction to Acupuncture)

Perhaps the most tangible impact of the new developments are the emergence of a new breed of physicians who are uncomfortable with the notion that medicine can be practiced out of a little black bag.

Prof. Norman Cousins (1987)

Ancient Wisdom in Acupuncture

What some Chinese physicians take out from their little black bag when they attend to their patients, are not a stethoscope, drugs and typical articles of trade of a western doctor, but a set of needles! What are these needles for? To treat their patients; they are acupuncturists.

Treating a patient by inserting needles into him is astonishing enough. But the most astonishing is that acupuncture is a self-contained medical system: using needles and nothing else, an acupuncturist can treat almost any disease! Moreover it is one of the oldest Chinese therapeutic methods. Acupuncture has been being successfully practiced in Chinese societies since pre-historic times!

Hence, acupuncturists (as well as other specialists in Chinese medicine), do not use sophisticated instruments of high technology not because these instruments are expensive and complicated, but because simple tools like needles have served their needs effectively for millennia.

Of course sophisticated instruments, despite their cost and complication, serve very useful purposes. No one seriously suggests that we should discard them. But problems arise when we become over-dependent on them, when we seem to reverse the role that they are tools and we are masters. Situations may sometimes become not only hilarious but limiting.

For example, even though people have been carrying on their normal lives without any medical complaints for years, some doctors still insist that they are sick, just because sophisticated instruments say that the measurements of some of their bodily conditions (like blood pressure and cholesterol) are above threshold levels.

On the other hand, despite overwhelming evidence to show the effectiveness of certain therapeutic methods, some doctors conveniently discard, even mock at, these methods as unscientific or superstitions, just because their instruments fail to measure variables imposed by them, sometimes irrespective of whether these variables are relevant, or worse still, because these methods are based on a paradigm different from theirs.

Our instruments have become so sophisticated and expensive, that we, often unwittingly, regard them as all-powerful and all-knowing, that we simply cannot accept the possibility (or reality) that our instruments may not be so powerful or knowing after all, that many of the things propounded by ancient wisdom do not show objectively on our instruments or in our paradigm because we are not sufficiently knowledgeable to understand this wisdom.

We frequently forget that ancient wisdom is accumulated over three millennia, whereas modern science actually has a history of less than three centuries. A small part of this ancient wisdom is found in acupuncture.

Some Startling Modern Accomplishments

If we wish to understand acupuncture properly and hopefully learn some useful lessons from it to enrich our own medical system, the first thing is to be open-minded, that is, we must realize that there are other ways of viewing health and medicine besides the western perspective and that it is futile forcing western medical principles and practices into acupuncture.

Perhaps we may feel more assured if we remember that the effectiveness of acupuncture as a therapeutic approach is beyond doubt, or else it would not have survived more than 30 centuries, practiced by societies who had reached very high levels of civilization! Archaeological findings, including a great deal of stone needles, show that acupuncture was already used in China during the stone age.

But you would be mistaken to think it is primitive, or whatever progress to be made in acupuncture has already been made. There has been continuous development in the long history of acupuncture. For example, regarding the number of energy points or acupuncture points, only 160 were known 2000 years ago, 354 about 1000 years ago and more than 1700 now.

Modern acupuncturists have discovered a whole range of important acupuncture points on the outer ear that are linked by the meridian network to all parts of the body.

Chinese researchers, using western research methods and instruments, have discovered some startling facts. For example, the amount of white cells in a person's blood can be influenced by acupuncture.

By manipulating the acupuncture points of hegu (Li 4), dazhui (Gv 14) and zusanli (S 36), a person's white blood cells could be increased by as much as 94.7%; whereas by manipulating taixi (K 3) and allowing the needle to stay in that acupuncture point for ten minutes, the white cells could be reduced by 44.2%!

Acupuncture treatment can increase our defence system against microbes. In an experiment, the microbe count in a dysentery patient before acupuncture treatment was 434; after treatment it dropped to 235, indicating that his defence ability increased by 83.8%.

Acupuncture can even be applied for birth control. Researching into the validity of an acupuncture classic that says "Applying acupuncture or moxibustion on the shimen (Cv 5) vital point of a woman will cause her to be sterile", acupuncturists did that to 127 fertile women and discovered the success of this birth control method was 79%.

On the other hand, by manipulating energy points like guanyuan (Cv 4), zhongji (Cv 3) and sanyinjiao (Sp 6), women who had stopped menstruation prematurely, had their regular menstruation and fertility recovered.

In another experiment on 160 men whose sperm count was low, by applying acupuncture on points like qugu (Cv 2) and sanyin-jiao (Sp 6), and moxibustion on guanyuan (Cv4) and mingmen (Gv 4), 98.95 of them had their sperm count increased tremendously; 71.85 of them later fathered children.

This experiment, however, was not conclusive because most of the men also took Chinese herbs.

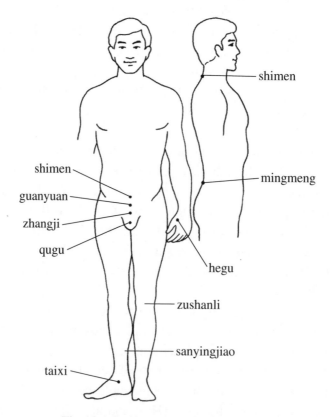

Fig 19.1 Relevant Energy Points (1)

If you are bewildered, as most readers would, by the names of the energy points whose translation into romanized Chinese renders them into strange, meaningless sounds, their international symbols in English, given in brackets behind their names, will be useful. The letters indicate the meridians and the numbers their positions on their respective meridians.

For example the symbol for hegu is Li 4, meaning that it is the 4th point along the flow of the large intestine (colon) meridian. Gv 14 for dazhui means that it is the 14th point along the governing meridian.

The international symbols in French and German for hegu and dazhui are GI 4, DI 4 and VG 13 (not 14), LG 14 respectively.

There are hundreds of energy points, too many to be shown in this book, but they are readily found in most acupuncture books. Those that are mentioned in this and the next chapter are illustrated in the accompanying diagrams.

Although the international symbols are convenient, unfortunately the meaning and poetry of the energy points are inevitably lost. All the energy points are meaningfully and poetically named. Hegu, for example, means "meeting at the valley", which poetically indicates both its location and its significance. It is located between the bones of the thumb and the index finger, described as a valley and is the meeting point of the streams of energy from the lung meridian and the colon meridian. Dazhui means "big vertebra". It is located below the seventh cervical vertebra, which is a big vertebra in the spinal column.

In 1958 the world was greatly surprised when Chinese acupuncturists successfully used acupuncture as anaesthesia in major surgical operations. The most amazing aspect was that the patients, while under anaesthesia, were perfectly conscious and could cooperate with the surgeons, all their internal organs functioned normally, their immune and defence systems were enhanced and their recovery was faster!

This and other outstanding medical breakthroughs in acupuncture will certainly bring much benefit to world medicine. There were, nevertheless, three setbacks in acupuncture anaesthesia, namely the anaesthetic effects was sometimes not thorough, some patients showed strong reaction when their internal organs were handled and the patients' muscles were not sufficiently relaxed in abdominal operations.

Overcoming these setbacks should not be the exclusive privilege nor responsibility of the Chinese. Western medical scientists, with their advanced technology, can contribute much towards this goal. An understanding of acupuncture is of course a prerequisite. Acupuncture is an extensive discipline; this chapter and the next are necessarily only a brief introduction.

How Does Acupuncture Work?

Acupuncture seems irrational only if we see it from the viewpoint of western medical philosophy; if we see it from the Chinese medical viewpoint, which is a logical thing to do as acupuncture was mainly developed and practiced by the Chinese who made no pretensions to western medical concepts, it becomes sensible and meaningful. The central idea of acupuncture is the meridian system. If you are still not clear about the meridian system, please refer to Chapters 8 and 9 . The meridian system is responsible for the circulation of vital energy and for harmonizing yin-yang. Man is able to live healthily, and to adjust himself to the ever changing environment internally and externally because the meridian system is functioning normally.

Man is constantly involved in these two dimensions of life-sustaining activities: he must maintain a meaningful exchange of energy for all his physiological and psychological functions (like transporting nutrients to and toxic waste from his cells and regulating a continuous exchange of mental impulses between every part of his body); and he must react effectively to a perpetual interference of endogenous and exogenous pathogenic agents (like grief and anxiety, microbes and changing climatic conditions).

If interruption to energy flow or disharmony of yin-yang is slight, or for a short time, the body is able to bear it, though it may not be functioning at tip-top conditions. This situation applies to most people, who, for example, may have organs working at partial abilities and become stressful even over simple everyday problems.

If the interruption or disharmony is severe or prolonged, owing to the failure of their meridian function, sicknesses will surface. The failure of particular meridians is manifested in pathogenetic conditions which can be transmitted to the body surface and manifested as pathogenetic symptoms.

The purpose of acupuncture is to diagnose the cause of the sickness, define the meridians where energy is interrupted or yin-yang is disharmonious and by means of manipulating appropriate energy points with acupuncture needles, reinvigorate its natural energy flow and harmonize yin-yang, thereby restoring the patient to health.

For example, if a hypertension patient consults an acupuncturist, after careful diagnosis, the physician will discover that the sickness was caused by rising yang energy from the liver due to deficient yin energy of the kidneys. By manipulating the appropriate energy points, the acupuncturist reestablishes smooth energy flow and harmonize yin-yang, lowering the yang liver energy and replenishing the yin kidney energy, thus restoring the patient to health.

It is interesting to note the difference of approach between the Chinese and the west in their treatment of hypertension. The Chinese do not treat the high pressure at the blood vessels, which they regard as a symptom; they treat the root cause at the liver and the kidneys. Western medical scientists who are still puzzled why hypertension happens, will certainly benefit by testing the Chinese premise.

If "heat-evil" (which corresponds to microbes in western terminology) is retained in the lungs and the meridian system fails to provide sufficient defence-energy to overcome the heat-evil, this pathogenetic condition is figuratively described as excessive heat, which is expressed as excessive yang, in relation to the yin body defence. The job of the physician is to restore this yin-yang imbalance by dispelling heat.

This can be accomplished in acupuncture by manipulating certain energy points to "cleanse" away the heat. (In western terms, the enhanced body defence that results from manipulation of certain acupuncture points, overcomes the microbes, therefore "dispelling heat".) Again the difference of approach between the Chinese and the west is striking. The Chinese physician does not classify heat-evil into various types (or in western terms, he is not concerned with the exact type of microbes that attacked the lungs); his main concern is to clear the heat-evil, whatever its name western bacteriologists may call it.

This of course does not imply that study of microbes is not useful; but it is not necessary in this case.

Diagnostic Methods in Acupuncture

Besides the four diagnostic methods used by all Chinese physicians, the acupuncturist has a wide range of additional diagnostic techniques related to the meridians. As the normal functioning of meridians is responsible for health, symptoms of particular diseases due to failure in certain meridians can be readily found in those meridians. The following are some of these techniques.

Because of their particular functions, energy points are of various kinds. The "shu" and the "mu" energy points, found at the back and the front of the body respective, are where the energy of the respective internal organs are focused.

For example the energy of the lungs and of the kidneys is focused at their shu energy points, known respectively as feishu (B 13) and shen-shu (B 23); and that of the triple warmer and of the intestine at their mu energy points, known respectively as shimen (Cv 5) and guanyuan (Cv 4). These shu and mu energy points can be used in diagnosis.

If a person feel "sour" and painful when his feishu (B 13) is touched, it indicates that his lung system is not functioning properly. If he feels "sour" and painful when his guanyuan (Cv 4) is pressed, there is disorder at his urinary or sex organs.

From years of experience, masters have recorded that certain illnesses can be indicated by a feeling of tenderness at certain energy points. For example, tenderness at zhongdu (Liv 6) and at the liver-section of the outer ear indicates an infectious disease at the liver; tenderness at liangqiu (S 34) and zusanli (S 36) indicates stomach disorder; tenderness at zusanli (S 36), yinlingquan (Sp 9) and diji (Sp 8) indicates ailments at the intestine or colon.

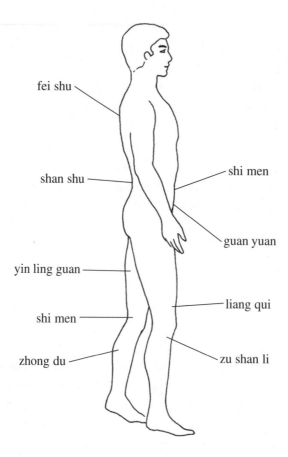

Fig 19.2 Some Relevant Energy Points (2)

While the human body is regarded as a microcosm of the universe (because the flow of vital energy in the body is a miniature of the flow of cosmic energy of the universe), various parts of the body like the palm, the ear and the foot, are microcosms of the body. Different parts of a palm, for example, reflect different parts of the body. In other words, by pressing a certain part of our palm, we can affect its corresponding part in our body. Fig 19.3 shows this correspondence on the palm.

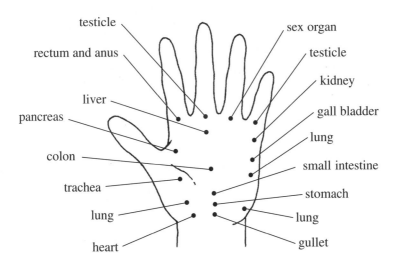

Fig 19.3 Correspondence of Internal Organs on Palm

By stroking his palm or thumb systematically on the patient's palm, the physician may have an idea of the conditions of the patient's internal organs. The type of response also indicates the type of disorder, such as "feeling of swelling and pain" indicates inflammation and feverish conditions, "sour, numb sensation" indicate chronic illnesses, and "numb feeling" indicate obstinate diseases. For example, if your friend feels sour when you press at the base of his index finger, it suggests that he may have piles, prolapse of the rectum, or any chronic ailment at the anus.

Among the many energy points along a meridian, the point from where arises the source of energy for that particular meridian, is called the "jing" (meaning "well" or "spring") energy point of that meridian. The jing energy points of the twelve primary meridians are sometimes employed in diagnosis. As primary meridians are in pairs, there are two jing energy points for each pair of meridians.

Place a lighted joss-stick (or lighted match-stick, heated metal piece or any suitable tool) close to a jing energy point and note the time in seconds the patient feels the heat or any particular sensation like an ant-bite or needle-prick. Then place the joss-stick close to the other jing energy point. Repeat this procedure with the remaining meridians. Calculate the average time of reaction.

The jing energy points with less than half the average time for its reaction, indicates "solid" illness at that meridian; more than twice the average time indicates "empty" illness. (A solid illness is one where the cause is easily discernible, like a structural defect or a bacterial attack; in an empty illness the cause is not obvious, like a functional disorder or some hormonal imbalance.)

When the two jing energy points of the same meridian show discrepancy in their reaction, it indicates that illness is present at that meridian.

Another diagnostic method is to move a finger along meridians. Certain illnesses are manifest themselfs as a lump of congested energy near particular energy points. For example, patients with migraine may have a lump the shape of a pea near the fengchi (G 20) and the tianzhu (B 10) energy points; those with infection in the lungs may have a lump like an olive seed at the feire energy point (newly found, at third throcic vertebra at back); and those with chronic liver inflammation may have rod-like lump near ganshu (B 18) and ganre (newly found, at fifth thoraric vertebra).

So if you happen to find a lump beneath your skin, do not start worrying, it is not necessarily cancer; even if it were, it could be cured!

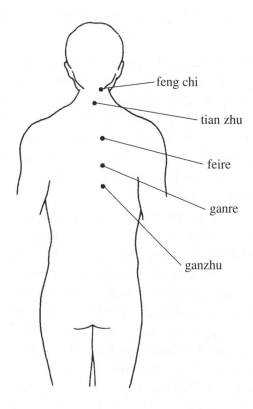

feng chi

tian zhu

feire

ganre

ganzhu

Fig 19.4 Relevant Energy Points (3)

Therapeutic Functions of Energy Points

A herbalist cures his patients by prescribing suitable herbs (including all types of materia medica) for them to take in orally. Inside their bodies, these herbs are transformed into healing energies to be transported by their meridian systems to affected parts of the body to "eliminate evil" (that is, eliminate pathogenetic agents like stress and microbes) and "restore good" (that is enhancing the natural self-curative and regenerative functions of the body).

The acupuncturist accomplishes the same goal using needles. By inserting needles into selected energy points and manipulating them in certain ways, he generates healing energies to eliminate evil and restore good.

Which energy points should he select for particular diseases? Just as the herbalist benefits from the experience of past masters who have left behind a rich legacy of herbs and their healing properties, the acupuncturist also benefits from a wealth of knowledge concerning energy points and their therapeutic functions.

There are hundreds of energy points that the acupuncturist can use for treatment. To help him remember them, they are classified in many ways, such as according to their meridians, according to their location at different parts of the body and according to the syndromes or diseases which they are effective for. Space constraint, obviously, permits us to examine only some of these points briefly as examples; interested readers will have to refer to suitable acupuncture books for detailed study.

For the convenience of modern users, in the description below names of diseases are often given in modern (instead of traditional) terms, which are mostly borrowed from the west. Instead of acupuncture, the physician may use moxibustion, which is burning moxa leaves or other medicinal material in the form of cones or sticks over selected energy points.

Baihui

Meaning:
Meeting of hundred meridians.
International symbol: Gv 20.

Classical note:
Situated at the crown of the head where all meridians meet.

Meridian:
Du mai, or governing meridian; meeting point of governing meridian with all the six yang meridians, namely meridians of the colon, stomach, intestine, urinary bladder, triple warmer and gall bladder.

Other names:
Sanyang, wuhui, tianman, niyuangong.
Main therapeutic functions: headaches, dizziness, prolapse of the rectum, hypertension, insomnia, sound in the ear, energy collapse, paralysis, unconsciousness and mental disorders.

Application:
Slant insertion forward or backward for about 1 to 3 cm; local tension discernible; moxibustion 5 to 7 cones; caution for children and those with fluid retention in the head.
(As early as the time of the Nei Jing, it has been stressed that acupuncture must *not* touch the brain and the spinal cord.)

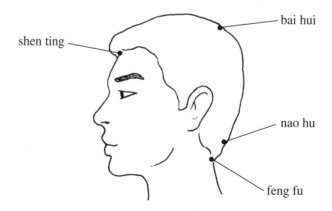

Fig 19.5 Location of Baihui

Zhongwan

Meaning:
  Middle of the stomach.

International symbol:
  Cv 12.

Classical note:
  Commander of the spleen and stomach, controlling the flow of nutrient energy.

Meridian:
  Ren mai, or conceptual meridian; mu energy point for stomach energy.

Other Names:
  Weimu, weiwan, taichang, zhongguan.
  Main therapeutic functions: All acute and chronic gastrointestinal disorders, like prolapse of the stomach, gastritis, indigestion, vomiting, abdominal flatulence, diarrhoea, constipation and acute colic congestion, as well as hypertension and nervous disorders.

Application:
  Direct or slant insertion for about 3 cm; local sensation of swelling or bowel movements; moxibustion 5 to 10 cones.

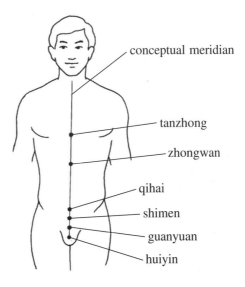

Fig 19.6 Location of Zhongwan

Neiguan

Meaning:
Inner conjunction.

International symbol:
P 6.

Classical note:
It is linked to the heart and pericardium and to the pathway of blood flow.

Meridian:
Pericardium meridian; junction-point that links with the conceptual meridian and the yin wei (or in-protective) meridian through collaterals.

Other names:
Shouwan.

Main therapeutic functions:
Cardiovascular diseases, heart pains, palpitations, gastritis, abdominal pains, vomiting, migraine, fever, malaria, rheumatic pains at shoulders and elbows, asthma, chest disorders, depression, hysteria and mental derangement.

Application:
Direct insertion between 1 and 6 cm (through to the waiguan at the other side); feeling of electric impulses at local site, fingers, elbow, armpit and chest; moxibustion 5 to 7 cones.

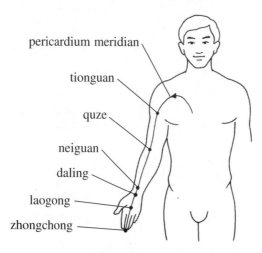

pericardium meridian

tionguan

quze

neiguan

daling

laogong

zhongchong

Fig 19.7 Location of Neiguan

Sanyinjiao

Meaning:
Meeting-point of three yin meridians.

International symbol:
Sp 6.

Classical note:
This is where the taiyin, xueyin and shaoyin of the leg meet.

Meridian:
Spleen meridian; meeting-point of the spleen, liver and kidney meridians.

Other names:
Taiyin, dayin, xiasanli, chengming.

Therapeutic functions:
Disorders of the gastro-intestinal system, disorders of the urino-genital system, female hormonal imbalance, numbness and rheumatic pains of the lower limbs, measles and urticaria.

Application:
Direct insertion between about 3 to 6 cm; "sour" sensation at site, sole, calf and knee; moxibustion 3 to 6 cones; must **not** apply on pregnant women, as it may lead to miscarriage.

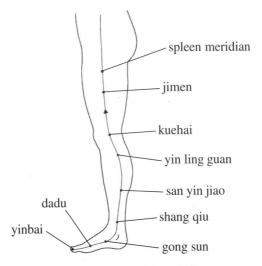

spleen meridian

jimen

kuehai

yin ling guan

san yin jiao

dadu

shang qiu

yinbai

gong sun

Fig 19.8 Location of Sanyinjiao

Theory of Healing

Some readers may be surprised at some of the above information. How can manipulating the same energy point, for instance, cure diagonally opposite diseases like diarrhoea and constipation? How can the acupuncturist cure such infectious diseases like measles and malaria without the use of antibiotics or even any medicine?

While these are pertinent questions in western medicine, they become irrelevant in the Chinese system, because the Chinese uses a different paradigm. It is like asking how one could speak Chinese if he does not know singular and plural nouns or past simple tense and present continuous tense — which is actually the case in Chinese!

The same energy points can be used to cure diagonally opposite diseases, as well as other greatly varied diseases, because of different ways of manipulating the inserted needle. Manipulation of energy points and other important aspects of acupuncture will be explained in the next chapter.

If we are to oversimplify the operation so as to illustrate the underlying principle better, we can say that in treating diarrhoea we manipulate the zhongwan (Cv 12) energy point to reduce stomach energy, whereas we manipulate the same point to increase stomach energy in treating constipation. Here, the energy point is the same, but the manipulation is different. You will read something more fantastic in a later chapter on qigong, where exactly the same therapeutic exercise is used to cure diagonally opposite diseases!

An acupuncturist is able to cure infectious diseases without using antibiotics or even without using any materia medica, because he restores the healthy internal environment and natural curative functions of the patient to overcome the infection himself.

Many of us are so used to current western medical thinking, especially treatment by chemotherapy, that we often forget we ourselves can overcome hostile microbes many, many times more efficiently than the best medicine man has ever produced. We are in fact doing exactly this every day of our lives, overcoming billions of microscopic pathogens that otherwise may cause disorders ranging from the common cold to the most deadly diseases perhaps still unknown to man.

What actually happens to the microscopic pathogens when an acupuncturist or any other Chinese physician re-establishes harmonious energy flow or yin-yang balance in the patient? The Chinese do not have advance instruments like radioactive tracers or microscopic camera to show objectively the exact situation at the cellular level inside the patient's body.

Nevertheless, some speculations can be offered. These speculations are not wild guesses, but are based on principles and practices that have been proven correct over many centuries — speculations that may provide us with inspiration and ideas for some unexpected breakthroughs in the search for solutions to overcome many of the medical problems presently afflicting western societies.

The hostile microbes were probably killed by the patient's natural defence system, which has been enhanced by acupuncture treatment and are flushed out of the patient's body in natural ways like sweating, breathing out, excretion and urination. Or they are kept in check in some manners that they cannot cause harm to the host. Why, then, were they not killed or kept in check in the first place?

There are four sensible possibilities. One, this defence-energy is prevented by blockage from flowing to the site of microbe attack. The causes of blockage can be many and varied, such as negative energies due to negative emotions or stress, or "climatic" conditions like heat and dampness that are unfavorable to the flow of defence-energy.

We must remember that at the subatomic scale, the quanta of negative energy in the form of sub-atomic particles (as explained by Max Plank's discovery of quanta), and the subatomic particles of the molecules that cause heat or dampness are formidable physical obstacles to defence-energy flow. The acupuncturist's needle stimulates and marshals defence-energy from other parts of the body, so that with increased amount and momentum, it can break through the blockage to the disease site and overcome the hostile microbes.

Two, there may not be a formidable blockage, but the microbes are concentrated in particular areas. This pathogenetic condition can be due to taking in contaminated food leading to microbe concentration at the gastrointestinal system, breathing in pestilent air leading to microbe concentration in the respiratory system, or suffering from a septic wound leading to microbe concentration at the circulatory system. Because of their concentration, the microbes collectively become too potent for the local defence-energy to handle, thus resulting in an infection.

By manipulating relevant energy points to promote energy flow, the acupuncturist spread the microbes over a wider area, thereby thinning their virulence. In this way the patient's natural systems can overcome the otherwise hostile microbes, killing them, holding them as prisoners, tricking them into doing useful work, or handling them in ways still unknown to us.

Thirdly, there may be a temporary breakdown in the patient's feed-back or "intelligence" system, with the result that other essential systems like the immune system and the defence system do not operate as they should because they are not fed the right information. Hence, the microbes which could be easily kept under control in normal, healthy conditions, now become hostile and have a gala time.

The breakdown of the patient's intelligence system may be caused by stress, which figuratively or subatomically hardens the meridians (or nerves, in western terminology), along which information-energy (or electrochemical impulses) flows, or blocked by toxic wastes which may be in a gaseous state and which the body failed to dispose off efficiently. By manipulating the right energy points, the acupuncturist stimulates vital energy flow (in the form of bio-electric current), loosening the "hardened" meridian and clearing the blockage, thereby restoring the patient's intelligence system and health.

The fourth possibility is that the patient is weak, or temporarily weakened sufficiently for microbes to attack. The hostile microbes may have been in the patient's body all the time, or they may have just entered his body. The temporary weakening may be caused by negative emotions or stress, or drastic change of environmental or climatic conditions. It may also be caused by the consumption of certain kinds food that upsets the normal chemical balance of the body.

By manipulating suitable energy points, the acupuncturist corrects this abnormal condition of the patient. He may open up the flow of reserved energy from the secondary meridians; strengthen the functions of the spleen and the stomach, or the liver and the kidneys for increased production of energy and blood; or activates various energy fields (which correspond to endocrine glands in western terminology) to produce the necessary energies (or hormones) to meet exigencies. As the patient is strengthened he is able to overcome the hostile microbes.

The above description provides a theoretical framework to explain how acupuncture as well as other branches of Chinese medicine cure patients of not only infectious but also all other types of diseases. The two fundamental principles of invigorating energy flow and harmonizing yin-yang operate in all cases.

20

MANIPULATING ENERGY FLOW

(Principles and Methods of Acupuncture)

How does it (acupuncture) work? It is fair to say that nobody knows — at least not in terms that can be understood by us in the West. But work it certainly does.

Dr Andrew Stanway.

Hurricane Inside Our Body

Some of us may doubt the ability of flowing energy in our body to relieve illnesses, and wonder how it can accomplish this task, if it ever does. To extend the concept of man as a microcosm of the universe, let us compare man's illnesses with disasters in nature, such as hurricanes, droughts or gigantic fires. Indeed at the cellular level inside our body, our diseases are like these disasters to our body cells, and Chinese physicians figuratively describe such comparable micro-disasters as wind-evil, dryness-evil and fire-evil respectively.

The causes of the macro-disasters could be intrinsic such as imbalance of air pressure and tectonic movements, or extrinsic such as large-scale pollution or warfare. Similarly, the causes of the micro-disasters in our body could be endogenous like psychological disorders and physiological malfunctions, or exogenous like toxification and microbe attacks. Let us look at two hypothetical approaches in meeting the disasters.

First we quantify the damage and identify the trouble-makers. Then we rectify the damage topically. Often we are helpless when the causes are overwhelming or not clear, like a hurricane caused by difference of air pressure, or a gigantic fire where the arsonists are unknown. But if we know who the trouble-makers are, we are usually good at shooting them, though we often kill our own men in the process.

Another approach is to focus on the recovery, without bothering who exactly the trouble-makers are nor measuring objectively the rate of damage. By adjusting the air pressure, the hurricane is overcome; by moisturizing the air the drought is relieved; and by bringing rain or letting forth a torrent of mountain stream, the fire is put out. We can do all these things at the cellular level using acupuncture.

This analogy may be far-fetched, but it suggests a picture of what the operation of acupuncture is like to microscopic creatures in the patient's body. It also illustrates that just as we ourselves can be helpless against the power of moving air, at the cellular scale where a microbe's life span is only a few seconds, and whose size is so small that literally millions of them can fill this full stop, will have no match against the manipulation of energy flow by a skillful acupuncturist.

Principles of Energy Point Selection

As in all other branches of Chinese medicine, after applying the four diagnostic methods and other additional techniques to find out the symptoms, and the eight diagnostic principles to generalize the syndromes, the acupuncturist classifies the disease according to the patient's pathogenetic conditions. Then he works out a strategy for treatment. He does not merely apply certain energy points to treat diseases that these points are said to be effective for, as may be done by amateurish healers and which may sometimes even result in spectacular cures!

A professional acupuncturist treats his patients holistically, aiming at restoring health rather than just relieving symptoms. Like a herbalist who combines different herbs, he combines different energy points to achieve maximum effects, and he is guided by the following three principles, namely the principles of same meridians, of different meridians, and of opposites.

In the "principle of same meridians", the acupuncturist selects energy points along the meridians where the illness is located. This is obvious, and most basic. If the kidney meridian is lacking in vital energy, for instance, the acupuncturist manipulates the kidney meridian to increase the energy there. If there is dampness in the small intestine meridian, he manipulates this meridian to clear the dampness. There are two approaches in this principle: local selection, and distant selection.

In local selection, the acupuncturist chooses energy points that are located at the site of the illness, or in the case of illnesses concerning internal organs, at the corresponding surface area of those organs. For example, to treat a nose problem, yingxiang (Li 20), which is the energy point found at the base of the nose, and which has branch-meridians flowing to the nose, is selected. To treat stomach pains, zhongwan (Cv 12), which is the energy point directly above the stomach, and where the stomach energy is focused, is chosen.

Note that although the nose is under the lung system, the branch-meridians where the nose problem is located come from yingxiang (Li 20) which lies on the colon meridian. Similarly, zhongwan (Cv 12), which is on the conceptual meridian, is used to treat stomach pains instead of other points on the stomach meridian, because its energy flows directly into the stomach.

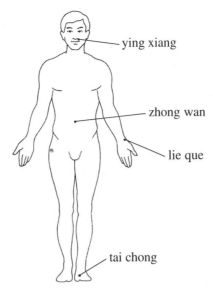

Fig 20.1 Relevant Energy Points (4)

In distant selection, energy points that are far away from the site of disease, but along the same meridian, are selected. For example, to treat cough due to disorder of the lung meridian, lieque (L 7) which is located at the wrist on the lung meridian is selected; to treat headaches caused by hypertension, taichong (Liv 3) which is located above the second toe along the liver meridian is selected. But why do we select lieque (L 7) and taichong (Liv 3), and not other energy points on the same meridians which are also distant from the disease sites?

This is because lieque (L 7) is a luo-xue, or "junction energy point", where a branch-meridian joins the lung meridian to the colon meridian. When this junction is opened by manipulating it, the "fire-evil" (such as microbes) that causes the cough at the lungs, will be killed or inhibited and carried along by increased energy flow generated by manipulating other energy points in suitable combination, can be drained into the colon meridian, and consequently to the colon to be flushed out of the body. Manipulating other points wrongly may aggravate instead of relieving the lung disorder.

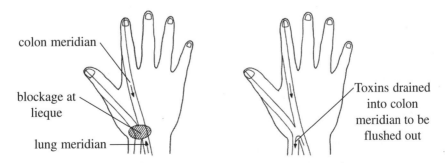

Fig 20.2 Opening the Gate to Flush out the Evil
(Diagrammatic)

Taichong (Liv 3) on the liver meridian is selected because it is a yuan-xue, or "source energy point", where the source of the energy flowing in the liver meridian is located. But why choose the liver meridian? Because rising liver energy causes hypertension which in turn causes headaches. Suppose a factory is over-supplied with electric power, and is becoming risky.

To reduce its power (either its amount or its voltage), you need not go to the factory; you do it at the power station which is usually distant from the factory. Taichong (Liv 3) is the power station regulating energy to the liver meridian.

This "distant selection principle" explains why needles inserted at the knees and elbows are able to provide anaesthesia for abdominal operations, as they are connected by the same meridians. Because of space limitation, it is not feasible to explain below every principle involved in choosing energy points. Only brief comments are given for some examples.

Far From the Disease Site

In the "principle of different meridians", the acupuncturist inserts needles into energy points along meridians that are not directly afflicted with the illness. There are many approaches in this principle: "same side", "both sides", "all around", "near", "far", "corresponding", "meeting-point", "external-internal" and "connecting-meridians".

In the "same side approach", the acupuncturist chooses energy points on different meridians but on the same side as the disease. For example, if a patient complains of toothaches on his right side, the acupuncturist may choose jiache (S 6) of the stomach meridian, and hegu (Li 4) of the colon meridian on the same right side. Jiache (S 6) is a crucial point at the jaw, with branch-meridians to the teeth. Hegu (Li 4), which is located at the outer palm, is an important energy point for stopping pain, and the one end of its colon meridian is linked to the mouth.

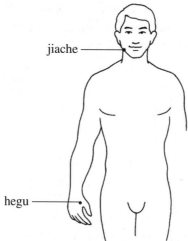

jiache

hegu

Fig 20.3 Relevant Energy Points (5)

In the "both sides approach", energy points on different meridians on both sides are selected. For example, to treat coughs with a lot of phlegm, besides choosing lieque (L 7) and taiyuan (L 9) on the affected lung meridian, the acupuncturist may also choose on both sides hegu (Li 4) on the colon meridian, and fenglong (S 40) on the stomach meridian. Taiyuan (L 9), meaning "big and deep", is the power station for the lung meridian; fenglong (S 40), meaning "abundance with nutrient energy", is the junction linking the stomach and the spleen meridians.

The acupuncturist may manipulate energy points all around the disease site, as in the "all around approach". For example, to treat an eye complaint, he selects jingming (B 1), tongziliao (G 1), sibai (S 2), cuanzhu (B 2) and sizhukong (T 23), which are all around the eye but on different meridians. Although the eye belongs to the liver system, energy points on other meridians are chosen because their branch-meridians directly affect the eye.

In the "near approach" and the "far approach", the acupuncturist chooses from different meridians energy points which are near or far away from the disease site respectively. For example, in treating cold and fever, which is mainly an illness of the lung meridian, two major energy points among others the acupuncturists inserts his needle into, are dazhui (Gv 14), on the governing meridian near the lungs, and hegu (Li 4), on the colon meridian near the base of the thumb.

In the "corresponding approach", the acupuncturist selects shu or mu energy points of the zang and fu organs (the viscera), or the corresponding major energy points of other organs. The interesting fact is that these shu and mu energy points, where the energy of the organs is focused, are not located on the meridians of the respective organs. The shu energy points are found along the urinary bladder meridian, and the mu energy points are found mainly along the conceptual meridian.

To treat a disease of the spleen, for example, the acupuncturist may manipulate the corresponding shu energy point for the spleen, which is pishu (B 20).

To treat the tongue (which does not have a shu or a mu energy point because it is not a zang or fu organ), he may manipulate its corresponding major energy point where the tongue energy is focused, and this point is known as fengfu (Gv 16), and is situated along the governing meridian.

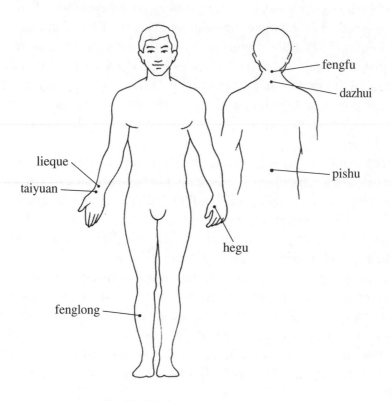

Fig 20.4 Relevant Energy Points (6)

There are some energy points, known as "jiaohui-xue" or "meeting-points", where two or more meridians meet. They are particularly important for the six of the eight secondary meridians, other than the conceptual and governing meridian, because these six secondary meridians do not have energy points for their own.

Sanyinjiao (Sp 6), which is a meeting point of the spleen, kidney and liver meridians, is a very important acupuncture point and is frequently used in the "meeting-point approach" to treat many different diseases.

In the "external-internal approach", the acupuncturist chooses the yin or yang part of the affected meridian. For example, if the disease is located at the stomach, instead of selecting energy points on the stomach meridian for manipulation, he selects points on the spleen meridian, which has much influence over the stomach energy, and which is the yin or internal counterpart of the stomach meridian.

Or, if the illness is found at the heart meridian, instead of manipulating energy points on this meridian, which may cause repercussions to the heart, he chooses points on the small intestine meridian, which is the yang or external counterpart of the heart meridian.

When disease occurs in a particular meridian, the acupuncturist may treat the preceding or the subsequent meridians using the "connecting-meridians approach". For example, if there is insufficient energy in the liver meridian, he may manipulate energy points at the preceding gall bladder meridian to channel more energy to flow to the liver meridian; or if there is excessive energy at the liver meridian, he may open points at the subsequent lung meridian so that the excessive energy can be drained away.

The Principle of Opposites

The third principle of selecting energy points involves the selection of "opposites", irrespective of whether these opposite energy points fall on the same or different meridians. There are five approaches, namely left-right, up-down, diagonal, front-back, and yin-yang.

In the "left-right approach", the acupuncturist selects energy points on the opposite side of the disease location. For example to treat a patient suffering from numbness on the left of his face, he may chooses appropriate energy points like cuanzhu (B 2), jing-ming (B 1), chengqi (S 1), sibai (S 2), yingxiang (Li 20), dicang (S 4), daying (S 5) and jiache (S 6) on the patient's right side.

Why is this so? If you are driving along an expressway (British system) and wish to turn to your right via an overpass, you have to move to the left lane; and if it is blocked here, you cannot travel to your right.

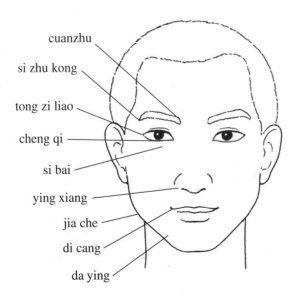

Fig 20.5 Relevant Energy Points (7)

It is fascinating to learn that an illness located at the top part of the body is more effectively treated if we manipulate its opposite point at the bottom, and vice versa, as in the "up-down approach". For example, for relieving hypertension, we manipulate yongquan (K 1) which is situated at the sole of the foot; to stop vomiting, we manipulate gongsun (Sp 4) at the ankle; and to cure prolapse of the rectum, we manipulate baihui (Gv 20) at the crown of the head!

How does this work? These far apart places are connected by meridians. They work the same way as your turning off a ceiling light by pressing the switch at the door.

To make it more interesting (and effective), we may use the "diagonal approach", which is a combination of the left-right and up-down approaches. For example, to relieve a patient of palpitation or insomnia, we can manipulate his left shenmen (H 7) at the wrist and right sanyingjiao (Sp 6) at the leg, or his right shenmen (H 7) and left sanyinjiao (Sp 6).

So do not be surprise, when you complain of pain at your right ribs, your acupuncturist manipulates energy points on your left foot.

The selection of energy points can be based on front-back opposites. This principle is often used in combination with the "local" or "near" approach and the "distant" or "far" approach. For example, renzhong (Gv 26) located between the nose and the upper lip, is an effective point for resuscitating a patient from coma and high fever, and it is often combined with dazhui (Gv 14) located at the back.

For asthma, a useful combination is tiantu (Cv 22) below the throat, and feishu (B 13) at the back. Renzhong (Gv 26), described by classical masters as connecting heaven and earth, is a life-saver; dazhui (Gv 14) is a major point on the spinal column; tiantu (Cv 22) controls the wind-pipe; and feishu (B 13) is where lung energy is focused.

Another approach which is often used but may appear puzzling to the uninitiated is the yin-yang opposites. Basically, the acupuncturist chooses energy points on a yin meridian to supplement those on a yang meridian, and vice versa. This approach is related to, but not the same as, the "external-internal approach".

In treating cold and fever, for example, the acupuncturist combines lieque (L 7) on the affected lung meridian, with hegu (Li 4) on the colon meridian. The yang colon meridian is the external counterpart of the internal yin lung meridian. When lieque (L 7), the junction-point or gate, is opened for the "lung-evil" (pathogens causing cold and fever at the lung meridian) to pass into the colon meridian, hegu (Li 4), the source-point or power station of the colon meridian situated behind lieque, provides the energy to flush out the "lung-evil".

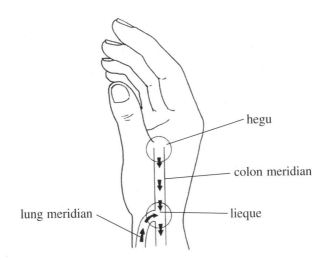

Fig 20.6 Cooperation between Lieque and Hegu
(Diagrammatic)

The above explanation is of course only a brief introduction for general readers. An acupuncturist must have a sound knowledge of hundreds of energy points and their properties, like a herbalist knowing hundreds of herbs. He must also understand thoroughly man's internal cosmos, that is, the meridian system and the internal organs, as well as medical fundamentals so that he can select and combine suitable energy points for manipulation with his needles to restore health.

Main Manipulative Techniques

Selecting and combining energy points is only the preliminary, albeit very important, part of the healing operation. The other part, which brings about the desired therapeutic effect, is manipulation of the selected points. Acupuncture is not merely inserting needles into energy points. Even if the right points are chosen but manipulation is not done correctly, one may obtain an effect opposed to what was desired.

There are many types of acupuncture needles. As early as the Warring State period (3rd century BC), there were "nine types of needles". The one popularly used today is one of these nine types, known as "hao zhen", or thin long needle. It is usually made of silver or stainless steel, and may range from 3 cm to 15 cm. All needles and other tools must be properly sterilized before and after use.

There are three modes of inserting the needle: vertical, which is most common; slanting at about 45 degrees, which is employed to avoid bones or internal organs; and horizontal at about 20 degrees, often used at the head and face.

When a needle is inserted correctly in an energy point, the patient may feel "sour", "numb", "swelling", "heavy", "heated" or "gently electrified". This is known as "arresting energy", and is crucial for the success of the acupuncture treatment. The acupuncturist is able to know when this condition is attained, as he will feel the needle being firmly gripped by the arrested energy. If he feels that the needle is loose, light, slippery, or empty, as if inserted into a bean curd, then energy is not "arrested" and no significant therapeutic effects will be obtained.

When a needle is correctly inserted, and "arresting energy" is felt, there are three main modes of manipulation. The acupuncturist may repeatedly push in and pull up the needle (but not out of the skin) in a technique known as "pull-push"; repeatedly rotate the needle a complete circle clockwise then anti-clockwise in a "rotation" technique; or he may leave the needle motionlessly in a "retention" technique.

There are many supplementary manipulating techniques. If "arresting energy" is not satisfactory, the other non-needle hand may gently tap around the energy point to help energy to be arrested. The acupuncturist may also tap or stoke along the relevant meridian to stimulate better energy flow. To increase energy sensation, he may stroke or tap on the inserted needle, or cause it to vibrate to and fro. To enhance effect, he can, with the insertion point at the skin as pivot, move the exposed end of the needle in circles, causing the other pointed end to move in circles too inside the patient's body.

Enhancing and Cleansing Energy

While there are countless manipulative techniques to achieve various therapeutic effects, they can be generalized into four key words: xu, shi, pu, xie, which means empty, solid, enhance and cleanse. Basically, if an illness is empty, enhance the energy and if the illness is solid, cleanse it (where "it" can mean the illness or the energy!). Enhancing is also used when the patient is weak, and the illness is "cold". Cleansing on the other hand is used when the patient is strong and the illness "hot". When neither enhancing nor cleansing is emphasized, the technique is termed "even", which is another commonly used technique.

An "empty" illness is caused by the weakening of the body, and where the illness is not obvious. For example, because of energy deficiency, a person's organs function far below their optimum, though conventional medical tests may not register him as clinically ill — such as poor memory, being easily irritated, chronic body pains, or inability to conceive. The basic principle when treating empty illnesses is to enhance the patient's vital energy.

A "solid" illness is caused by the victory of disease-causing agents over the body's defence or reaction, and where the illness is obvious. It is usually caused by the "six external evils" like drastic climatic changes or microscopic organisms.

In Chinese medical philosophy, these exogenous agents inside the patient's body are refereed to as "evil energy". The basic therapeutic principle is to cleanse this evil energy.

Enhancing or cleansing energy can be achieved in the ways described below. When the two aspects are equal, like pulling and pushing with equal effort, or rotating clockwise and anti-clockwise in equal pro-portion, the effect is even.

In the "pull-push" technique, pushing heavily but pulling lightly, or pushing more and pulling less, results in enhancing energy. The reserve results in cleansing.

In the "rotation" technique, if the clockwise rotation is greater or more than the anti-clockwise rotation, energy is enhanced. Reversely, energy is cleansed.

The "retention" technique by itself does not enhance nor cleanse energy, but it strengthens the effect. For example, after rotating anti-clockwise more than clockwise, then retain the needle for a while, for a greater cleansing effect.

The rate of manipulation can have an enhancing or a cleansing effect: slowness enhances, speed cleanses energy. Slowly insert the needle. When energy is arrested, rotate the needle a few times. Withdraw the needle to below the skin and retain it there for a short while. Then swiftly take out the needle. This procedure enhances energy. The reverse procedure cleanses energy. Insert the needle quickly. Rotate the needle more times. Draw out the needle slowly.

Breathing in and out can also be used as an enhancing or cleansing technique. After arresting energy, observe how the patient breathes. Pushing or rotating clockwise as he breathes out, pulling or rotating anti-clockwise as he breathes in, enhances energy. The reverse has a cleansing effect.

The manner of withdrawing the needle from the body is also significant. Withdrawing the needle swiftly, and closing the energy point quickly with a finger and massaging it gently, has an enhancing effect. Withdrawing slowly, shaking the needle sideways in the process to enlarge the hole, and exposing it to let out evil-energy has a cleansing effect.

"Burning the volcano" and "cooling the sky" are two interesting techniques to enhance and cleanse energy respectively. Insert the needle to a shallow position as the patient breathes out. After arresting energy, push in heavily thrice, then slowly pull the needle (but not out of the body) once. Repeat this procedure two times. Finally draw out the needle as he breathes in, and swiftly close the energy point with a finger. This is "burning the volcano" and the patient feels warm all over.

To cleanse energy, insert the needle deeply as the patient breathes in. After arresting energy, pull up heavily three times (but not out of the body). Then push in slowly once. Repeat this procedure twice. Finally as the patient breathes out, withdraw the needle and expose the energy point. This is "cooling the sky", and the patient has a cool and refreshing sensation.

Other Needles and Other Techniques

Instead of using the hao zhen, or thin long needle, the acupuncturist can achieve similar effects by using other types of needles and methods, though their application is not as extensive, versatile or popular, and the energy points selected are often different. One of these types is known as plum-flower needles, which is a collection of small needles grouped together used for hitting onto the skin of the patient to stimulate blood circulation and defence-energy. Hence, they are sometimes called "skin needles". Another type is called "flesh needles". They are small short needles or pins, to be left on the patient's body for a day or two.

Another special type is the spear-headed needle, which is used to pierce into the skin to let some blood flow out. Blood-letting, which was a major therapeutic method in western medicine for many centuries in the past, is still useful for some therapeutic purposes like waking a patient from coma or unconsciousness, dispelling heat and draining dead blood like those caused by internal hemorrhage.

As one particular organ is also a microcosm of the whole body, some acupuncturists operate on only a selected external organ, like the ear, nose, palm, sole, or the whole head. You may find, for example, an odd sight of a patient with his ear, and no where else, covered with needles.

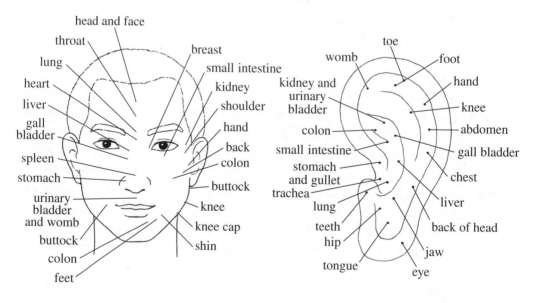

Fig 20.7
Head Acupuncture for Whole Body

Fig 20.8
Ear Acupuncture for Whole Body

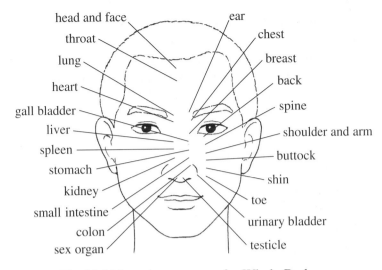

head and face
throat
lung
heart
gall bladder
liver
spleen
stomach
kidney
small intestine
colon
sex organ

ear
chest
breast
back
spine
shoulder and arm
buttock
shin
toe
urinary bladder
testicle

Fig 20.9 Nose Acupuncture for Whole Body

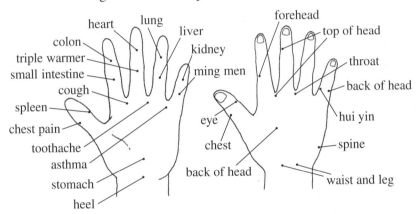

heart   lung   liver
colon   kidney
triple warmer
small intestine
cough   ming men
spleen
chest pain
toothache
asthma
stomach
heel

eye
chest
back of head

forehead
top of head
throat
back of head
hui yin
spine
waist and leg

Fig 20.10 Palm Acupuncture for Whole Body

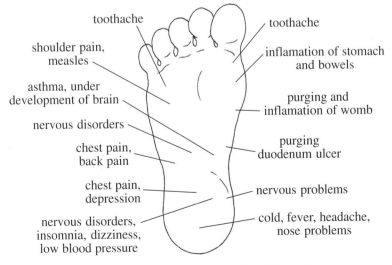

toothache
shoulder pain,
measles
asthma, under
development of brain
nervous disorders
chest pain,
back pain
chest pain,
depression
nervous disorders,
insomnia, dizziness,
low blood pressure

toothache
inflamation of stomach
and bowels
purging and
inflamation of womb
purging
duodenum ulcer
nervous problems
cold, fever, headache,
nose problems

Fig 20.11 Sole Acupuncture for Whole Body

Moxibustion is sometimes used instead of acupuncture. Moxa leaves or other medicinal ingredients are made into cones or sticks, and are burned at selected energy points. The energy points and principles involved are the same as those in acupuncture using the thin long needle. Cupping, i.e. placing a suitable vessel with partial vacuum over an afflicted area to suck out evil-energy, is sometimes used to supplement moxibustion.

Treating the Patient, not the Disease

Acupuncture masters have recorded their experiences and knowledge for posterity. The following is an example. It is worthwhile to note that unlike western medicine, even for an infectious disease the Chinese focus not on the microbes which they know are exogenous pathogens, but on restoring the healthy conditions of the patient. They classify dysentery into three types not according to the kinds of microbes that causes the disease, but according to the reaction of the patient to it.

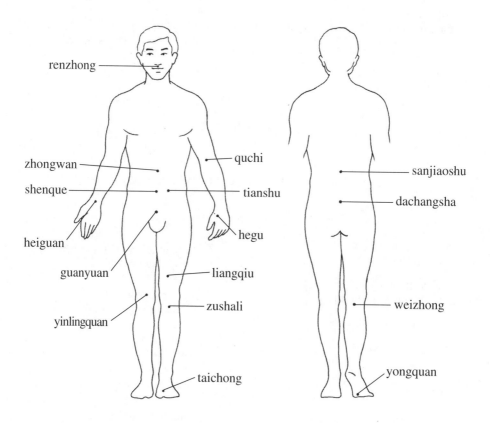

Fig 20.12 Energy Points for Treating Dysentery

Disease:
  Purging due to pestilent-evil, or dysentery.

Symptoms:
  Pestilent evil infecting the whole body, abdominal pains, tenesmus (or ineffectual and painful straining of defecation), frequent purging of bloody and mucus faeces, feeling of nausea and vomiting.

Causes:
  Taken contaminated food with pestilent-evil attacking the spleen and stomach, resulting in disorder of spleen and stomach energy, and retention of dampness in the gastrointestinal tract. The disease may be classified into three types according to pathogenetic conditions.

Dampness-Heat Type:
  Fever and chilliness, headaches, tiredness, thirst, abdominal pains, nausea, vomiting, purging more than ten times daily beginning with liquid faeces, later with mucus and blood, tenesmus (ineffectual and painful straining in defecation), short yellowish urine, yellow fur on tongue, and smooth rapid pulse.

Therapeutic Principles:
  Dispel heat, invigorate energy flow, clear dampness, and use the cleansing principle.

Main Energy Points:
  Tianshu (S 25), zhongwan (Cv 12), zusanli (S 36) and hegu (Li 4).

Cold-Dampness Type:
  Slight fever, tiredness, chest congestion, abdominal flatulence, pain at the limbs, no thirst, slight abdominal pain, nausea, vomiting, frequent purging more than ten times a day with liquid faeces and mucus, slight tenesmus, clear or slightly yellowish urine, oily fur on tongue, and rapid weak pulse.

Therapeutic Principles:
  Warm middle warmer, disperse cold, clear dampness, use the even principle.

Main Energy Points:
  Tianshu (S 25), sanjiaoshu (B 22), yinlingquan (Sp 9), guanyuan (Cv 4), and dachangshu (B 25).

Virulent Type:
Chilliness, high fever, headaches, abdominal pains, acute tenesmus, drowsiness, coma, convulsion, crimson tongue, yellowish dry fur, and smooth and rapid or weak pulse.

Therapeutic Principles:
Clear heat, cool blood, and disperse pestilent-evil.

Main Energy Points:
Shixuan (tips of ten fingers) or Weizhong (B 40) — prick to let blood flow, zusanli (S 36), tianshu (S 25), and dachangshu (B 25). If the illness has deteriorated to become life-threatening, with symptoms like cold limbs, impalpable pulse, and coma, use the principle of "recovering yang and rescuing collapse" by applying acupuncture on renzhong (Gv 26), neiguan (P 6), yongquan (K 1), and zusanli (S 36), and use moxibustion or shenque (Cv 8).

Useful Combination:
Quchi (Li 11) for fever; neiguan (P 6) for vomiting; hegu (Li 4) and taichong (Liv 3) for convulsions; additionally, liangqiu (S 34) and dachangshu (B 25) for abdominal pains.

Explanation:
Acupuncture on tianshu (S 25), zhongwan (Cv 12) and guanyuan (Cv 4) can dispel cold and dampness in gastrointestinal tract. Moxibustion on guanyuan (Cv 4), shenque (Cv 8) and dachangshu (B 25) can activate yang and clear dampness; and combined with acupuncture on sanjiaoshu (B 22) can disperse fire-evil. Acupuncture on hegu (Li 4), quchi (Li 11), and yinlingquan (Sp 9) can clear heat and dampness; on neiguan (P 6) can clear congestion at the middle warmer and stop vomiting; on hegu (Li 4) and taichong (Liv 3) can relieve convulsion; on renzhong (Gv 26) and yongquan (K 1) can reestablish yang (meaning resuscitation). Bloodletting at shixuan (ten finger tips) and weizhong (B 40) can clear heat-evil and recover consciousness. Acupuncture on liangqiu (S 34) can stop pain. For acute cases, use rotation and retention of needle technique.

Other techniques:
Ear acupuncture — insert needles at colon, small intestine, triple warmer, spleen and stomach regions, and retain needles for 2 to 3 days. Can be combined with body (orthodox) acupuncture. Cupping — tianshu (S 25), zhongwan (Cv 12), guanyuan (Cv 4) and dachangshu (B 25) for relieving abdominal pains.

Note: The above methods may be used or modified for acute inflammation of the gastrointestinal tract, whose symptoms are abdominal pains, vomiting and liquid faeces but tenesmus is not obvious.

The above methods, of course, are not the only ways in acupuncture to cure particular diseases. Because there are many energy points and different combinations to choose from, different acupuncturists who have a thorough understanding of the meridian network, therapeutic principles and relevant concepts, can achieve similar results by using other points.

Indeed, some Chinese physicians do not even use needles to achieve similar effects; they use their bare hands as in massage therapy, which will be explained in the next chapter.

21

HEALING WITH FINGERS —
AND WITH NOTHING ELSE!

(Chinese Massage Therapy)

Although western medicine has attained very high levels in the localistic and reductionist study of man, it is till far from the core of the mysteries of life. Yet the thinking and accomplishments of Chinese medicine, despite having a layer of traditional philosophy, lead people to believe that it is closer to the core of life's mysteries.

Wang Fu, master massage therapist, 1984.

Your Healing Fingers

When they go for house calls, a traumatologist brings along a bag full of splints, bandages and medicine, an acupuncturist brings along his set of needles, while a massage therapist brings along only his fingers. But do not be mistaken that Chinese massage, unlike some other massage systems, is just for a tonic body rub.

Chinese massage therapy, which is a major branch of Chinese medicine like acupuncture and traumatology, has its comprehensive philosophy and methods, and can be applied to a wide range of illnesses.

There are, nevertheless, some diseases that are not suitable for massage therapy, such as burn, scald, skin infections, acute contagious diseases, malignant growth, serious illnesses of the heart and the liver, and serious mental derangement.

Chinese researchers using modern scientific methods have found that massage improves the natural functions of our body. For example, it can increase the amount of white blood cells in people who are deficient in them, but reduce it in those who have too many; increase the amount of antibodies to strengthen our immune system; and adjust the right amount of acids and other chemicals in our muscles.

Massage therapy is one of the oldest, if not actually the oldest, Chinese therapeutic approaches to cure diseases. All great Chinese ancient masters, like Bian Que, Hua Tuo and Zhang Zhong Jing used massage therapy as well as acupuncture and internal medicine in their practice.

During the Tang Dynasty (618-907) massage therapy became a speciality on its own. The depth and range of this Chinese healing system can be seen from the fact that the Tang government officially designated massage therapists into four ranks, namely practitioners, specialists, masters and professors.

In ancient China, massage was known as "an-mo", which literally means "pressing and stroking", the first two major techniques in Chinese massage therapy. Since the Ming Dynasty (1368-1644), it has been more popularly called "tui-na", meaning "pushing and gripping", which are the next two major techniques.

This change of name was due to a shift in technique emphasis, because during the Ming period massage therapy was widely used to treat children, and the pushing and gripping techniques were particularly effective.

The oldest known and regarded by many physicians as the most authoritative Chinese medical text, Nei Jing or Inner Classic of Medicine, described "an", "mo", "tui", "na" as the four fundamental techniques in massage therapy. It also laid down some essential principles. This overwhelming dependence on almost all important principles and methods in Chinese medicine on a text written more than 2000 years ago may understandably cause many people to imagine Chinese medicine to be passive or stagnant.

This could be valid if no significant developments were made since the time of the classic. This, of course, is not so, as the history of Chinese medicine (Chapters 3 and 4) has shown continuous progress, with may discoveries made well in advance of the west. In massage therapy, for example, against the four fundamental techniques of Nei Jing, we now have more than thirty.

Therefore, we are left with the other premise, that is, what was said in the Inner Classic is true, and has been continually verified for over 2000 years. The Inner Classic, though attributed to Huang Di, the Yellow Emperor of antiquity, was actually the crystallization of all the medical achievements of the Chinese people since the unknown past until the Zhou Dynasty (1066-221 BC), after which the classic has been revised and edited in subsequent dynasties. From the viewpoint of western medicine, with a history of only a few centuries, 2000 years is a long time; but from the perspective of the Chinese who have the longest continuous medical tradition known to man, 2000 years ago marked the accumulation of a medical legacy stretching back to millennia.

Looking back at the time span since man first knew medicine as he existed on this earth, 2000 years being a fraction of one percent of the time he has been on this planet, is exceedingly recent.

How Does Massage Therapy Cure Illnesses?

Most people are ready to accept that a good massage can loosen our tired muscles and promote blood circulation; but many would find it hard to believe that massage therapy can cure diseases ranging from a simple headache and diabetes to hernia and infantile convulsion.

If you happen to have frequent headaches and are weary of taking too many pain killers, you can test the claim of massage therapy by trying the therapeutic methods described in this chapter, for unlike other branches of Chinese medicine, in massage therapy it is quite safe to practice many of its methods on your own, though of course to be a massage therapist you would need years of specialized training.

And to understand how we can use only our fingers, without using any materia medica or instruments, to cure a wide range of diseases, you must put aside medical prejudices and explore the exotic world of Chinese medical philosophy.

The modern master, Wang Fu, explains that man, like the cosmos of which he is a microcosm, is manifested in two complementary yet opposing aspects of yin and yang. When he is sick, the disharmony of yin-yang affects not only him but the whole cosmos.

This is the fundamental holistic concept of Chinese medicine. While there is this common factor among all people, there are also individual differences. In the same environment, because of individual differences such as in their immune system, some people may succumb to illnesses, while others do not. This is the Chinese medical concept of "limitless variety", and is the starting point of the Chinese view on physiology and pathology.

The Inner Classic of Medicine says:

Yin-yang is the way of heaven and earth; the principle of all phenomena; the parent of change; the source of life and death; the house of gods.

In modern language, it means that the concept of yin-yang can explain the operation of the cosmos including man; everything, be it object or idea, is subjected to its operation; it is the basic factor of all transformations in the world; it is the root cause of man's health and illnesses; it can lead to the very core of the mysteries of life.

Once we understand and appreciate this concept of yin-yang (Chapter 5), simple in its fundamental meaning, but profound in its myriad manifestations, we can understand the hitherto incredible and seemingly inexplicable theories and cures in Chinese medicine.

The most basic principle explaining the workings of massage therapy, or any branch of Chinese medicine, is restoring the harmony of yin-yang. For example, if a patient has excessive microbes in his body, expressed as excessive yang, the massage therapist can reduce the excessive yang by using appropriate techniques; if his illness is symbolized as "cold" or yang deficiency, such as inadequate metabolic process, the therapist can restore yin-yang harmony by increasing yang.

To supplement the concept of yin-yang, Chinese medical philosophers use the concept of the five elemental processes (Chapter 6). Because these concepts can express complex ideas concisely, and are not often explained to the public, many people, including the Chinese themselves, erroneously think they are primitive and unscientific. The irony is that they actually contain gems of wisdom which modern science is only beginning to rediscover.

Many massage techniques are applications to correct physiological or psychological malfunction of the patient according to the concept of the five elemental processes. For example, a patient with hypertension is symbolically described in Chinese medical terms as "excessive yang wood due to insufficient yin water".

This is because the illness is due to rising liver energy as a result of deficient kidney function; and the liver and the kidneys correspond to the elemental processes of wood and water respectively. To treat hypertension, the massage therapist manipulates in such ways to bring the excessive yang energy down from the head to the feet, and to increase the kidney energy. Both the flow of excessive yang energy and the kidney energy correspond to the water process. The therapist in this case is employing the principle of "water nourishing wood" to overcome hypertension.

The third important concept to explain how massage therapy works, is the concept of man's internal cosmos (Chapter 7), i.e. his internal organs and the functions of energy and blood.

Chinese masters have discovered some startling knowledge concerning the relationship between man's physiological conditions and disease, and have recorded this information in principles like "When the heart and the lung are diseased, its energy is retained at the elbow", "When the liver is diseased, its energy is retained at the armpits", "When the spleen is diseased, its energy is retained at the thigh", "When the kidney is diseased, its energy is retained at the back of the knee", "The liver corresponds to muscles and tendons", "The spleen affects the flesh of the whole body", "The lung corresponds to the skin and hair", and "The kidney affects the bones".

Such knowledge is very useful for diagnosis and therapeutics. For example, when a massage therapist finds that the patient's energy is locked at his elbow, it suggests that his illness is located at the heart or the lung systems; the logical treatment is to release this locked energy at the elbow.

When he finds that his patient's flesh is poorly formed, it suggests that his spleen system is diseased; the logical treatment is to massage his spleen meridian to improve his spleen function.

The fourth important concept is the meridian system (Chapters 8 and 9), which includes the twelve primary meridians, the eight secondary meridians (especially the conceptual and the governing meridians), the twelve meridian-extensions, the twelve meridian-muscle systems, the twelve skin regions, and the fifteen branch-meridians including collaterals and sub-collaterals which are blood capillaries.

The Chinese discoverd that the muscles of our body are related to the meridians. For example, the muscles at the index finger, the flexors of the hand and wrist at the outer edge of the ulna, the lateral and anterior deltoids at the upper arm, and the sterno cleido at the side of the neck are affected by the colon meridian.

Different regions of our skin are also controlled by different meridians. Fig 21.1 illustrates the major skin regions. Massaging suitable skin regions can stimulate sub-collaterals to spread defence-energy to the required disease locations.

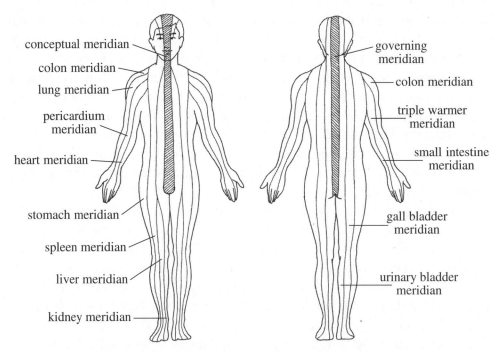

Fig 21.1 Skin Regions and Corresponding Meridians

Meridians not only transport nutrient-energy to and remove waste products from all body cells, they coordinate all physiological and psychological functions of the body as a holistic organism. Illnesses occurs because of interruption to the harmonious flow of vital energy in the meridians. Hence, a thorough understanding of the meridians and their energy points is essential for the therapist to massage the appropriate parts of the body to restore harmonious energy flow. Massaging hegu (Li 4) of the colon meridian, for example, can relieve headaches, toothaches, cold and fever, and loss of speech due to stroke; massaging sizhukong (T 23) of the triple warmer meridian can relieve migraines, facial numbness and various eye problems.

These four concepts — yin-yang, five elemental processes, organ systems and meridian network — are applicable to all branches of Chinese medicine. They are perhaps most striking in massage therapy where, without the aid of any materia medica nor instrument, health can be restored by correcting deviated functions according to the above concepts. The manipulative techniques to correct deviated functions are described in the following section.

Thirty Techniques in Massage Therapy

Initially there were only four generalized techniques, namely an, mo, tui and na. According to a tradition, Bodhidharma, the great Indian monk who initiated Shaolin Kungfu and founded Zen Buddhism at the Shaolin Monastery in China, extended the techniques to ten: an, mo tui, na, cuo, chui, gun, nian, rou and dan.

We now have many more, with variations for each technique. Thirty of the most popular techniques and their therapeutic functions are briefly described below. The same techniques may be called by different names by different therapists.

1. An, or Pressing.
Press with a finger, knuckle, fist, palm or elbow on a selected energy point or diseased area. Cleanse meridians and activate energy flow, reduce or stop pain, increase blood circulation, improve the digestive system, enhance defence-energy, promote sweating and improve nerve function.

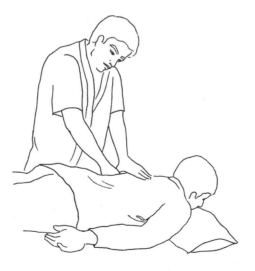

Fig 21.2 An or Pressing Technique

2. Mo, or Stroking.

Move the fingers or palm over and over the patient's body. Harmonize energy flow and blood circulation, relieve fever, dispel cold, reduce internal blood clot, swelling and pain, improve sweating, and enhances nerve function.

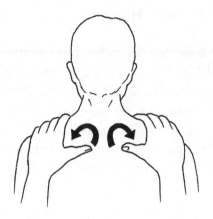

Fig 21.3 Mo or Stroking Technique

3. Tui, or Pushing.

Move the fingers, palm or fist forward along the patient's skin. Loosen muscles, regulate skin temperature, dispel stagnant energy, clear internal blood clot, cleanse blockages, enhance or cleanse energy and blood flow, and promote nerve function.

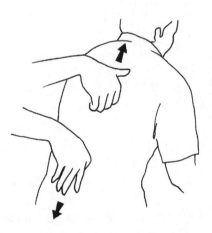

Fig 21.4 Tui or Pushing Technique

4. Na, or Gripping.

Firmly hold the muscles or energy points of the patient. Cleanse meridians and eliminate internal blood clot, harmonize energy flow and blood circulation, and produces anaesthetic effects.

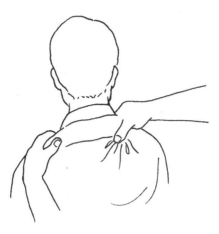

Fig 21.5 Na or Gripping Technique

5. Cuo, or Rolling.

Use one or both hands to roll the patient's body or limbs. Regulate skin temperature, cleanse meridians and promote blood circulation, harmonize sub-meridians, stops pain, and invigorate vital energy.

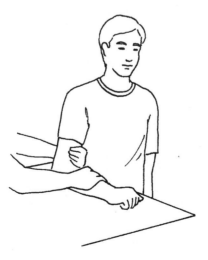

Fig 21.6 Cuo or Rolling Technique

6. Chui, or Pounding.
Hit or pound gently on the patient with a fist or palm. Cleanse meridian and promote blood circulation, harmonize yin-yang, clear blockages and internal blood clots, relieve mental depression, dispel wind and cold, relieve fever, disperse toxins, strengthens the liver, kidneys and muscles, arouse consciousness, and can be used as a first aid measure against heart attacks.

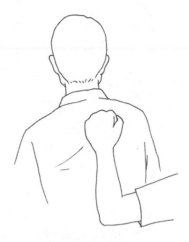

Fig 21.7 Chui or Pounding Technique

7. Gun, or Rounding Technique.
Round the knuckles or back of the curved palm on the patient. Cleanse meridians and activate energy flow, mobilize stagnant energy, dispel cold, stop pain, promote digestion, increase defence-energy, and enhances nerve function.

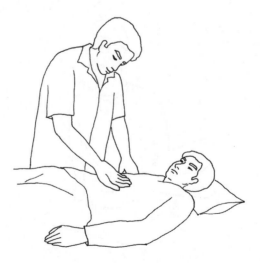

Fig 21.8 Gun or Rounding Technique

8. Nian, or Holding.

Gently hold and press the thumb and another finger on the patient. This technique is often used on the patient's fingers where energy tends to stagnate. By pressing gently, the stagnant energy is made to flow, and the technique is sometimes called "opening collaterals at joints".

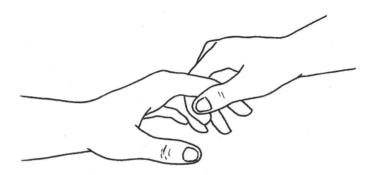

Fig 21.9 Nian or Holding Technique

9. Rou, or Rotating.

Place a finger or palm on the affected area and rotate or shake it without moving from its position. Eliminate swelling, clear internal blood clots, loosen muscles, relieve headaches, improve digestion, and clear constipation.

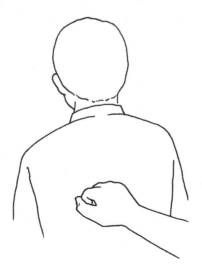

Fig 21.10 Rou or Rotating Technique

10. Dan, or Springing.

Hook a finger against the thumb, then suddenly release the finger so that it springs onto the patient's energy point or disease site. Effective for opening energy blockage. This technique is reputed to be invented by Bodhidharma. A master with internal force can focus it at the springing finger, and channel it into the patient that not only affects the part in contact with the springing technique, but is transmitted all over the patient's body to open all his blockages! There are records of such accomplishments in Chinese medical texts.

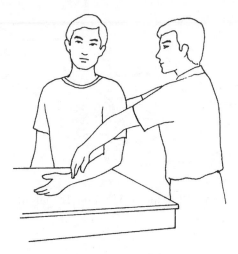

Fig 21.11 Dan or Springing Technique

11. Qia, or Piercing.

Place a finger or an energy point or disease site, and press hard. For unconsciousness and coma, dispel "evil", relieve numbness, and stop pain.

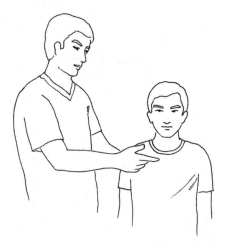

Fig 21.12 Qia or Piercing Technique

12. Nie, or Pinching.

With the thumb and another finger, raise a small part of the patient's skin or flesh. Dispel stagnation, clear blockage, and relieve numbness.

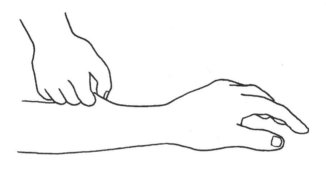

Fig 21.13 Nei or Pinching Technique

13. Ca, or Rubbing.

Move a thumb, finger, palm or fist over the patient's affect part producing some friction. Improve blood circulation, eliminate internal blood clot, and stop pain.

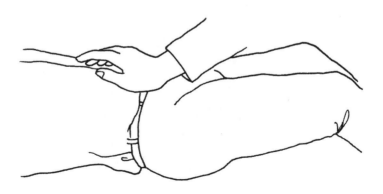

Fig 21.14 Ca or Rubbing Technique

14. Ci, or Poking.

Use one or more fingers to poke onto the patient's affected part. When five fingers are used, this technique is like the plum-flower acupuncture needles. Spread defence-energy, stimulate blood flow, and arouse nerve function.

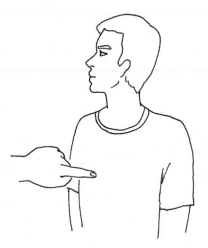

Fig 21.15 Ci or Poking Technique

15. Pai, or Tapping

Use the open palm to hit the affected part. Disperse poison, clear blockages, relieve numbness, stop pain, enhance energy and blood flow, and improve nerve function.

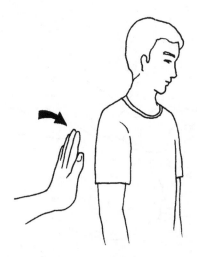

Fig 21.16 Pai or Tapping Technique

16. Luo, or Pulling.

Hold the patient's affected part and pull. It can be applied to a part of the flesh or to a whole limb as in setting a fracture or dislocation. Dispel cold, loosen muscles, and cleanse meridians.

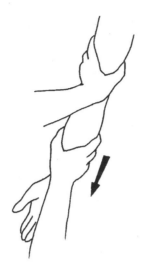

Fig 21.17 Luo or Pulling Technique

17. Yao, or Circulating.

Move the patient's fingers, toes, limbs, head or body in circles or from side to side. Clear blockages, disperse stagnant energy, loosen muscles, set fractures and dislocation, and check proper movements.

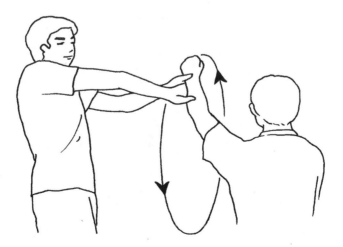

Fig 21.18 Yao or Circulating Technique

18. Dou, or Jerking.

Circulate the affected part or limb, then suddenly pull hard. Stimulate energy and blood flow, relieve numbness and spasms, and loosen muscles. By jerking the appropriate fingers or toes, the therapist can invigorate energy of the respective organs, because the meridians flow to them. For example, by jerking the big toe, he can influence the energy of the spleen and the liver, because meridians at the toes are linked to these organs; by jerking the middle finger he can improve over-all blood circulation, as the meridian here is link to the pericardium.

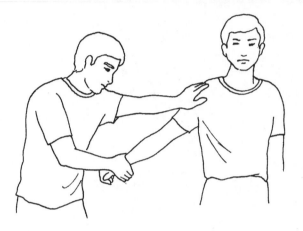

Fig 21.19 Dou or Jerking Technique

19. Fen, or Separating.

Move fingers or palms of both hands apart to opposite directions on patient's affected area. If the area is small, use two fingers of the same hand. Clear internal blood clots, loosen muscles, stop pain, and cleanse meridians. Useful for headaches, hernia, spasms and convulsions.

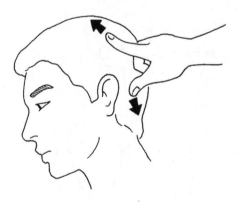

Fig 21.20 Fen or Separating Technique

20. He, or Uniting.

Move fingers or palms together on the patient's affected area. Enhance vital energy, nourish kidney energy, promote digestion, warm spleen system, and dispel cold. This is the counterpart of the separating technique. While the separating technique is principally cleansing, this uniting technique is mainly enhancing.

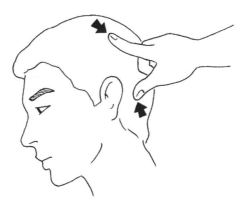

Fig 21.21 He or Uniting Technique

21. Zhen, or Vibrating.

Vibrate, or quickly move, a finger or palm on a selected energy point or affected area, without moving the finger or palm from the point. Reduce swelling, relieve spasms, loosen muscles, and for therapists with internal power, transmit vital energy into the patient.

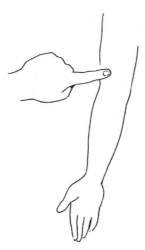

Fig 21.22 Zhen or Vibrating Technique

22. Zhuan, or Turning

Hold the patient's head with both hands and turn it from side to side. Loosen muscles, set neck dislocation, and relieve stiff or twisted neck, and other illnesses concerning the neck.

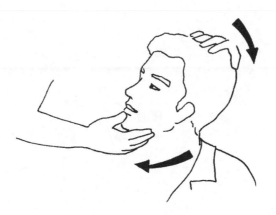

Fig 21.23 Zhuan or Turning Technique

23. Tai, or Raising.

Move the affected limb, head or any body part gently, then suddenly raise it. Loosen tendons at joints, improve joint movement, set fractures and dislocations.

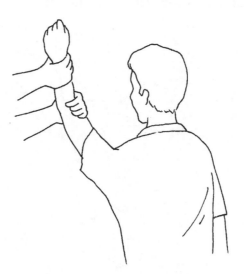

Fig 21.24 Tai or Raising Technique

24. Qu or Bending.

Bend the affected finger, limb, trunk or head gently. Loosen muscles and tendons, promote joint movement, clear stagnant energy, set fractures or dislocations.

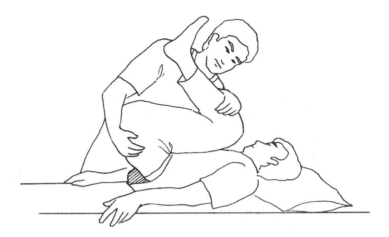

Fig 21.25 Qu or Bending Technique

25. Chen, or Stretching.

The chen or stretching technique is usually used in conjunction with the qu or bending technique. After bending, the affected part is stretched; sometimes it is also pulled. Enhance energy flow, strengthen muscles and tendons, and promote joint movement.

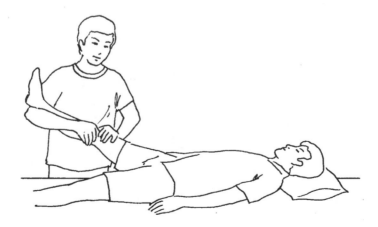

Fig 21. 26 Chen or Stretching Technique

26. Ba, or Moving.

Place one finger against the affected joint, and with the other hand move or rotate the finger, toe, limb or the rest of the whole body. Facilitate joint movement, loosen muscles and tendons, and stimulate energy and blood flow, reduce swelling and pain, and set dislocation.

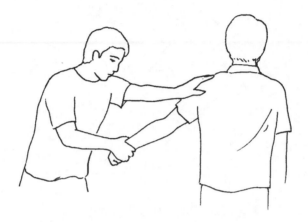

Fig 21.27 Ba or Moving Technique

27. Dian, or Dotting.

Tap or dot a finger gently along a meridian. Stimulate energy and blood flow, clear blockages, and enhance or cleanse energy.

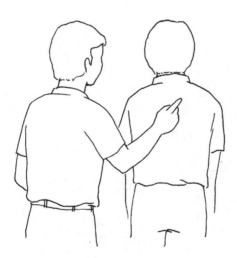

Fig 21.28 Dian or Dotting Technique

28. Bei, or Carrying.
Carry and rock the patient with his back on your back. Loosen the spinal vertebrae, and useful for various back ailments.

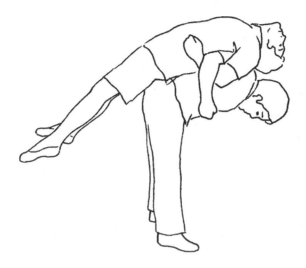

Fig 21.29 Bei or Carrying Technique

29. Bao or Lifting.
Stand behind a seated patient and with your arms under his armpits and lift him. This technique is suitable for various illnesses concerning the back and the spine.

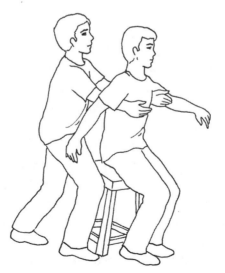

Fig 21.30 Bao or lifting Technique

30. Cai or Stepping.

Step with one or both legs on the patient who is in a lying position. It must be performed with care as great pressure is involved. It is usually applied on the patient's lumbar region. Remove pain, loosen muscles, and stimulate energy and blood flow.

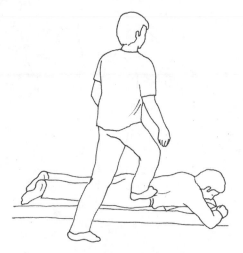

Fig 21.31 Cai or Stepping Technique

Enhancing, Cleansing or Even Effects

Like acupuncture, manipulative techniques in massage therapy can be enhancing, cleansing or even. The enhancing principle is used to strengthen the patient, and is suitable for "empty" illnesses, i.e. illnesses due to the weakening of the patient's natural functions. Cleansing is used to eliminate pathogenetic causes, and is suitable for "solid" illnesses, i.e. illnesses where the disease-causing agents are obvious.

When neither enhancing nor cleansing is emphasized, the effect is even. The "even principle", which is often used, is applicable when both enhancing and cleansing effects are required, or when neither are specially needed.

When massage techniques are used in line with the flow of the meridians, the result is enhancing. For example, when employing the "an" or pressing technique on any energy points along the lung meridian which flows from the shoulder to the thumb, the therapist applies pressure towards the thumb, and the effect is enhancing, as it increases the energy flow.

If his pressure is directed towards the patient's shoulder as he presses on an energy point, i.e. his manipulative technique is applied against the flow of the lung meridian, the effect is cleansing, because the energy flow is reduced. If he presses vertically downward, neither in line nor against the meridian flow, the effect of his technique is "even".

The same principle applies to all other manipulative techniques. For example, when using the "tui" or pushing technique on the spleen meridian, which flows from the foot to the body, the therapist pushes along the meridian towards the body, i.e. in line with the meridian flow, the effect is enhancing. If he pushes towards the leg, i.e. against the meridian flow, the effect is cleansing.

However, if a meridian flows the other way round, like the stomach meridian which flows from the body to the foot, the effect is reversed, i.e. pushing towards the body is cleansing, and pushing towards the foot is enhancing.

Another way to achieve the enhancing or cleansing effects is the nature of applying the techniques. If a technique is performed gently, lightly and fast, the effect is enhancing. If it is done forcefully, heavily and slowly, the effect is cleansing.

A third method uses the waist as a guideline to achieve enhancing or cleansing effects. Massaging movements towards the waist has an enhancing effect, those from it are cleansing. For example, when using the "mo" or stroking technique, if the therapist strokes towards the waist, the effect is enhancing; if he strokes away from it, the effect is cleansing. When using the "na" or gripping technique, if the gripping moves towards the waist, the effect is enhancing, away from it, the effect becomes cleansing.

Application of Massage Therapy

As there are many different techniques and sites for operation to achieve similar therapeutic principles, different massage therapists may use different methods for similar illnesses. For example, in treating gastric pains, first of all the therapist has to find out whether it is a solid illness (shi zheng) or an empty illness (xu zheng).

A solid gastric illness, like diarrhoea, is caused by "real" agents such as microbes, whereas an empty gastric illness, like gastritis, is caused by "apparent" factors such as weakening of stomach function. In a solid illness, the main objective is to "eliminate evil", which in the case of diarrhoea is cleansing the evils of dampness and heat. In an empty illness, the main objective is to "restore good", which in the case of gastritis is enhancing stomach energy.

Whether it is cleansing evils or enhancing energy, the massage therapist has a choice of techniques and sites to operate on. When cleansing evils of the stomach, for example, he may use pai, gun or fen (tapping, rounding or separating techniques) directly on the abdomen, or he may use tui, nie or dian (pushing, pinching and dotting techniques) on the stomach meridian at the leg.

When enhancing stomach energy, he may use an and mo (pressing and stroking techniques) on the abdomen, or he may use the enhancing effect of an and rou (pressing and rotating techniques) on pishu (B 20), weishu (B 21), sanjiaoshu (B 22), dachangshu (B 25), guanyuanshu (B 26) and xiaochangshu (B 27) on the gall bladder meridian at the patient's back.

Let us see how headaches are treated by a massage therapy master, Wang Fu.

Introduction:

Headaches are one of the commonest complaints, and its causes are many and varied. Chinese medical thinking believes that it can be due to external as well as internal causes. External causes include the evils of wind and cold, wind and heat, and wind and dampness. Internally it can be caused by rising yang energy from the liver, contaminated phlegm, energy or blood deficiency, and deficiency of kidney energy.

Generally new headaches are caused by exogenous agents, and is a "solid" illness; whereas chronic headaches are caused by endogenous agents, and is an "empty" illness. Clinically, headaches may be classified into various kinds according to its pathogenetic conditions.

Using the Six Syndromes classification (see Chapter 12), front headaches belongs to yangming illness, side headaches belongs to shaoyang illness, back headaches belongs to taiyang illness, headaches at the crown belongs to jueyin illness, and headaches extending to the spin belongs to a disease at the governing meridian.

Therapeutic Principles:

Treatment depends on the different types of headache. Generally, a "solid" headache should be cleansed, with the patient sitting during massage therapy treatment; whereas an "empty" headache should be enhanced with energy, with the patient lying down during treatment. If there is a mixture of "solid" and "empty" syndromes, treatment can be both enhancing and cleansing, or "even".

Front headaches:

An (press) yangbai (G 14). Tui (push) from yintang (third eye) to shenting (Gv 24), in a technique known as "opening heavenly gate", for about two minutes. If necessary, rou and an (rotate and press) some of the following points: cuanzhu (B 2), hegu (Li 4), taiyang (temples), shangxing (Gv 23), and baihui (Gv 20). If there is blocked nose or running nose, an (press) yingxiang (Li 20); if there is cold phlegm, an, rou, mo and ca (press, rotate, stroke and rub) feishu (B 13) and lieque (L 7).

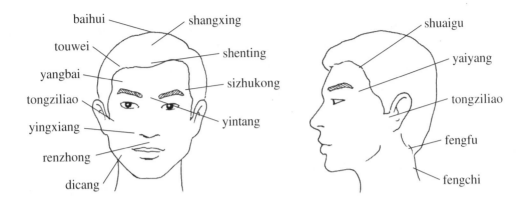

Fig 21.32 Relevant Energy Points at the Head

Side Headaches:

Mainly an and mo (press and stroke) taiyang (temples), tui and na (push and grip) the back of the head, and rou (rotate) fengchi (G 20) until the head perspires slightly. If necessary, an and rou (press and rotate) the following energy points: touwei (S 8), tongziliao (G 1), sizhukong (T 23), and yanglingquan (G 34); and tui (push) from baihui (Gv 20) towards the spine.

Back Headaches:

Mainly tui and an (push and press) fengchi (G 20) and fengfu (Gv 16). Other points like touwei (S 8), shangxing (Gv 23), shuaigu (G 8), and hegu (Li 4) may be used in combination.

Top Headaches:

Mainly an (press) baihui (Gv 20) and yongquan (K 1). Manipulating yongquan (K 1) can channel energy to flow towards the leg, thus relieving headaches. Other points like dicang (S 4), hegu (Li 4), renzhong (Gv 26),touwei (S 8) and jiache (S 26) can be manipulated in combination.

Headaches Extending to Spine:

Tui (push) from the crown of the head down the spin, then an and tui (press and push) dazhui (Gv 14). Nie (pinch) cuanzhu (B 2) and yintang (third eye). Na (grip) jianjing (G 21); gun (round) the muscles at the back; an and rou (press and rotate) the painful spots; then mo (stroke) the back.

Headaches due to Hypertension:

Mo (stroke) with cleansing effect both taiyang (temples), then with the side of the palm tui (push) down the spin from dazhui (Gv 14) to changqiang (Gv 1), followed with techniques of an and rou (press and rotate) on yongquan (K 1), and na (grip) on kunlún (B 60) at the ankle and fengchi (G 20) behind the neck. If necessary, combine with manipulation of yintang (third eye), touwei (S 8), lieque (L 7), and hegu (Li 4), applying the cleansing effect.

Headache dues to Weakness of Nervous System:

This type of headaches are usually slight, and accompanied with dizziness, mainly at the forehead, top and temporal regions. However, the whole head is not comfortable. It is usually an "empty" illness, and the main therapeutic principle should be enhancing. Tui, an, rou and na (push, press, rotate and grip) the following points: yintang (third eye), taiyang (temples), yangbai (G 14), fengchi (G 20), and hegu (Li 4). Then nie (pinch) cuanzhu (B 2). Using both thumbs, apply the fen (separate) technique from yintang (third eye) to sizhukong (T 23) at the outer corner of the eye-brows. Then ci (poke) with ten fingers on the forehead. Use the side or back of the palm to chui (pound) gently on the whole head. In between various manipulative movements, use ten fingers to ca (rub) the head as if combing hair. This will arouse the spirit, activate the senses, clear the head and eliminate pain.

Severe Headaches due to Disorder of the Nerves:

The pain, which is spasmodic, can be excruciating, like being slashed by sharp weapons, being burnt or electrified. The pain is usually at the sides of the head, and is caused by wind-evil, fire-evil, contaminated phlegm or internal blood clot. It is a "solid" illness. Treatment by massage therapy is not as speedy as by acupuncture, though relieve and recovery can be achieved. Manipulation is generally heavy, applying techniques of tui and na (push and grip) on hegu (Li 4), jiache (S 26), xiaguan (S 7), dicang (S 4), neiting (S 44), and zulinqi (G 41). Some readers would be surprised to find that neiting and zulinqi, two important energy points for relieving severe headaches due to nervous disorder, are located respectively at the base of the second toe and a short distance behind the little toe! Also apply the an (press) technique on "a-shi" points.

These interesting "a-shi" points are not established, regular energy points; they are topical and located at the spots where when a physician presses on them, the patient would cry out "a" or similar sounds. These points prove to have effective therapeutic values. They are therefore called "a-shi" or "ah-yes" points, meaning that "when a patient cries out `ah', yes that is the point to manipulate on".

Chinese medicine, as you have found, is not only effective but exceedingly fascinating. You must be ready for interesting surprises when you explore this exotic yet practical world of Chinese medicine.

In the next chapter, you will read something you will probably not believe, but you have the opportunity to test it yourself if you are game for some pleasant and beneficial experiences.

22

DANCE OF HEALTH AND LONGEVITY
(Health Exercises and Preventive Medicine)

Better to hunt in Fields, for Health unbought,
Than fee the Doctor for a nauseous Draught.
The wise, for Cure, on exercise depend;
God never made his Work, for Man to mend.
John Dryden.

Medicine or Health?

It is indeed nauseous to reflect that doctors, almost beyond their control, prosper on account of people becoming sick. Must this necessarily be so? While some may be anxious that improving health can affect their income, most doctors and medical scientists, I believe, would like to advance to a stage like what Thomas Edison said:

The doctor of the future
will give no medicine,
but will interest his patients
in the care of the human frame,
in diet, and in the cause
and prevention of disease.

Chinese physicians have believed in this philosophy throughout their medical history. The Nei Jing has mentioned many times that:

Mediocre medicine cures diseases;
Superior medicine prevents them.

Chinese physicians also believe that good medicine, whether it is preventive or curative, must have three qualities: it must be cheap, effective and easily available. This contrasts clearly with the expensive instruments available only in centralized, specialist hospitals and the costly set-ups of exclusive health centers in western societies.

If it was because of money that Chinese physicians practiced medicine, many would not have chosen this profession, and great physicians in ancient China would not have rejected emperors' offer of a luxurious life in imperial courts, so as to serve common people many of whom could not afford to pay medical fees.

Chinese physicians were mostly poor; even in modern times they are usually not rich. Social and economic historians may like to find out whether the relative poverty of Chinese physicians has anything to do with the philosophy they hold.

Chinese medical philosophy demonstrates Dryden's belief that "God never made his Work, for Man to mend". The Chinese believe that man is made perfect and as health is his birthright, he never needs to be sick so long as he maintains his proper energy flow and yin-yang harmony. Throughout the ages, there have been countless exercises to help man to maintain good health, which in the Chinese concept means not just being free from illnesses, but physical, emotional, mental and spiritual well-being.

Different Types of Health Exercises

Chinese archaeological records show that health exercises were practiced by the Chinese in prehistoric times. The importance of these exercises in curing illnesses as well as promoting health and longevity were stressed in many ancient medical texts. Chinese health exercises can be divided into three convenient groups, namely physiotherapy, qigong exercises and kungfu exercises.

Physiotherapy is mainly used for curing chronic and degenerative illnesses and for augmenting other therapeutic methods like traumatology and massage therapy. They are not suitable for acute diseases. Some of the ancient physiotherapy exercises were in the form of dance. When correct breathing constitutes an essential part of the physiotherapy exercises, they approximate qigong therapy.

Qigong, pronounced as ch'i kung, is a profound and extensive discipline in itself and will be explained in greater detail in the next two chapters. One important dimension of qigong concerns health and medicine, and is known as health qigong and medical qigong. One incredible health qigong exercise will be explained later in this chapter, as an example of Chinese health exercises. Medical qigong, or qigong therapy, which is meant for curing illnesses, will be explained in the next two chapters.

Kungfu, or Chinese martial art, is actually meant for fighting, but because it is also excellent for promoting health, many people nowadays practice kungfu primarily for health, even to the extent of neglecting its paramount combative functions. There are many different styles of kungfu, the most popular being Shaolin Kungfu and Taijiquan.

However, it is regrettable that many people who practice kungfu nowadays perform only the outward form, missing the essential inner aspects of energy flow. Although the outward form of kungfu can still promote health, the essence is lost if the inner aspects are not included.

While there is a discernible difference between health and medicine in the western perspective, which is generally topical and reductionist in nature, this difference is not significant in the Chinese, because the Chinese view health and medicine holistically. In this holistic, organic paradigm, health and medicine, prevention and cure are not categorically separated; they are merely convenient descriptions along a continuum ranging from severe illnesses to excellent health without any rigid division.

Hence, people who are not sick may take herbs to enhance their energy, like Chinese women regularly taking the "Eight Precious Herbs Decoction" after their menstruation flow to replenish themselves.

Chinese health exercises, in comparison with therapeutic approaches like herbal medicine, acupuncture and massage therapy, belong to the higher end of this continuum. If you are sick these health exercises can help to relieve your sickness, though you will get faster result from therapies located at the lower end; but the main purpose of health exercises is to promote you to the health side of the continuum and are excellent in preventing all forms of illnesses from pulling you down the scale.

Within the health exercises, the graduation is from physiotherapy which aims more at curing, through qigong exercises which are both curative and preventive, to kungfu exercises which provide radiant health. There are many and varied forms of health exercises, but because of space constraint only two examples are described below.

Chinese Physiotherapy

Treatment by Chinese physiotherapy is holistic because it involves the whole body. It is natural as no materia medica or instruments are used. It is active as the patient must take the initiate in his treatment.

Chinese physiotherapy is most suitable for the following kinds of illnesses: chronic and degenerative diseases, especially of the respiratory, circulatory and digestive systems; ailments concerning macular and joint movements; disorders caused by habitual bad posture; and dyskinesia or paralysis due to nervous impairment.

The following set of physiotherapy exercises is effective for relieving disorders caused by "wind and dampness evils affecting the joints", which corresponds to arthralgia, myalgia, rheumatism and arthritis. It consists of ten exercises, which can be practiced individually, in sequences of a few selected exercises, or as a complete set. The exercises can be performed in different order. The number of times for performing each exercise depends on the needs and conditions of the patient, and a rough guide is about 5 to 10 times if practiced with other exercises, about 20 to 60 times if practiced alone. An important principle is that the patient must *not* be exhausted after the exercise. All the exercises are to be performed *without* exerting any force.

1. Stand upright and relaxed, with feet slightly apart, and arms hanging loosely at the sides. Vigorously and continuously rotate both wrists a complete circle in one direction, then in the other direction.

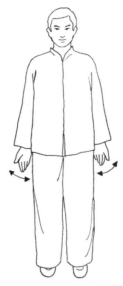

Fig 22.1 Rotating Wrist

2. Continuously swing your arms forward about 45 degrees and backward about 45 degrees, with your arms and fingers fairly straight. Perform this exercise more times than the other exercises, at least 20 times (forward and backward as one time) if practiced in combination with other exercises, 100 times if practiced alone.

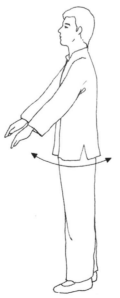

Fig 22.2 Swinging Arms

3. Hang your arms at your sides. Keep them straight but not locked. Without moving your arms, move your palms forward so that your fingers point to the front. Then move the palm as far back as you can, with the fingers pointing backward.

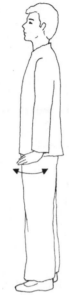

Fig 22.3 Flicking Palms

4. Move your hands up from sideways and try to touch your shoulders with your fingers. Drop your arms, and repeat.

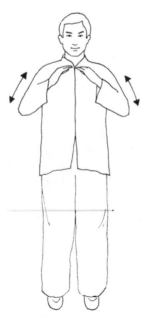

Fig 22.4 Touching Shoulders

5. Move your arms upwards from the front and place your palms together with fingers pointing skyward. Drop your arms, and repeat.

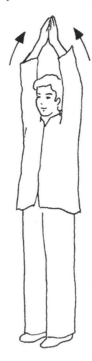

Fig 22.5 Fingers Pointing Skyward

6. Clasp your hands behind your head, then straighten your arms sideways so that your palms face skyward and your fingers point to both sides.

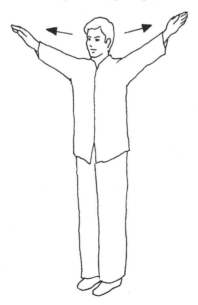

Fig 22.6 Clasping Hands And Straightening Arms

7. Raise your heels and stand on your toes. Then carefully drop your heels and raise your toes, standing on your heels.

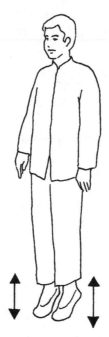

Fig 22.7 Standing on Toes and Heels

8. Move your right leg about two and a half shoulders' width in front, bend your right knee forward to a position above your right toes, and straighten your back left knee. Hold your two fists at your waist. This is the bow-arrow stance. Repeat with the other leg.

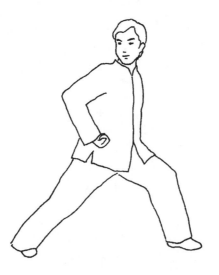

Fig 22.8 Bow-Arrow Stance

9. Raise your straight arms in front to shoulders' height with palms facing downward and fingers pointing forward. Squat down by bending your knees and raising your toes. Then stand up and drop your arms and heels.

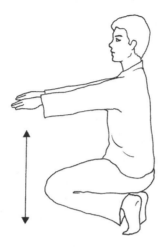

Fig 22.9 Squatting with Raised Heels

10. Stand with feet about a shoulder's width apart. Extend your straight arms sideways to shoulders' height, with palms facing downward and fingers pointing to both sides. Squat down without raising your heels. Stand up and repeat. This exercise is called "Three Levels to the Ground" in Shaolin Kungfu.

These exercises may appear simple, but if you can practice them properly and conscientiously, i.e. once or twice daily for at least three months, you will say good-bye to all aches not only at your hands and legs, but your whole body.

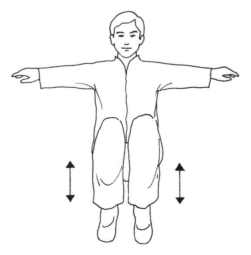

Fig 22.10 Three Levels to the Ground

Incredible Qigong Exercises

Would you believe that some qigong exercises can make you roll on the ground, shout loudly, walk like a bear or dance like a monkey and they are not of your own volition? Almost nobody would believe that; but the best thing is you can now test it yourself by following the exercise explained below. This opportunity was not available until recently, not even among most Chinese, because in the past qigong, the art of developing energy, was taught only to selected disciples.

Fortunately, the change of attitude from the feudalistic concept of "what is good should be kept for oneself" to the modern philosophy of "what is good should be shared with all people" has enabled this wonderful art of qigong to reach other people irrespective of race, culture and religion.

This form of qigong exercise is known as "Five-Animal Play", and was formalized by the great second century physician, Hua Tuo. Initially people thought that Hua Tuo imitated the movements and significance of the tiger, bear, deer, bird and monkey, to devise a set of exercise for health and longevity. However, recent research suggests that these movements were not pre-selected, but manifested spontaneously while the performer is in a qigong state of mind.

But why are there five animals, not four, six or any other number? Why do the movements resemble those of a tiger, bear, deer, bird and monkey, and not those of other creatures? And why do these movements manifest involuntarily?

The number is five because there are five different kinds of energy from the five "zang" or storage organs — lungs, kidneys, liver, heart and spleen. The energy of the pericardium, the sixth "zang", is similar to the heart energy. The energies of the six "fu" or transformation organs — colon, urinary bladder, gall bladder, small intestine, stomach and triple warmer — are similar to their corresponding "zang" organs.

Because of the different nature of the organs, as symbolized by the five elemental processes, different organ energies behave differently. When these organ energies are manifested outwardly as external body movements, they constitute five archetypes of movements. Hua Tuo and other masters used the five animals to symbolize these five archetypical movements.

When lung energy, for example, flows strongly and makes a person moves, the way he moves is different from the kind of movement made by kidney energy or energies from any other organs. As lung energy is generally powerful, it may make the person roar ferociously; as the outlet of the lung is the nose, it may make him snort fiercely. Different persons may roar or snort differently, or may perform other actions, yet these movements generated by vigorously flowing lung energy can be stylized into an archetype, and ancient masters used the tiger to represent such movements.

Movements caused by kidney energy will have different characteristics. As the kidney is responsible for the nourishment of the skeletal structure, vigourously flowing kidney energy may flow to the bones and make the performer walk upright like a bear. Liver energy affects the muscles, and may cause him to shape his fingers like the antler of a deer. Heart energy is related to joy, and its outlet is the tongue, making him twittering like a bird. Spleen energy is expressed through the mouth, causing the performer to make funny faces like a monkey. The movements described here are stylized; the actual movements of a performer may not be so clearly categorized.

If we are to ask why does kidney energy affect the bones and liver energy affect the muscles, and not the other way round, or why these functions are not performed by other organs, it is like asking why does the heart pump blood and the lungs operate breathing, and not the other way round, or why the circulatory and respiratory functions are not performed by the stomach or the gall bladder. The obvious answer is this is the way our body works.

The difference, nevertheless, is that western science has not discovered this knowledge about kidney and other organ energies which the Chinese have successfully used in their medical practices for ages. Western scientists, with their advanced technology, can contribute much to world knowledge if they care to test this information.

Can these energies make us move involuntarily, and sometimes in funny patterns? Yes, if we allow them, and generate them in appropriate qigong exercises. They are powerful and wonderful.

In fact these and other energies in our body are responsible for changing the air we breath and the food we eat into suitable nutrients, keeping millions of microbes in check which might otherwise make us lie in a hospital, regulating muscles in our eyes and nerves in our brain so that we know what we are reading, and performing countless other things to maintain a system of activities which we call living. If these energies are blocked or disharmonious, we will become ill.

The objective of the "Five-Animal Play" or similar exercises in a qigong genre known as "the art of self-manifested movements" or "induced qi flow", is to clear energy blockages and harmonize energy flow. How do we know where the blockages are or where the flow is not harmonious? They are where the illness is.

The most useful aspect of the exercise is that we do not have to know the exact spots of illness — indeed, in many instances we do not even realize that the illness exists; the flowing energy of the induced qi flow will cure that illness without our knowing!

Energy flows from areas of high energy to areas of low energy, and illness is located where energy level is low. To ask why is this so, is like asking why water flows from high levels to low levels. The answer in both cases is that is their natural properties.

For example, there may be many immediate causes of a liver disorder, such as stress, hardening of liver tissues, disruption of nervous impulses to and from the liver, microbe attacks, and other reasons still unknown to western medicine. But the root cause, from the Chinese medical perspective that views the disorder holistically, is disharmonious energy flow of the liver.

If energy flow is harmonious, negative emotions that produces stress will be flushed out, liver tissues will be bathed with nourishing energy that can "soften" diseased tissues, blockages will be cleared to allow smooth nerve function, harmful microbes will be killed or inhibited by defence-energy, and the natural abilities of the patient will be restored to overcome whatever abnormal conditions that cause illness. Induced qi flow exercises will harmonize the energy flow, thus curing the disorder.

The "Five-Animal Play" and similar induced qi flow exercises are invaluable; they are suitable for almost all diseases, except obvious improbabilities like a bullet in the stomach or a severed limb where surgery is needed. The following "Five-Animal Play" is expounded by the modern qigong master, Liang Shi Feng.

The Five-Animal Play

It is very useful, especially for beginners, to know the following points before attempting the "Five-Animal Play":

1. You will probably be very surprised at what you will do.
2. It is definitely non-religious.
3. Your self-manifested movements are caused by your enhanced energy flow, which is natural like your blood circulation, and not by such factors as benevolent or evil spirits as some imaginative people may like to believe.
4. Follow the instructions and advice carefully. Deviated practices may result in side-effects such as dizziness, palpitation and nausea. But do not be unduly worry; side-effects happen in every therapeutic method if it is improperly done. "Five-Animal Play" is probably safer than taking antibiotics or injection.
5. Let people who are likely to see your funny movements, if any, know that these movements are part of the exercise, so that they would not be alarmed. Ensure that your practice site is safe, such as far away from a steep drop, drains and sharp objects.
6. You may need many practices before you experience discernible involuntary movements, and the movements may not necessarily be as spectacular as a tiger's roar or a monkey's jump. On the other hand, before you are familiar with the exercise and have good control over it, it is advisable not to let your movements be too vigourous. Many people just sway gently like a happy willow.

7. The term "involuntarily" is used here relatively. Actually you are in control all the time; you can stop the exercise anytime you want, but you allow the movements to go on "involuntarily" because they are beneficial and you enjoy the experience.
8. Do not let anyone disturb you during the exercise.
9. Whatever the reason, do not stop the exercise abruptly. Always bring your movements to a gentle and graceful stop.
10. Many people find the exercise such a memorable experiment that they could not have dreamt it possible before. Now let us enjoy the "Five-Animal Play". Stand upright and relax. You must keep away all irrelevant thoughts throughout the exercise.

For men, use the left middle finger to press on the navel 49 times. Then drop the finger, and use the right middle finger to massage baihui, i.e. the energy point at the crown of the head, 10 times. For women, use the right middle finger on the navel and the left middle finger on baihui for the same numbers of times. Drop both arms at the sides after that.

Close your eyes gently and repeat the following a few times to yourself inside your heart:

> So calm and peaceful I become
> Drifting in clouds I'm so free
> Harmoniously my energy flow
> And I enjoy a spontaneous spree

Experience the sensation of what you say to yourself. Feel physically and mentally relaxed, that your vital energy is flowing smoothly without blockage all over your body, that it is so comfortably and naturally pleasant. Then gently think of your energy field at your abdomen (or, if you are not sure of what an energy field is, just think of your abdomen).

Then think of your vital energy at the crown of your head, flowing down like a cascade of waterfall all over your body. Think of the vital energy flowing and opening meridians (or energy pathways) from your head downward to your feet. Enjoy the tinkling sensations of energy flow, if any. Do this thinking or visualization three times.

Then think of your yintang (third eye) for about two or three seconds, followed by thinking of your two yongquan, i.e. the two energy points at the soles, for about six or seven seconds. (If you are not sure where the two yongquan are, just think of your soles.)

Your normal eyes are still close. Keep them close throughout the exercise, but later when you are familiar with the exercise, you may open your eyes if you like.

Gently focus your attention on your abdominal energy field (or on your abdomen). See your navel in your mind's eye. Forget about your normal nose breathing, and breath with your navel! This can be done by thinking of cosmic energy flowing into you through your navel. As your navel breaths in cosmic energy, you navel is being sucked backward. Do not do this physically; this should be done in visualization, or mere thinking. Think of your navel breathing five times, and by the fifth time, your navel is psychically sucked to the back of your waist, though it may not have moved physically.

In your mind's eye, see your navel pressing against your mingmen, i.e. the energy point at the back-middle of your waist. Focus your attention at the mingmen for about 6 or 7 seconds.

Then breathe with your navel again five times, with your navel psychically pushing forward as it breathes out. If you are puzzled by this concept, just think of energy flowing out from your body through your navel, and each time it flows out, your navel moves forward from the imagined position at the back. By the fifth breath, your navel has psychically returned to its original position (though physically it may not have moved at all).

Gently focus all your attention at your navel. Your mental eye looks at the navel; your ears listen to the navel, and your mind thinks of your navel, to the exclusion of all other sensations. Remain at this tranquil position focusing on the navel for about fifteen minutes, then complete the whole exercise.

However, if at any time during this fifteen minutes of focusing on your navel, you begin to move on your own, gently follow the movements. The movements are gentle at first, then gradually building up to active movements. You may move away from your original position, and even perform antics not of your volition. Some people may shout, laugh or cry, which are means of emotional release. Most people sway gracefully.

If your movements become vigourous and you are at the beginner's stage, it is advisable to slow down your movements. This can be simply done by an act of will. Just mentally instruct your movements to go slowly. If you have been intrigued by expressions like "mind over matter", this experience will show that you yourself have this ability.

After about 15-30 minutes of induced energy flow, gently tell your movements to slow down, then bring the movements to a graceful stop. Stand still for a few seconds, gently thinking of your abdomen. Complete the exercise by rubbing your palms together, then placing your warm palms on your eyes, dabbing them and opening them. Walk about briskly for about thirty steps, and feel how fresh and invigorated you are.

This "Five-Animal Play" is a priceless gift from Hua Tuo, who first devised it in the 2nd century, and from the modern qigong master, Liang Shi Feng, who generously revealed its secrets. It is one of the best answers from Chinese medicine to explain Jakob Henle's query concerning rheumatism, hysteria and cancer. (Please see the Preface.)

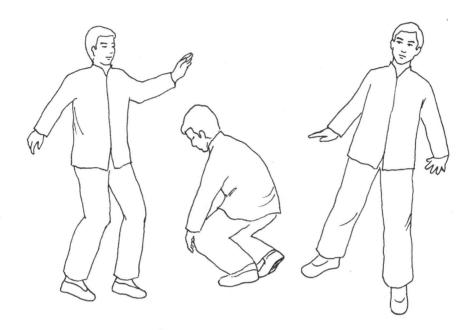

Fig 22.11
Some Spontaneous Movements from Five-Animal Play

According to Chinese medical thinking, rheumatism is caused by energy stagnation in or between body cells. "Five-Animal Play" is excellent for curing rheumatism as it promotes energy flow. People known to be hysterical, improve noticeably by practicing this or other qigong exercises, as enhanced energy flow helps to stabilize emotions. "Five-Animal Play" restores natural self-healing and regenerative abilities, thus contributing to the remission of cancer patients.

But even when you have this precious gift, you have to practice it properly and conscientiously, i.e. once or twice daily for at least three months, to obtain its benefits. It is understandable that many readers will find the exercise and its claim to promote health and longevity and cure almost any disease incredible; whether they would accept this generous offer is, of course, their own prerogative.

Many people, including Shakespeare, have said that there are more strange things in our world than in the stars. If you are keen to know some of these strange things, and benefit from them, the next two chapters on qigong will provide more examples.

23

THE ART OF ENERGY AND VITALITY
(Introduction to Qigong and Qigong Therapy)

The terms vitality and energy often feature in our language when we feel healthy and have a sense of well-being. If we observe animals and birds in their natural state a sense of strong energy or vitality is often apparent. What is this energy and where does it come from? Where does this energy go when we feel ill and listless? Is the experience of vitality a by-product of good health or is it the basis for health?

Judy Jacka.

The Wonders of Qigong

Chinese medicine all along has addressed itself to the questions in the above quotation, which we shall answer in this chapter. Energy, which the Chinese call "qi" (pronounced as "ch'i") is the basis of Chinese physiology, psychology, pathology, diagnosis, pharmacology, therapeutics, prognosis, and all other aspects of Chinese medicine. Every branch of Chinese medicine without exception deals with energy, and the one that is most directly concerned with energy is qigong therapy, which is an important aspect of qigong.

Qigong (pronounced as "ch'i kung") is an ancient art of developing energy, particularly for health, martial arts, mental training and spiritual fulfilment, irrespective of culture, race or religion. Until recently, qigong has been kept highly secretive, taught only to carefully selected disciples. In the past qigong was known by various names, such as the art of vitality and longevity, the art of inner force, and the art of wisdom. One major aspect or dimension of qigong which is specially used for preventing and curing illnesses, and promoting vitality and longevity, is known as health qigong and medical qigong, or qigong therapy.

Medical qigong or qigong therapy may be sub-divided into two types for convenience: one, where a qigong therapist treats a patient by such means as manipulating the patient's energy points and transmitting his own vital energy into the patient; and two, where the patient practices selected qigong exercises on his own for treatment. If we wish to be particular in classification, we can say that qigong therapy is used when a therapist is actively involved, medical qigong when the patient cures himself using qigong exercises, and health qigong when the purpose is not for curing diseases but for preventing illnesses, maintaining health and promoting longevity.

Nevertheless, as there is no rigid compartmentalization in the Chinese concept of the continuum from sickness and medicine to health and longevity, these three terms are often used interchangeably. In this way, qigong is an excellent unique health system in the world. Where else can you find the same art which can cure your diseases if you are sick, prevent you from succumbing to future illnesses if you are currently healthy, increase your energy and vitality so that you can appreciate your health in your daily work and play, and maintain this energy and vitality to your ripe old age — not only at the physical, but also at the emotional, mental and spiritual levels?

Enjoying these wonderful benefits, often unbelievable to the uninitiated, is one significant reason why I chose to specialize in qigong instead of traumatology, the speciality of three of my four masters.

However, the original reason for choosing qigong, I am ashamed to admit, was selfishness on my part. My master, Sifu Lai Chin Wah, who is better known as Uncle Righteousness, often cured patients free of charge; another master, Sifu Ho Fatt Nam, reminded me that traumatology patients were usually poor, as rich people were seldom exposed to injuries that result from hits and falls.

On the other hand, diseases that are usually and effectively treated by qigong therapy, like cardio-vascular diseases, diabetes and asthma, commonly afflict the affluence. Even in my idealistic younger days, I had the pragmatism to reason that if I would practice a healing art, I might choose one where patients could pay.

However, practicing qigong therapy have not made me financially rich, but I have become rich in many other ways. I can now understand why my masters, although they did not have a lot of money, led very rewarding lives, and I even have an inkling of why great physicians in ancient China like Hua Tuo and Zhang Zhong Jing would renounce luxurious lives as imperial physicians to practice medicine among poor people.

Through qigong I have helped literally hundreds of people to be relieved of their so-called incurable diseases, ranging from simple migraines and insomnia to severe illnesses like sexual impotency and cancer.

The joy of seeing patients recovering from their so-called incurable diseases, especially when impersonalization, mechanization and expensive fees are absent, is something that money cannot buy, something that contributes to making medicine a noble profession.

Yin-Yang Harmony in Qigong

How qigong can achieve the wonderful benefits of curing and preventing illnesses, promoting health and longevity, is closely connected with Judy Jacka's questions in the quotation above.

The energy that qigong develops is the very same energy that sustains and operates life. It is the energy that coalesces into subatomic particles which constitute all your body cells, that transmits all impulses to and from every part of your body for precise and delicate cooperation, that controls microbes that may cause you trouble, that regulates all your necessary emotional and mental activities, and does all the myriad jobs that you are normally unaware of, but that are essential for you, me and everyone else to be alive. It is our vital energy or life force.

Where does this vital energy come from? Normally, about eighty percent of it comes from the air we breathe, and twenty percent from the food we eat.

In Chinese terms, this process is known as transforming heaven energy and earth energy into vital energy. Heaven energy is absorbed by the lungs from the air, and earth energy provided by the stomach from food and drinks. "Fire" energy from the heart, and "water" energy from the kidneys are necessary for the transformation process.

We do this all the time, but practicing qigong will greatly enhance this natural ability, and qigong therapy will restore this natural function should it get out of order sometimes.

This means that, according to Chinese medical philosophy, even if you have a lot of fresh air, and a lot of food, if your heart and your kidneys are not functioning properly, you still cannot produce the vital energy efficiently.

On the other hand, even if the heart and the kidneys are functioning well, but if the lungs or the stomach are not processing the heaven energy or the earth energy, then the production of vital energy is also affected. When any one of these four types of energy — heaven, earth, fire or water —is not available in the proper proportion, the Chinese refer to this unnatural situation as yin-yang disharmony.

The aim of qigong, as well as all other branches of Chinese medicine, is to restore and maintain this yin-yang harmony.

Yin-yang harmony applies to countless other situations. In the production of vital energy from heaven and earth energy, toxic waste, figuratively known as "polluted energy", is also produced. If this polluted energy or toxic waste is not disposed of efficiently, it will affect the smooth flow of vital energy.

Translated into conventional medical terms, this means, among other things, polluted energy may affect the flow of electric impulses along the autonomous nervous system, thus affecting the feed-back system, which may result in organic disorders.

This unnatural situation is also known as yin-yang disharmony; but whereas in the earlier example, yin refers to earth energy and water energy, and yang to heaven energy and fire energy, here yin refers to meridians carrying impulses from various organs to the "heart" or mind, and yang from the "heart" or mind to the various organs. Qigong is an excellent way to clear energy blockages, including blockages caused by toxic waste, thereby restoring yin-yang harmony.

Such energy blockage, which disrupts the smooth functioning of the autonomous nervous system, explains where energy goes to when we feel ill and listless. The vital energy is blocked from going to where it should naturally go, which may result in infectious, organic or psychiatric diseases.

For example, disorders like cold, migraine, rheumatism and hysteria, may occur. Energy blockage hampers the flow of vital energy to cleanse away cold viruses. Energy blockages at the head may result in pains, causing migraine, or resulting in emotional oppression, causing hysteria. Energy blockages in or between cells in the body causes rheumatism.

When the blockages are cleared, by qigong or other means, the disorders will be cured. Why this is so will be discussed in some detail after we have answered Jacka's questions.

There are also two other possibilities explaining our lack of energy when we feel ill and listless. Besides energy blockage, which may be expressed as excessive yin at the site of blockage, the patient may not have much energy to start with in the first place, which is known as insufficient yang. In both cases, the yin-yang disharmony is due to yang deficiency, which is a common cause of most diseases.

Secondly, the patient may have a lot of energy, but it is not properly balanced. In a hypertension patient, for example, there is too much rising liver energy but insufficient kidney energy, which can be expressed as excessive yang on top and insufficient yin below. The therapeutic principle is to readjust the energy balance by bringing down excessive yang energy, and enhancing insufficient yin energy.

It is worthy to note that yin-yang harmony is natural. This is a statement not of metaphysics or speculative philosophy, but referring to medicine and health. By nature, our body in its countless, almost divine ways, maintains health and vitality. Every moment of our life, our body successfully fights hostile microbes, repair wear and tear in all our tissues and organs, and ensures that we are in control of our emotions and mental faculties. It is only when one or more of our body parts fail to function naturally, that illnesses occur. Yin-yang disharmony describes a temporary unnatural situation in our body. Qigong directly employs energy flow to restore or maintain yin-yang harmony.

Hence, the experience of vitality, which is the manifestation of harmonious energy flow, is the basis for health. Health is the product of vitality, not vice versa. When our vital energy is flowing smoothly, when yin-yang is in harmony, which is a natural phenomenon, health is the direct result. If the flow of vital energy is disrupted, if yin-yang becomes disharmonious, illnesses will appear. It is not the other way round: it is not that as the result of an illness, energy flow becomes disrupted and yin-yang becomes disharmonious.

Restoring or maintain yin-yang harmony can be accomplished in many different ways. Some of these ways and their underlying principles, as in herbal medicine, external medicine, traumatology, acupuncture, massage therapy and health exercises, have been discussed in previous chapters.

It is significant to note that unless we have a sound knowledge of Chinese medical philosophy, it is easy for us to be misled by descriptions like "The Chinese believe that all kinds of illnesses can be overcome by restoring yin-yang. Yin refers to whatever is negative, dark, cold, internal and retrogressive; yang refers to all that is positive, bright, hot, external and progressive."

The harm is aggravated when the above statement about Chinese medicine is actually true; but the danger is that without background knowledge, a great profound truth can be made to appear ridiculous.

In the same way, it can be quite ridiculous to a Chinese patient who knows little about western medicine to be told that to cure his illness he is to have a huge needle containing some unknown liquid injected into his thigh, or various frightening wires connected to his body so that some electricity will be charged into him.

Just as the loss will be more to this ignorant patient than the doctor who prescribes such medication; in the case of misleading information on Chinese medicine, the loss will be more to western societies who would be denied a proper understanding of an effective medical system, than to Chinese medicine which would continue to serve its followers effectively irrespective of how misinformed writers may describe it.

Qigong Therapy and Infectious Diseases

Although the specific reasons why or how qigong therapy cure diseases may be complex, they can nevertheless be summarized into two main principles. These two principles apply to all other branches of Chinese medicine — herbal medicine, external medicine, traumatology, acupuncture, massage therapy and health exercises — but it is most obvious in qigong therapy.

The two principles, which are interrelated and have been mentioned in the preceding section, are cleansing meridians (which means clearing blockages to ensure smooth energy flow) and harmonizing yin-yang. Of course, if quoted out of context, this statement can be quite ludicrous.

Using the conventional classification of diseases into infectious, organic and psychiatric, let us see how cleansing meridians and harmonizing yin-yang can cure illnesses. Infectious and organic diseases are discussed below, leaving psychiatric disorders to a later chapter.

By nature we can cure ourselves of all kinds of infectious diseases. If this premise were false, mankind would have been wiped out by pathogenic micro-organisms long, long ago. Why, then, some of us at some time fall prey to infectious diseases? In Chinese medical thinking, which comfortably forgets about the exact species of microbes involved (since we can naturally overcome all kinds of microbes, it does not really matter what particular kinds of microbes are involved), this can be due to deficient yin or excessive yang.

Yin deficiency is caused by a general weakening of the body, and may be brought about by numerous factors like worry, grief, lack of sleep, exercise or proper food, and stressful living. Whatever is the contributing factor, the immediate cause is insufficient defence-energy to contain hostile microbes.

Yang excessiveness is caused by an increase of micro-pathogens, in amount or potency. This may be the result of taking in contaminated food, inhaling air with virulent microbes, or sustaining a cut in the skin that allow microbes to penetrate the body. The ultimate factor is that the microbes have become too powerful for our defence-energy at the infected site to handle.

In qigong therapy, like in acupuncture and massage therapy, the therapist opens relevant energy points of his patient to stimulate defence-energy to flow to the infected site, readjusts energy levels of the patient to attain yin-yang balance, or spread the concentration of infectious microbes over a wider area, so that the body's defence system can overcome them more easily, and then flush them out through breathing, sweating and other means.

The therapist may also transmit his own vital energy into the patient to enhance the latter's energy. In medical qigong, the patient attempts to realize the same objectives on his own by means of appropriate qigong movements, breath control and meditative exercises.

Research has shown that the qi or energy transmitted by a qigong master on to disks of cultured cells of influenza, gangrene and cancer, killed 80%, 30% and 50% of these cells after five minutes of qi transmission. Other researches show that practicing qigong improves the immune and defence systems tremendously.

However, unless a person is already advanced in qigong (in which case he is unlikely to be inflicted with infectious or any diseases), employing qigong therapy or medical qigong to cure infectious diseases is a very slow process. Hence it is not suitable for acute illnesses, which, leaving aside the question of side effects from antibiotics, is probably best treated by western medicine if a cure is available.

Practicing qigong, however, is an excellent form of preventive medicine. If your vital energy is powerful and flowing harmoniously, infection cannot develop even though sufficient infectious micro-organisms that would have caused sickness in another person, are present in your body.

Qigong and Organic Diseases

The forte of qigong is in curing and preventing organic or degenerative diseases, the top killer in the world today, surpassing even wars and motor accidents. In every minute and in all of us, cholesterol is being deposited on the inner walls of blood vessels, calcium is forming into stones in our urinary bladder and kidneys, pollutants are choking our lungs, acids are pouring into our stomach, sugar is continuously added to our blood stream, poison is clogging our body and brain cells.

Yet, we do not normally get high blood pressure, bladder or kidney stones, asthma, gastritis, diabetes, rheumatism and migraine. Why? Thanks to our natural systems. As soon as the cholesterol, calcium, pollutants, acid, sugar and various poisons reach a critical level, intricate reactions in our body will trigger off the production of the relevant chemicals to neutralize the excess residues.

This is possible only if our vital energy is flowing harmoniously; if energy blockage disrupts the flow of vital energy, our natural yin-yang harmony will be affected. In other words, if there is disruption to our intricate feed-back system, our body systems may not function naturally.

Chinese physicians regard hypertension as the result of excessive rising liver energy due to insufficient kidney energy, an explanation understandably difficult for those not familiar with Chinese medical philosophy. Let us now use a different perspective, a viewpoint from western medical philosophy, to examine how qigong can cure this major medical problem in western societies.

The following description is my theory, my attempt at an explanation. As such it may be wrong; what actually happened may or may not be what is explained below. Nevertheless, the theory is derived from sound Chinese medical principles, and is based on numerous cases of hypertension patients relieved of their illness after practicing qigong from me.

I use the terms "cure" and "relieved" subjectively, in a sense that these former patients now no longer suffer from hypertension, and there are no relapses over many years. There were no scientifically controlled experiments, no quantitative records, because such measures are beyond my knowledge and competency.

If any research scientists are interested and would like to investigate my theory, I will be most happy to contribute, and there is reasonable optimism to believe that if the theory is valid, it may lead to some exciting medical discoveries.

Blood vessels are linked by meridians to the "master-mind", which is usually referred to as the "heart" in Chinese medical philosophy. In classical Chinese, the term "heart" often refers not to that tough organ which pumps blood, but to the mind.

There are two sets of meridians, conveniently called yin-meridians and yang-meridians, which correspond to the parasympathetic and sympathetic autonomous nerves. Yin-meridians flow from the blood vessels to the "heart" (or, perhaps, brain), whereas yang-meridians flow from the "heart" to the blood vessels.

The yin-meridians continuously carry impulses from the blood vessels to the "heart", informing it of the exact situation at the blood vessels. When the deposition of cholesterol at the blood vessels reaches a critical level, the "heart" on receiving the information, will send out signals along the yang-meridians to instruct the blood vessels (or any relevant parts of the body) to produce the necessary chemicals to neutralize the excess cholesterol.

This goes on subconsciously all the time in all of us. If there is an excess of, say, 50 units of cholesterol in your blood vessels, 50 units of yin impulses will flow along your yin-meridians to your "heart", which will send 50 units of yang impulses along the yang-meridian to the blood vessels, giving instruction to produce 50 units of neutralizing chemicals. This is expressed as yin-yang harmony.

Hence, so long as your body systems function normally, the more excess cholesterol you have in your blood vessels, the more chemicals will be produced to neutralize it. The Asian diet is traditionally rich in cholesterol, yet their incidence of high blood pressure is not proportionately higher than that of the Americans or the Europeans.

Problem arises when this yin-yang harmony is disturbed, like when the energy flowing along the yin-meridians or the yang-meridians is affected. This happens when "polluted energy" — which may result from metabolic waste not efficiently cleared out from the body, from negative emotions due to stressful conditions, or from other factors — accumulates and stagnates along the meridians.

Let us say energy blockage occurs along the yin-meridians. Blockage, here, does not necessarily mean that no energy at all passes through the meridians, in which case that person may die; it means that smooth flow of energy is significantly interrupted. For example, if 20 units of yin impulses are blocked, then only the remaining 30 units reach the "heart", giving a false picture that there are only 30 units of excess cholesterol at the blood vessels when actually there are 50. Please refer to Fig 23.1.

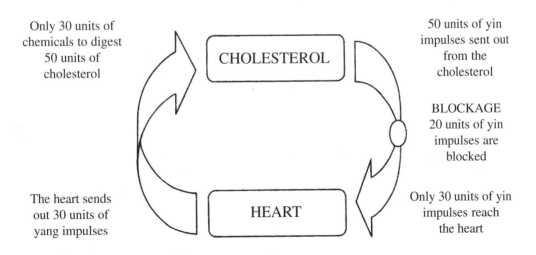

Only 30 units of chemicals to digest 50 units of cholesterol

50 units of yin impulses sent out from the cholesterol

CHOLESTEROL

BLOCKAGE 20 units of yin impulses are blocked

The heart sends out 30 units of yang impulses

HEART

Only 30 units of yin impulses reach the heart

Fig 23.1 Yin-Blockage Causing Hypertension
(Diagrammatic)

The "heart" therefore releases only 30 units of yang impulses along the yang-meridian, which will result in the production of only 30 units of chemicals to neutralize the excess cholesterol. 20 units of cholesterol are not neutralized, and as this excess accumulates in time, it will constrict the blood vessels, causing high blood pressure.

Similarly, yin-yang disharmony will result if energy blockage occurs in the yang-meridians instead of the yin-meridians. On receiving the right information from the yin-meridians, the "heart" transmits 50 units of yang impulses as signals for the production of the right amount of chemicals to neutralize the excess cholesterol. If, say, 15 units of yang impulses are blocked along the yang-meridians, then only 35 units reach the blood vessels, resulting in the production of 35 units of chemicals when 50 units are needed. In time, hypertension will occur.

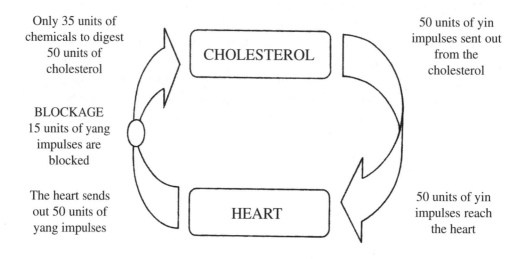

Fig 23.2 Yang-Blockage Causing Hypertension
(Diagrammatic)

If we take a drug to dilate the blood vessels, we merely treat the symptom, not the cause. If we take a cross-section of the blood vessels, there is no doubt that it will show the vessels are constricted. But this structural defect is a symptom; the cause is a functional disorder. Even if we rectify the structural defect, it will inevitably recur unless the malfunction is corrected.

This explains why there is much dissatisfaction over western medicine in its treatment of organic or degenerative diseases, because all its expensive instruments are geared to diagnose the structural defects of these organs, and all consequent therapeutics treat the symptoms.

THE ART OF ENERGY AND VITALITY

Qigong therapy attacks the problem at its cause. It clears the energy blockage so that vital energy can flow smoothly, thereby restoring the yin-yang harmony. When yin-yang harmony is restored, our body will produce the right amount of chemicals to neutralize the unwanted cholesterol, and recovery from hypertension becomes a matter of course, without the need for any medication nor surgery.

The above theory is necessarily simplified so as to bring out its salient principles, which are similarly applicable to other organs. If the meridians are connected to the lungs, for example, the medical problem becomes asthma, hay fever and other lung disorders. If they are connected to the kidneys, the problem may be kidney stones or kidney failure.

This explains that the same set of holistic qigong exercises can be used to cure a wide range of organic diseases, including some diagonally opposite disorders! For example, people who are obese or underweight, or suffering from illnesses like indigestion and gastritis can be relieved of their complaints by practicing the same set of qigong exercises. According to Chinese medical thinking, obesity is more a problem of hormonal balance than diet and exercise. Obese persons may take little food, yet their mass continue to grow. Excessive vigourous exercises to burn away extra mass is not only a waste of energy, but may be injurious to health.

In Chinese terms, both obesity and skinniness, or indigestion and gastritis, are due to yin-yang disharmony. In the case of obesity and indigestion, there is insufficient production of the right chemicals to break down excess mass in the body or excess food in the stomach; whereas in skinniness and gastritis, once production of the appropriate chemicals is in process, the respective glands do not know when to stop. The root cause for these disorders is a failure of harmonious energy flow, or the feed-back system.

Often, it does not matter very much where the disruption of energy flow occurs; sometimes it may occur far away from the identifiable disease location at another end of the meridian network. For example the energy blockage that affects blood vessels may not be found at or around the vessels, but perhaps at the intestines or the legs connected by meridians. Yet, once the harmonious energy flow is restored, the right chemicals of the right amounts will be produced at the right time and place. Hence, the same set of holistic qigong exercises that promotes harmonious energy flow for the whole body, can be effective for different diseases. On the other hand, a particular disease can be cured by many different qigong exercises.

Thematic and Holistic Approaches

Qigong therapy is of two major types: thematic and holistic. In thematic qigong therapy, the therapist, like an acupuncturist, has to know in great detail the complex working of the meridian network and related systems so that he can manipulate with his fingers where an acupuncturist would use needles, the appropriate energy points to influence his patient's energy flow to accomplish desirable results. He has an advantage over the acupuncturist in that he can channel his own vital energy into his patient (something many readers have to see to believe), or instruct the patient to perform particular qigong exercises for specific needs — therapeutic means that are not normally available to the acupuncturist.

In holistic qigong therapy, the therapist is sparred the trouble of memorizing and accurately locating hundreds of energy points, for he can induce his patient's vital energy to flow in a general way (like the induced qi flow exercise in the previous chapter), that can cure an incredibly wide range of diseases. Alternately, he can prescribe holistic qigong exercises which have holistic curing effects.

In practical situations, however, especially if they depend on patients' fees for a living, some qigong therapists will often need the thematic approach, not that it is necessarily better, but that besides not wanting their clients to have the impression that they use only one general method for all diseases, it is also easier to justify collection of fees each time their patients consult them.

This conflict of interest between a therapist as a healer and as an entrepreneur can be strikingly brought to the fore in an excellent holistic qigong exercise like the "Five-Animal Play" described in the previous chapter.

If performed properly and regularly, this qigong exercise is worth at least as much as what a patient would have to pay for an expensive surgical operation, for it can enable him to be cured, without having to endure surgery, organic diseases which many people may think surgery is indispensable! But for a qigong therapist, giving only oral instructions and personal supervision for a few sessions, without the need to provide supportive, symptomatic medication over a long period, nor the necessity of expensive surgical technology, it is difficult for him to charge expensive fees even if he wanted to.

This incidental comment is meant not to show the difficulty of becoming wealthy through practicing qigong therapy, but that an inexpensive yet effective medical alternative readily available may sometimes be passed over by some healers for economic rather than professional reasons.

Actually, in Chinese medical thought the cardinal criteria for good medicine are that it must be cheap, effective and easily available. Medical qigong fulfils these criterias excellently, for once you know the method, it is free, effective and can be practiced almost anywhere.

Medical Qigong Exercises

The following medical qigong exercises are meant for relieving high blood pressure. While having the service of a qigong therapist, such as for opening relevant energy points, channelling energy and correcting technical mistakes, will certainly speed up recovery, patients can still obtain remarkable results practicing on their own. They must, however, practice daily for at least a few months. It is expected that readers not familiar with qigong therapy may find the exercises odd.

Stand upright and relaxed with feet about a foot apart, and arms hanging loosely at both sides. (Weak or old patients can perform the exercise sitting down.) Close your eyes gently and smile from the heart. Take your own time to relax yourself along the following three linear regions:

1. Relax both sides of your head, then think of the relaxation moving slowly down both sides of your neck to both your arms to the tips of your ten fingers.
2. Relax the front of your head, then let the relaxation move slowly down your face, down the front of your body, down your legs to your ten toes.
3. Relax the back of your head, then let the relaxation move slowly down the back of your neck, the back of your body, down the back of your legs to your soles.

Repeat the relaxation process three times. You may, whenever you like, pause or linger at any part of your body for a few seconds, thinking of that part being totally relaxed.

After performing the relaxation down the three linear regions thrice, gently think of your qihai vital point, which is located about three inches below your navel, for about five minutes. Qihai means "sea of energy". This energy point is the seat of the middle energy field, known as "zhong dan tian" in Chinese. Do not worry about your breathing throughout the exercise, but it is very important that your thinking of this energy field must be done gently.

Then rub your two palms together to warm them, and place them on your eyes. Dab your eyes with your palms as you open your eyes. Then massage your face gently and walk about briskly for about twenty steps. This completes the first part of the exercise. Perform the whole process in the morning, evening and at night for about two weeks, then progress to part two.

In the second part, the whole exercise is the same except that instead of focusing your mind gently at your abdominal energy field, you gently think of your two soles. At each of your sole there is an important energy point known as yongquan, which means "gushing spring". Practice the second part three times a day in the morning, evening and at night for about two weeks. By then, you may feel energy gushing out at your yongquan energy points like springs.

After about two weeks, you can proceed to part three. Repeat the exercise, but focus your mind at your mingmen vital point, which is in the middle of your waist at your back. Mingmen means "gate of life", giving us an indication of how important this energy point is. Practice daily for about two weeks. In all these three parts, just let your breathing be spontaneous or natural.

Part four is the exercise proper and should be attempted only after you have spent about a month and a half on the preliminary three parts. After relaxing your three linear regions thrice, think of your yongquan or "gushing spring" for a few seconds. Then slowly raise both arms from your sides, with palms facing skyward, until they meet high above your head. Please refer to Fig 23.3. Next, turn the palms so that they face downwards. Slowly lower your palms together from high above your head down your face, the front part of your body, then down your two legs, bending your knees and squatting down as your palms pass down your legs. Then slowly stand up.

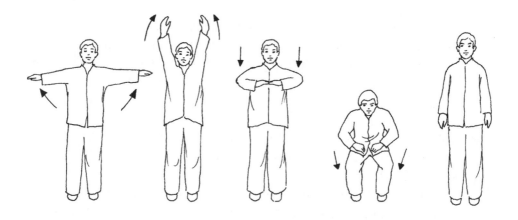

Fig 23.3 Medical Qigong for Hypertension

Breath control is used in part four to facilitate energy flow. It is very important that the breathing must be done gently. As you raise your arms, gently breathe in through your nose. As you lower your palms from up above your head to your feet, gently breath out through your mouth. As you stand up, gently relax your breath, without breathing in nor out. Besides, as you lower your hands, gently visualize that you are bringing your energy down from your head to your feet. Repeat this about ten times.

As you progress, you may gradually increase to about twenty times. Complete the exercise by gently focusing your mind at your qihai, or yongquan, or mingmen. You may, if you like, take turns to focus your mind at these points during different practice sessions. As you progress you can increase the time for mind focusing.

There is no fixed time for the duration of the whole exercise, but a rough guide is between 15 to 30 minutes. You have to practice the exercise three times a day for few months if you want results.

Although this qigong exercise is a thematic healing method for hypertension, it is beneficial for relieving many other diseases. The deep relaxation at the start of the exercise, for example, is not only an effective therapeutic technique for almost all illnesses, including emotional and mental disorders, but is also very useful for stress management, for which qigong is excellent.

Hypertension and other cardiovascular diseases kill more people in western societies than anything else does. The second top killer is cancer. Qigong not only provides an effective cure for both these killer diseases, but more importantly an excellent preventive system as well.

It is understandable that many readers will be sceptical of this claim, but the next chapter will explain the principles and practice of qigong against cancer that may bring hope to cancer patients, new ideas to oncologists, as well useful information which may one day save your life.

CANCER CAN BE CURED!
(Cosmic Energy and Mind in Healing)

Why do some people get cancer and others do not? We spoke of the non-smoker who develops lung cancer and the heavy smoker who does not. Why are some people more at risk than others? The same question, of course, can be asked about any carcinogen. For all the millions spent on research, medical science has yet to come up with acceptable answers to these questions. None of the studies help us understand why we get cancer.

Dr. Frederick B. Levenson.

Treat the Patient, Not his Cells

The question of cancer, which the renowned oncologist, Dr D. W. Smithers, explains is "just a shortened way of saying something that cannot be simply defined", brings us to an important aspect of perspective. If we take the western perspective and called an unknown disease cancer, that describes the disease as incurable. But if we take the Chinese perspective, there is no such thing as an incurable disease.

The Chinese approach is, instead of desperately working on the unknown and undefined, to work on the known and established. In other words, instead of attempting to pinpoint the unlimited exogenous factors that may bring about symptoms collectively called cancer, the Chinese physician finds out which natural function or functions of the patient has gone wrong that caused his inability to react effectively against these factors, which in his normal condition he can handle them efficiently.

It is heart-warming to remember that exogenous causes of cancer and all other dreadful diseases affects everybody, but if their natural functions are operating normally, they can overcome these causes, usually without their knowing. We are free from cancer not because we are free from carcinogens, but because we have the natural ability to overcome them.

The more I read on cancer, the more it occurs to me that if western theoretical knowledge is right, Chinese qigong — not surgery, chemotherapy or radiotherapy — will provide the right treatment procedure. But, unlike in western science where incredible details about the cell and other related topics are known, such reductionist and quantitative information from the qigong perspective in its relation to cancer cure, is conspicuously lacking.

This lack is due to two main factors. The concept of cancer as it is normally known in the west, is not found in traditional Chinese medical philosophy. The nearest concept in Chinese medicine is "poisonous or malignant growth", which is not regarded as fatal nor incurable. The Chinese term for cancer is "ai", but it is translated from the western concept, and not a traditional Chinese term. Secondly, the Chinese explanation is holistic rather than particular; it relates the cause of disease to the patient as a whole person, instead of finding the cause in minute parts.

It is precisely for this reason, treating a cancer patient as a whole person instead of just attacking his misguided cells, that Chinese medical philosophy and practice have much to offer western oncologists. When it is the other way round, to investigate microscopic bodily units and their operation, the Chinese have a lot to learn from the west.

While western cancer research and conventional treatment that adopt the cell as the focus of their conceptual framework seems to me to be leading into a blind alley, I am particularly impressed with western efforts that attempt to cure people of cancer, instead of killing cancer cells in them. These efforts inevitably regard cancer patients as whole persons, with emphasis on the patients' state of mind rather than the cellular condition of his body; and they are generally successful.

As early as 1848, the tremendous influence of the patient's mind on his own body was demonstrated by Dr John Elliotson in his *Cure of a true cancer of the Female Breast with Mesmerism.* In our present time, Dr Alex Forbes, speaking from his experiences from treating about a thousand cancer patients at his Bristol Cancer Centre, says "of those who really do follow the method in all its aspects, all feel better and have a better quality of life than before". Dr Forbes' method involves the patient as a whole person, not just prescribing medication for his disease. Dr Bernauer Newton who initiated hypnotherapy on cancer patients in his Newton Centre of Los Angeles confirms that "it is the profoundly altered state of consciousness that is the single most important factor".

Despite their success and the fact that they were eminently qualified in conventional medicine, these brave pioneers were mocked by their mediocre colleagues, as it has been repeated so frequently throughout the history of western medicine. How would mediocre practitioners react to ideas coming from alternative medicine, although the so-called alternative medicine may be the norm in other cultures? In October 1983 the editorial of *The Lancet* aptly reminded doctors that "when so much medical practice is not supported by rigorous scientific testing, what right have clinicians to criticize the practitioners of alternative therapy?"

Basic Information Regarding the Cell

After spending millions of dollars and thousands of man-hours, western researchers have come up with an admirable explanation on the cause of cancer, though they are not so sure of its remedy. It is useful to understand their discovery, then examine if qigong makes any sense in the light of this knowledge.

According to western research, cancer is caused by the proliferated production of cells that have escaped the natural control of the body mechanism. An adult has about 100 trillion cells in his body. Cells die every second, but they are constantly replaced. Each day an adult produces about 300 billion cells to replace his cells lost. In a healthy person, cell production and cell loss are beautifully balanced; in Chinese medical thinking such a balance is called yin-yang harmony. Cancer happens when this balance is lost, or in Chinese term when yin-yang disharmony occurs.

Western geneticists provide a marvelous, detailed picture of cell production. There are forty six chromosomes in the nucleus of each human cell. In the chromosomes are molecules of DNA (deoxyribonucleic acid), which are arranged like "double helix" made up of four bases, coded as A (for adenine), G (guanine), T (thymine) and C (cytosine). Along one of the double strands of DNA, these four bases may be arranged in any order, but A is always matched with T, G with C, and vice versa, on the other strand. For example, if one strand consists of CGTACTAAA ..., the other strand will always consist of GCATGATTT .... These code letters represent only a very short portion of a strand; there are thousands of these four bases in the A-T, G-C combinations in a chromosome.

These bases are grouped into threes, known as triplet codons. Hence the above bases will form three triplet codons, CGT ACT AAA, in one strand of DNA, and GCA TGA TTT in the corresponding strand. These triplet codons are what we call genes, and are extremely important. They determine that the cells which are supposed to form your liver, for example, will form your liver, and not the stomach of an elephant. This is achieved by the processes of replication and transcription.

In replication, two strands of DNA "unzip" or separate, so that the corresponding bases will be synthesized. Hence the above portion CGT ACT AAA will have a new set of GCA TGA TTT attached to it, and the original GCA TGA TTT which has been separated from its original CGT ACT AAA, will have a new set of CGT ACT AAA in its corresponding strand. In this way the DNA reproduces its exact replica.

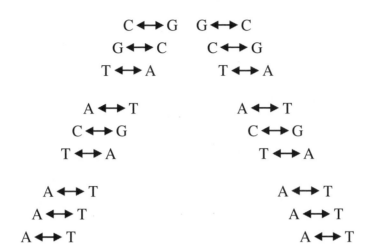

Fig 24.1 Replication of DNA

In transcription, the DNA transcribes its codes onto molecules of RNA (ribonucleic acid). The bases in the RNA are like those of the DNA except that T (thymine) is always replaced with U (uracil). Hence, the portion CGT ACT AAA of the DNA strain will produce the GCA UGA UUU portion in the RNA strain. RNA is usually a single strand, and it passes into the cytoplasm of the cell and acts like a template to reproduce other cells which will be exactly like the mother cell.

It is interesting to note that although traditional Chinese medicine knows almost nothing about DNA, RNA and cell division, their principles of yin-yang, wu xing (five elemental processes), and bagua (pakua or eight trigrams) can be used as philosophical frame-work to explain cell mechanism! The double strands of DNA and the A-T and G-C combinations are typical of yin-yang operation.

Western scientists, who are still uncertain about the underlying principles governing the formative order of the four bases, may derive some unexpected concepts leading to important discoveries if they apply the principle of the five elemental processes, which the Chinese insist are applicable at levels ranging from the subatomic to the galaxies. The triplet bases leading to the sixty four combinations perfectly fit the bagua principle, whose philosophy may provide western researchers with new insights.

Theory on the Cause of Cancer

As we produce billions of cells a day to replace cell loss (and for growth in children), it is not unreasonable that accidents may sometimes happen, i.e. some cells may have their DNA or RNA codes disturbed. Out of the billions of times of cell division a day, even if just one accident occurs, resulting in just one cell with a mutated DNA or RNA code, if left unchecked, it will be sufficient to cause cancer. But do not worry: we have unbelievably wonderful natural controls to check cancerous cells. The British Cancer Help Centre says:

> Cancer cells are common to us all. Many people are not aware that each one of us continually produces cancer cells in our bodies, cells which, for the most part, are kept in balance by the body immune system.

Even if cancer has surfaced, "if the body's own natural defence system can be brought back into action, healing will almost always follow," the centre assures us.

The Australian immunologist and Nobel Prize Laureate Sir Frank MacFarlane Burnet, confirming the established fact that mutations occur from time to time in both the body cells and the germ cells, says that "if a carcinogenic process is to succeed, these (immunological) controls must be eliminated."

Why then one in five persons in the United States and all other industrialized nations die of cancer? Cancer is not the problem only of the west. Dr Adel Zaatal, the medical superintendent of the Penang Mount Miriam Hospital, the only cancer hospital in South East Asia, says that one in three persons will develop cancer. Medical scientists suggest three main factors that cause cell mutation: chemical carcinogens, radiation and viruses.

The list of chemical carcinogens is so alarming that many oncologists wonder whether we are staying in an ocean of carcinogens. The following are only some of the common carcinogens: arsenic, asbestos, benzi-dine, benzpyrene, carbon tetrachloride, chromium compounds, lead, nickel compounds, oils, petroleum products, cigarette smoke, pitch, hydrocarbons, cobalt, soot and tar.

Dr Frederick B. Levenson gives an interesting report pertaining to two research scientists implanting quarters and dimes in rats' abdomens. Sure enough the rats developed cancer and died. The scientists concluded that "even close proximity to this highly toxic pollutant could be a risk and suggested that it should be removed from the environment. With almost reckless disregard for their own safety, they asked that everyone in the country to send their quarters and dimes, preferably in rolls, to them."

Yet, out of the 4 million cases of cancer between 1900 and 1950, only 500 were caused by chemicals. Professor Heinz Oettel wrote that "External chemical influences cannot — except for cigarette smoking — have anything like the significance ascribed to them as causes of human cancer."

Almost all oncologists agree that radiation is a serious cause of DNA or RNA mutation. The most notorious example is the very high incidence of leukaemia among survivors of the Hiroshima and Nagasaki atomic bomb explosions. Developing cancer is a perpetual occupational risk of radiologists and radiographers.

DNA or RNA mutation due to radioactive material may be caused by free radicals produced by our body. These highly radioactive free radicals are actually necessary in our body, and are used by our immune and defence systems to kill or neutralize hostile micro-organisms. However, if they escape the body's natural control systems, they may cause DNA mutation or give trouble to the brain.

Although it is extremely cruel, using viruses to induce cancer in experimental animals is one of the main procedures in cancer research. Luckily or unluckily, depending on one's attitude, cancer viruses, as far as our present knowledge tells us, cannot cause cancer in humans. Otherwise, cancer would become a fearful contagious disease. On the other hand, many virologists and immunologists regret that because it is not infectious in humans, they miss the opportunity to find a vaccine that can prevent cancer, though they would not be able to develop any antibiotics against it, because it is a viral and not a bacterial infection.

However, they have probably ignored the fact that we already have some unidentified but wonderful natural vaccines or antibodies against cancer viruses. About a hundred prisoners in Ohio volunteered for a daring experiment where they were injected with animal cancer viruses. Tumours developed but later subsided and never returned. When cancer viruses were injected into some volunteers the second time, they recovered much faster, demonstrating the marvelous effects of our immune system.

There are more than thirty different types of adeno-viruses which cause the common cold in man. In 1962 Sir John Trentin proved that Type 12 of these viruses could cause cancer in hamsters.

In the same year Dr Robert J Huebner found that Type 18 also caused cancer in these poor experimental creatures. Later Type 7 and 31 were added to the list. In 1965 adeno-virus 3 was added, but it took a long time to cause cancer, after 275 days in new-born hamsters. It is of great significance to note that these viruses that cause cancer in hamsters only cause the comparatively harmless common cold in us.

So, the next time you have a cold, it could be a blessing; it may be your self defence and immune systems overcoming the cancer viruses.

As chemical carcinogens, radiation and viruses only answer why some people develop cancer, but not why most other people who should have it actually do not, we have to look for a better explanation elsewhere. Many experts presently believe that our mind has a tremendous influence on whether we get cancer or not. An accumulating body of evidence now suggests that psychological factors can induce cancer or promote its growth and proliferation. Dr Frederick B. Levenson, who proposed the unified theory of cancer, stressed the significance of the emotional factor. He says:

> What is more significant is that these people (who developed cancer because of emotional factors) breathe the same air, drink the same fluids, eat the same foods, and are exposed to the same viruses as the rest of us. Why do they run a higher risk of cancer?

The answers to Dr Levenson's and other relevant questions can be found in chi kung. Chinese methods in handling emotional problems will be discussed in greater detail in the next two chapters. But before we look at qigong's answers and Chinese psychiatry, let us briefly examine the conventional treatments for cancer and why they are unsatisfactory.

Dissatisfaction over Conventional Treatments

The three main conventional treatments for cancer are surgery, chemotherapy and radiotherapy, or what Dr Levenson refers to as cutting, poisoning and burning.

Surgery is regarded by many oncologists as the most effective, if the cancer is at the first stage and part, i.e. if the malignant tumour has not grown nor spread much. Not only is the therapeutic method irreversible (a removed part cannot be put back again), when cancer is identified, especially if it is inside the body, it is usually past its first stage of growth and first part of metastasis or spreading. Even if the cancerous part is discovered very early, its surgical removal is no guarantee that cancer will not develop in other parts of the body.

As it is obvious if we have studied the theory of cancer discussed above, the manifestation of cancer in a particular part is just a symptom of some faulty control mechanism in the body. If this control system is functioning normally as in the great majority of us, cancer will not develop in the first place, or even if it has occurred, it will be checked and remedied usually without our knowing. Many people are unaware that even if the surgery itself is successful, which it usually is with the advancement of modern surgical technology today, if just one cell starts to mutate and is not kept in check, cancer will develop again.

Many people are also unaware that although chemotherapy seems to have only slight side effects in illnesses like contagious diseases, it is probably the most drastic of the three conventional treatments in cancer. This is because the powerful drugs that are taken in to kill cancerous cells, will kill other healthy and useful cells indiscriminately. Severe nausea, hair loss, weight loss, diarrhoea, fatigue and mental depression are common side effects. It is almost certain that the patient will never be the same person again. More seriously, though it may not be as obvious, is the tremendous weakening of the immune system, and general wearing down of the body's natural functions. The patient becomes a pitiful, visual reminder of what suffering from cancer is.

Yet, despite all these sacrifices, the recovery rate is low, if not nil although most doctors who prescribe chemotherapy for cancer would not admit it. It is virtually nil because the random killing of the powerful drugs inside the patient's body, treats the illness only symptomatically without attacking the root cause, which is cell mutation escaping control. This random killing probably aggravates the loss of the body's natural regulatory control over cell production.

Radiotherapy is as ineffective for similar reasons. Although there have been improvements in recent years in the targeting and the dosage of irradiation techniques, radiotherapy at its best is just treating the symptom, not the cause, of cancer. Even if irradiation can kill all current cancerous cells (and many, many more healthy cells), as long as the control system which the patient naturally and effectively had since birth until the onset of cancer, is not restored, cancer will continue.

In Chinese medical philosophy, the mass of dead cancer cells and dead healthy cells inside the body is as bad as, if not worse than, having a mass of living cancerous cells, for this dead mass seriously interrupts energy and blood flow, meaning that both the feed-back and the immune systems are further weakened. This of course aggravates the already failing cell regulatory control system.

What is worse, although it is indeed surprising that oncologists generally remain silent over this point, irradiation causes otherwise healthy cells to mutate. This probably explains why after radiotherapy, it is not uncommon that soon after cancer remission in one part of his body, the patient develops cancer in another part.

Conventional treatments are inadequate because they treat the symptom (the malignant cells) rather than the cause (the failure of the patient as a whole person to control cell production). This point, which constitutes a fundamental principle in Chinese medicine, is crucial. The failure to understand or appreciate this point, I believe, leads to deeper and deeper researches and treatments that go further and further away from the crucial point.

Indeed, it may be possible that cancer is a second line natural defence mechanism when the first line in checking cell mutation has failed. Suppose the cells are meant to become tissues of the liver. Because of some mistakes in the DNA or RNA, the newly produced cells resemble those of an elephant's stomach instead of liver cells.

To prevent the patient's liver from becoming like the stomach of an elephant, certain hitherto unknown defence mechanism rounds up these malignant cells and inhibit their innate function. Cancer, then, is a friend rather than an enemy. This suggestion is of course speculative, even ridiculous to some people, but many important and beneficial discoveries started as outlandish ideas.

Let us look at an analogy, that of a department in a factory manufacturing computers. The responsibility of this department is to regulate the number of workers for their various respective jobs. As the turn over of workers in this factory is enormous, mistakes are often made, such as supplying more of one type of workers, or supplying workers who do nothing besides getting their pay. (Or these malignant workers are mistakenly programmed to produce tyres instead of computers, in which case certain controls in the factory stop their functioning power.)

However these mistakes are rectified by an efficient team of controllers who patrol the factory and keep malignant workers in check. Problems really arise when the controllers fail in their function, when, for example, more and more unproductive workers are constantly supplied by the department. In time these excessive and malignant workers will proliferate the factory, taking away the space and also the salary meant for productive workers, forcing the factory to close.

What can we do about this sick factory? One way is to forcefully evict these malignant workers together with clearing away the factory space and equipment they are attached to. This may give the factory some remission, but if the controllers are not restored to their proper function, the unabated supply of malignant workers will cause similar problems probably at another site in the factory.

Another way is to shoot or poison workers indiscriminately, irrespectively of whether they are loyal and essential or malignant. This of course is a great drain on the factory, making it more sick than before. The problem remains unsolved as malignant workers keep turning up because the control system has not been restored.

A third way is to burn the workers and the affected part of the factory. Although great care is taken to burn only the malignant workers, many other workers are also affected, either directly or indirectly through heat. This irritates these workers, who were originally loyal and useful, and some of them mutiny.

Meanwhile much time and money is spent on research into every conceivable aspect of the department in question, of the malignant workers, as well as into improved methods of eviction, poisoning and burning. The information gathered from the research is accurate and amazing, such as if the departmental head smokes too much, he may start to give wrong instructions in his supply of workers;

malignant workers go through four stages in their life history; it may not be necessary to tear down part of the factory to evict malignant workers, it can be done through laser beams.

Yet, despite the remarkable advances made in the research, the basic problem remains unsolved. Why? Because we have forgotten at least two important factors: we have not regarded the factory as a holistic organic unit; and we have ignored the essential role of the controllers. As long as the research is based on a faulty premise, the resulting treatment will be faulty.

Are there any other alternative ways to deal with the problem? Of course, once we are ready to free ourselves from our stereotype perspective, many alternatives are possible. One promising approach is to forget about killing workers, and focusing our attention on their working conditions. Remember that the factory had been functioning normally all along. Find out what went wrong. For example, was the electricity supply normal, was the communication system functioning well, and were the workers getting their pay on time? Correcting one or more of these abnormalities will get the factory working properly again.

The weaknesses of conventional cancer research and treatment is so obvious to me that I cannot help wondering why most oncologists have not paid much notice to them. I can think of the following reasons. So much vested interest is involved in the current trend of cancer research and treatment that to suggest any change is tantamount to economic suicide.

Two, their pride, which is perfectly human, prevents the relevant and influential people to make any alteration from their established tradition.

Thirdly — as Dr Levenson has said: "the sophisticated cancer researchers, their eyes glued to their microscopes in the pursuit of answers, have failed to look up long enough to study the behaviour of their patients" — they have become so accustomed to their way of seeing things that they are genuinely unaware of or close to other possibilities.

The third reason, I believe, is most likely — at least for many doctors and researchers. It must be emphasized here that there is never any implication on my part that western doctors and researchers are inadequate.

In fact, they deserve much respect and admiration for their determination and sacrifice despite facing a seemingly hopeless situation. Oncologists, for example, suffer a higher incidence of cancer themselves than doctors who are specialists in other fields, although cancer is not contagious.

We can also imagine the anguish many doctors would face when, in between the devil and the deep blue sea, they have to prescribe some drastic treatment (rather than none at all) even though they know that its chances of curing the patient is not high and it would cause painful side effects.

How Qigong Can Cure Cancer

As Chinese medicine uses a different paradigm, it explains poisonous growth or cancer differently. Like any other diseases, the cause of cancer can be explained by using the etiology of "six evils" and "seven emotions", and its therapeutic principle summed up in the principles of yin-yang harmony and cleansing meridians.

It is interesting to note that the Chinese do not assign any specific cause or causes to cancer; any of the "six evils" and "seven emotions" can be causes, though the common pathogenic agents for poisonous growth are often "poisonous heat" and "false fire", and the meridian system involved is the liver meridian as it is closely connected with "cleansing blood" or detoxification.

Nevertheless, in the following explanation, Chinese principles will be explained by way of western conceptual framework.

The uncontrolled proliferation of cell growth, which western researchers regard as the cause of cancer, is referred to as yin-yang disharmony in Chinese medicine. While western medical scientists try to find the unknown factor or factors that are responsible for this malignant growth, the Chinese try to find amongst the known factors that maintain normalcy, which factors are amiss that result in abnormality.

In other words, the western scientists try to find the unknown factors X, Y, Z; the Chinese knowing that factors A, B, C, D, E, F ... are necessary for health, try to find which of these known factors are not functioning properly.

The west would be quite helpless if they fail to find the unknown factors. But because the Chinese are working with known factors, it is not difficult for them to find the factor that caused the malfunction; and the logical follow up is to provide the necessary remedy.

This difference of approach between the west and the Chinese is due to their fundamentally different ways of perceiving health and illness. Implicitly, western medical scientists assume that the ultimate cause of illnesses are from outside the patient, whereas the Chinese assume it is from inside.

The Chinese start with the premise that everyone is by nature healthy, and is capable of handling all the countless external disease-causing factors — unless, of course, they are extremely excessive, in which case it becomes suicide or murder. If he fails to handle them, it is because of some internal change.

In the case of cancer, the Chinese physician is not so concerned with external factors like chemical carcinogens, radiation, viruses, or any unknown factors which may have caused mutation of the DNA or RNA — after all, everyone is exposed to them. (This does not mean that knowing they are carcinogenic is not useful; it prevents us, for example, from becoming suicidal or murderous.)

The Chinese physician is concerned with finding out, with the help of the established and extensive system of diagnosis, why the patient's body fails to operate as it should. Once he has identified the known factors, which will be revealed through a thorough diagnosis, he will be able to restore the natural functions of his patient.

For example, he may find that the patient with poisonous growth at his neck has "poisonous heat" at the site of the growth, his liver energy is weak, vital energy stagnates at the meridians around the neck as well as at the liver meridian. Because of his particular way of training, he will describe a patient with a cancerous growth at the neck in this manner, i.e. poisonous growth due to poisonous heat at the neck, and weakness and stagnation of energy at the neck and the liver.

To a western doctor trained in a different paradigm, the same patient in the same situation will be described differently, such as having a carcinoma at the neck, where malignant cells have developed to a high degree of un-differentiation, and their DNA structure different from that of nearby healthy cells.

The Chinese physician may not know about cell differentiation and DNA structure, but when he has cleared the "poisonous heat", strengthened liver energy, and harmonized energy flow at the meridians around the neck as well as at the liver meridian, thereby restoring the patient's natural functions, western doctors will find the tumour subsiding, the cells at the affected area have become more differentiated, and the DNA structure of newly produced cells are normal.

The task of the Chinese physician is even simpler (but not necessarily easier) if he uses holistic qigong therapy or medical qigong for treatment. It is simpler because he does not have to be very specific or exact in his diagnosis, such as identifying that the causative "evil" is "poisonous heat" and not "false fire", and the energy stagnation is at the liver and not the spleen meridian.

This is permissible in qigong treatment because once vital energy has been induced to flow harmoniously, it will clear the "evil" irrespective of whether it is "heat" or "fire", and will cleanse the stagnation irrespective of whether it is at the kidney or spleen meridian.

However, the effect is slow, and may not be adequate if the patient is too old or weak. Hence, other approaches, like herbal medicine which requires specific diagnosis and prescription, can speed up the healing process.

Recent experiments using western scientific methods and instruments into qigong have produced some startling results which cancer researchers cannot afford not to investigate further. It has been found that the qi or energy transmitted by a qigong master onto cancer cells could kill 50% of them after five minutes!

Transmitted qi can also cause chromosomes that have been displaced to return to their proper alignment, and cause disturbed DNA to resume their normal structural patterns! Practicing qigong greatly enhances our defence and immune systems, as well as regulate our chemical balance.

The implications of these research results mean that practicing chi kung can correct accidental mistakes in the DNA or RNA, enhance the control system to check mutated cells, strengthen the defence and immune systems to overcome cancer viruses, kill malignant cells that escaped these controls without harming healthy cells, promote a better feed-back system for internal and external communications, and improve the transport system to clear away carcinogens and other toxins. Are oncologists and research scientists ready to test these claims even if they are considered unorthodox?

Some Wonderful Qigong Exercises

It is not necessary to prescribe specific qigong exercises to cure cancer, because firstly, most qigong exercises have holistic effects, and secondly, as there are different types of cancer with different pathogenetic conditions, a specific exercise is prescribed only if a detail diagnosis indicating specific pathogenetic conditions has been made. Most of my qigong students who managed to cure their cancer practiced general qigong from me.

The Five-Animal Play described in Chapter 22 is a helpful qigong exercise for relieving cancer and other organic or psychosomatic diseases. The following two qigong exercises are also holistic, which means that although they are specially described here for cancer patients, these exercises are equally effective for curing other diseases. They are as wonderful as they appear simple.

Stand upright and relax. Feel cheerful. Place any one palm on your abdomen, about two inches below your navel, and the other palm on top of it. Depress your abdomen with both palms and breathe out through your mouth slowly and gently. At the same time think of all the unwanted, negative things, including your illness or illnesses, flowing out. Pause for a short while, then release your pressure on your abdomen, so that the abdomen rises. At the same time, breathe in slowly and gently through your nose, while thinking of good cosmic energy flowing into you filling your every cell with vitality and life. Pause for a short while.

The whole process — breathing out, pause, breathing in, pause — constitutes one breath or breathing unit. Practice about ten breaths initially; gradually increase the number of breaths to about thirty six times over a period of about one month. Then continue at about thirty six breaths per practice session.

Practice once in the morning and once at night or evening for at least three months before you expect good results. It is important that your mind must be free from irrelevant thoughts, and the breathing out and in must be gentle. You may practice with your eyes either open or close.

This qigong exercise is called "Abdominal Breathing". Actually it is not easy for many people who are used to chest breathing, to perform abdominal breathing. So, if you find it difficult, you may perform the exercise with your normal breathing, except that your breathing out and in must be slow and gentle, and you need not press on your abdomen though you may still place your palms there. The crucial aspects of the exercise are your relaxed state of mind, and your thinking of illnesses flowing out and cosmic energy flowing in.

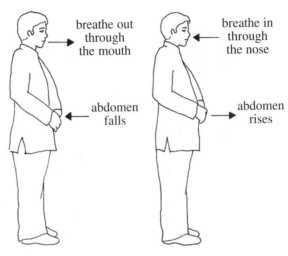

breathe out
through
the mouth

breathe in
through
the nose

abdomen
falls

abdomen
rises

Fig 24.2 Abdominal Breathing

The next exercise, known as Golden Shower, may be performed immediately after the above breathing exercise, or performed separately. Stand upright but relaxed with both arms hanging effortlessly at the sides, preferably in a quiet, pleasant, natural environment where nobody would disturb you. Close your eyes gently and feel cheerful.

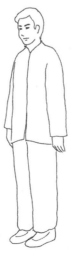

Fig 24.3 Standing Posture for Golden Shower

Remain motionlessly without any thoughts for a minute or two. Then feel that all your vital points and meridians are open. (You need not worry where these points and meridians are. If you are uncertain about vital points or meridians, just feel that all your "pores" and minute vessels in your body are open.)

Gently visualize beautiful, invigorating cosmic energy golden in colour flowing continuously down from the sky into you, through your head down your whole body to your soles and out into the earth. Feel the golden shower of this cosmic energy bathing your every cell, bringing life and vitality, and cleansing away illnesses and any unwanted material deep into the earth. (If you are a pious environmentalist, be comforted that the dispelled negative energy harmful to you will be useful to other things in the ground.)

The visualization must never be forced; it must be gentle and soothing. If you find it hard to visualize, just gently think of the process. Enjoy the golden shower for a few minutes.

Then gently focus your vital energy at your abdominal energy field (or just think of your abdomen) for a few seconds. Feel how relaxed and peaceful you are, and that all your natural systems are functioning properly. Then rub your palms together and place the warm palms on your eyes as you open them. Massage your face gently and walk about briskly for about thirty steps to complete the exercise.

For those too old or weak to stand, they may sit upright to practice this exercise. Practice twice daily for at least three months.

A useful procedure for daily practice is to start with Five-Animal Play, followed by Abdominal Breathing, and conclude with Golden Shower. If you find this program too long, practice any two of the three exercises per day, then change to another combination the next day, so that you can have the benefits of all these three different types of qigong exercises. If you find some of these exercises odd, it is because you are not yet familiar with them.

Although they have been practiced for centuries, until recently these exercises were taught exclusively to selected people only. There are also many other kinds of chi kung exercises besides the ones mentioned in this book that are effective for curing cancer.

Proposal for the Courageous

To say that cancer is curable through qigong does not mean that every case of cancer will be cured if the patient practices qigong, just as patients who suffer from definitely curable diseases like dysentery and bladder stone may still die if the illness has deteriorated beyond a critical stage or if complications have set in. It is also necessary to practice from a master or a qualified instructor.

Although qigong masters have accomplished remarkable results in cancer cure, because of the absence of proper control, many others who teach qigong today may not be skilful or knowledgeable in the art.

On the other hand, it is indeed surprising that cancer researchers generally have not been keen to investigate claims of cancer cure in qigong or other healing systems. They chose to concentrate their efforts on the cancerous cells instead of the cancer patients.

Isn't it odd, especially after so many unsuccessful efforts over the years, to cling on to the belief that the microscopic study of one cell could provide the key to a dreadful disease afflicting a living organism composed of 100 trillion cells, and exposed to myriad physiological and psychological influences independent of the cell? It is hoped that cancer researchers can be more flexible and open in their philosophical approach, and courageous enough to investigate other possibilities.

One area of promising possibilities lies in qigong. If the right people care enough for the suffering of cancer patients, it is not difficult to work our research programmes to test whether the claims made in qigong are true or false.

Needless to say the research programs must be based on sincerity, and not just disguised schemes to debunk their claims irrespective of the results.

25

UNITY OF ESSENCE, ENERGY AND SPIRIT
(Basic Concepts in Chinese Psychiatry and Neurology)

It is never surprising but always sobering to discover that much of what we cherish as contemporary achievement existed before, and much of what we deride as obsolete and shameful still plagues us.

Frederick Redlich and Daniel Freedman,
the Theory and Practice of Psychiatry.

Unity of Mind and Body in Chinese Medicine

As recent as fifty years ago the prevailing philosophy in western medicine was that mind had little or nothing to do with illness of the body. Gradually many western doctors suggested that the mental states of patients had some influence over his physical diseases, and the term psychosomatic was introduced. Now the situation is almost reversed. Some doctors went to the extent of believing, perhaps with the exception of injuries due to accidents, that disease is a function of the mind.

In Chinese medicine, the mind and the body, or the psyche and the soma, have always been regarded as one organic whole. Not only is a person's physical well being necessarily influenced by his mind, his mental state is also intimately connected with his body. A person's intellectual performance is affected if he is physically unwell; similarly, his physical health is disturbed if he is mentally or emotionally afflicted.

As the Chinese do not make a clear distinction between physical and psychiatric disorders, logically they do not categorically distinguish between diseases of the brain and of the heart, nor between mental and emotional illnesses. Neurological and psychiatric disorders are generally known as "diseases of the heart", as the heart in Chinese medical philosophy is both the seat of the mind and emotion.

Hence, although psychiatry, which also included treatment of neurological disorders, reached a very high level in Chinese medicine, psychiatrists did not exist as a professional group in ancient China. What is amazing is not that psychiatric (and also neurological) disorders were treated like any physical diseases by physicians, but that the treatment was generally successful.

While much of western diagnosis of psychiatric illnesses is guess work even in the present time, and many of their treatment uncertain, the Chinese have developed elaborate and effective systems for their psychiatric diagnosis and treatment. The west has much to benefit from a study of Chinese psychiatry.

Weaknesses in Western Psychiatry

Because of insufficient understanding of its working, many people have the misconception that Chinese medicine is unscientific or traditional, whereas western medicine is regarded as the epitome of scientific medicine. In this respect, a comparison of how Chinese physicians and western doctors typically diagnose and treat their patients is illuminating. Priest and Woolfson in their very influential book, "Handbook of Psychiatry", which has run to many reprints and revised editions, has this to say of western diagnosis in psychiatry:

> The way in which a diagnosis is made can be illustrated by imagining a female patient presenting to a doctor and complaining of palpitations. She also suffers from shakiness, muscular tension, apprehension and excessive perspiration. It will come to mind that she may be suffering from an anxiety state. It would be dangerous to jump to this conclusion at this stage without asking further questions. Suppose that as the interview continues she also confesses that she is in low spirits, has lost her energy, feels hopeless, has lost a lot of weight through lack of appetite, wakes early in the morning and suffers from suicidal ideas. Now the doctor will argue that the most likely diagnosis seems to be that of a depressive illness (in which anxiety symptoms are known to be quite common).

> He will change his ideas quite radically if she goes on to say that she hears hallucinatory voices addressing her in the third person and feels that all her actions are controlled by a mysterious machine located in the basement. In fact he may be convinced that she suffers from schizophrenia. This diagnosis would be acceptable as long as it were established that she suffered from a functional mental illness. However, any psychological symptom can be produced by organic brain disease. It would therefore be necessary to exclude the presence of brain disease before her particular hallucinations and passivity delusions were accepted as proof of schizophrenia.

Despite the emphasis on objectivity and quantitative data in western science, the above diagnosis is based totally on subjective judgement. Much of western psychiatric treatment is also full of uncertainties. The main forms of treatment for psychiatric disorders are psychosurgery, chemotherapy, electroconvulsive therapy (ECT), psychotherapy and behavior therapy.

Elton B. McNeil has the following to say about psychosurgery:

> This was a sad chapter to the history of somatic therapy, a chapter written by those who decided psychosurgery was necessary to 'cure' mental illness. Opening the skull to let the evil spirits out had been practiced since the beginning of civilized history; unfortunately it produced a sophisticated modern counterpart. ... In the brief period in which psychosurgery flourished (approximately 15 years), thousands upon thousands of patients were reduced to a state of damaged passivity that solved a cultural problem at the expense of the individual patient.

Since the 1950s the use of psychoactive drugs to control moods and mental disorders increased at a fantastic rate. However, "the hoped for one-to-one relationship between chemistry and behavior was to proven to be naive, for it quickly became evident that the behavioral effects of psychopharmacological compounds were often variable and unpredictable." If the side effects of these drugs are more widely known, many people would press for alternative treatment. For example, most phenothiazine and non-phenothiazine neuroleptics, which are major tranquilizers, cause amenorrhoea (stoppage of normal menstrual periods), infertility, and parkinsonism (progressive disorders of the central nervous system)! Even the tricyclic antidepressants, hailed as a major advancement in the treatment of depression, caused blurred vision, rapid heart beat, low blood pressure, fine tremour of limbs, and, in large or prolonged doses, heart attack.

Despite its many setbacks, electroconvulsive therapy, or electroshock as many would prefer to call it, is standard practice with many psychiatrists. In 1992 Medicare, the United States health insurance program for elderly and disabled people, paid for 101,854 sessions of electroconvulsive therapy, compared to 88,847 sessions in 1986. The National Institute of Medical Health of the United States estimated in 1992 that in America 110,000 people each year undergo electroconvulsive therapy.

Yet, "theories of exactly how an electroconvulsive shock works in treatment to alter human cognition, perception, emotion, and behavior are many, contradictory, and confusing." Besides, patients have to put up with side effects like amnesia (memory loss), and sometimes risk bone fractures and cardiovascular dysfunctions.

Psychotherapy, the off-shoot of Sigmund Freud's psychoanalysis, is basically talking to the patient until his emotional or behavioral disorders disappear. There are two inherent weaknesses. Patients with psychiatric problems are not likely to have the necessary linguistic and conceptual control nor clarity of mind to derive the insight needed to see the mistakes of their emotions or behaviors, thus overcoming them.

Secondly, the therapeutic strategy resembles a dressing up by the therapist of the patient's problems in less unpleasant light, so as to tempt the patient to accept what he could not accept earlier. If the patient could accept his unpleasant situations, they would not be his problems in the first place. Even if he is tricked by the therapist's clever camouflage into accepting the situations, it is only a temporary relief, and the problems will surface again later, because fundamentally they are unacceptable to him.

While psychotherapy is 'talk therapy', behavior therapy is 'act therapy', and has been developed only recently since the 1960s. Its development is a reaction against psychotherapy which some psychiatrists consider ineffective. Behavior therapists expostulate that what are considered as neurotic or psychotic disorders are actually distorted patterns of maladjusted or inappropriate behavior, and can be corrected through systematic relearning.

Although behavior therapy is currently a popular and expanding form of psychiatric treatment in western societies, its basic presumption is not necessarily or completely true. While some or even much behavior is learnt, it cannot be denied that physical factors like hormonal imbalance and cerebral defects are significant causes of mental and emotional disorders.

The model behavior set up by the therapists may be culturally biased, and the use of punishment as a powerful tool to correct unwanted behavior involves moral and ethical values.

Moreover, many psychiatrists question whether the treatment is merely repressing the patients' neuroses or psychoses with an imposed behavioral pattern, "like reducing a fever through the liberal use of aspirin. The fever is gone but the disease remains." Like psychotherapy, behavior therapy is ineffective against more serious types of psychiatric illnesses like schizophrenia and drug addiction, and organic brain syndromes like amnesia (loss of memory) and dementia (deterioration of intelligence).

With such weaknesses in western psychiatric diagnosis and treatments, and the increasing demand of modern stressful living, it is of no surprise that both the incidence and prevalence of psychiatric illnesses in western societies have become alarming.

The purpose of discussing the above weaknesses was not to belittle western psychiatry, but to show that a study of Chinese psychiatry, ironically thought by many people as non-existent, can be of much benefit to the west.

Basic Concepts in Chinese Psychiatry

It is useful to remember that while the Chinese recognize psychiatric disorders, they do not dichotomize them from physical illnesses. They also do not categorically differentiate psychiatric from neurological disorders.

Hence, all the knowledge and techniques used for treating disorders of the body, like yin-yang harmony and meridian systems, herbal medicine and acupuncture, are also applicable to treating disorders of the mind. The following concepts are important for a proper understanding of psychiatric (including neurological) health.

1. Unity of Soma and Psyche.

Chinese medical philosophers, as well as thinkers in other disciplines, have always emphasized the unity of some and psyche. Chinese masters have taught that the body is alive because of the mind, and the mind operates through the body. The Inner Classic of Medicine stresses that "to nurture the mind, we must understand the size, nature and physiology of the body."

2. Unity of Essence, Energy and Spirit.

Parallel to the unity of the mind and body, is the unity of essence, energy and spirit. Essence, or jing, refers to the finest material that constitutes the physical body. In modern western terms, it is the subatomic particles that make up all our bodily parts.

Energy, or qi (pronounced as "ch'i"), is the vital life force that operates all our internal and external movements, including all the minute, countless physiological and mental processes that we often take for granted.

Spirit, or shen, is the mind or consciousness that directs and controls our essence and energy. In metaphysical or spiritual context, it is the Real You. Essence without energy is just a mass of material; essence and energy together is like a working machine; it is spirit that makes a person human, almost divine. Essence, energy and spirit are not three separate parts of man cooperating together; they are three intimately related aspects of the same organic unity.

3. The Heart is the Seat of the Mind and of Emotion.

While some neurosurgeons wonder whether the mind exists as a separate entity or is just a function of the brain, the Chinese have no doubt that the mind is a reality, and its seat is at the heart, not the brain.

It is interesting to note that modern westerners are the only people in the whole history of mankind, and only at this point of time, to believe that the brain houses the mind, and implicitly houses emotion; all other peoples, including the Egyptian, Indians, Arabs, South Americans as well as the medieval Europeans, generally believe that the seat of the mind and of emotion is at the heart (though some people, like the Elizabethans during Shakespeare's time, considered it to be at the liver.) It must not be mistaken that these people were ignorant of an organ called the brain.

The Chinese, like other great peoples, had detailed and correct knowledge of the brain in ancient times, but on the whole they considered it to be some form of a magnificent computer, though there actually had been debates among the classical Chinese on whether the heart or the brain housed the mind.

4. Onus of Maintaining Health is on Nurturing Mind.

While Chinese medical philosophers and scientists since ancient times have realized the importance of the unity of psyche and soma, they emphasize the mind rather than the body in their approach to curing illnesses and promoting health. A medical axiom advises that "to regulate form, first regulate spirit; to nurture body, first nurture mind."

5. Importance of Virtue in Mind Cultivation.

Ancient Chinese masters, both religious and secular, emphasized that in cultivating our mind for achieving health and longevity, it is of utmost importance to cultivate virtue too. The Inner Classic advises: "Unwholesome desires cannot tempt his eyes; sexual temptations cannot move his heart; knowledgeable but not arrogant; unattached to materialistic gains; thus in accordance with the Tao, he can live to hundred years, yet his movements are not impaired and his virtue not stained."

These concepts provide the philosophical framework for Chinese psychiatry and neurology. Their belief in the unity of psyche and soma, for example, explains why the Chinese do not differentiate between psychiatric and physical diseases, and their doctrine of the heart as the seat of mind which controls all other organs including the brain, enables them to effectively treat neurological disorders like epilepsy and hemiplegia through the meridian system.

These concepts also provide useful insights to other aspects of health and medicine. Western researchers may find it rewarding to investigate whether the numerous unsuccessful attempts to find solutions to many of their medical problems, like cancer and degenerative diseases, is due to their failure to appreciate the inseparable unity of mind and body.

If we can accept this unity, then it becomes clear that the extremely reductionist and mechanistic approach in western medicine, like the detailed study of single cells (which is rewarding in its own right), instead of the patient as a unified organism with a mind, cannot be satisfactory in medical application because it is built upon a faulty premise.

On an optimistic note, many successes in Chinese medicine as well as in other alternative healing systems in curing so-called incurable diseases are possible because they take into account the tremendous influence of the patients' mind in recovery processes and health.

The fifth concept mentioned above, i.e. the importance of virtue in health and healing, may appear naive to some people. Perhaps if we know that the above advice in the Inner Classic was given by Chi Po (Qi Bo) to the philosopher-emperor Hwang Ti (Huang Di), we may be less arrogant in deriding ancient wisdom as obsolete, and begin to realize that many of our modern psychiatric and physical problems like depression, phobia, hypertension and ulcers, are actually our succumbing to unwholesome desires, sexual temptations and materialistic attachment.

On the other hand, Chi Po did not ask us to be puritanical; what he and other masters advised was that we should be moderate and virtuous in our daily living.

Etiology of Psychiatric and Neurological Disorders

Although there may be countless different causes of illnesses, psychiatric and otherwise, they can be classified into three groups, namely external causes of "six evils", internal causes of "seven emotions", and neither-external-non-internal causes. (Please also see Chapter 10.)

External causes like "cold" and "heat" may respectively lower a person's immune system or increase his metabolic processes, causing psychotic states like depression and hysteria. In more serious cases, "wind" and "fire", for instance, may cause neurological disorders like apoplexy and dementia.

Neither-external-nor-internal causes like abnormal lifestyles and insufficient sleep may lead to a paranoid state and illusion. Nevertheless, the internal causes of "seven emotions" are the most significant as far as psychiatric and neurological disorders are concerned. They are also connected with psychosomatic diseases, like hypertension, ulcers and sexual inadequacy.

The "seven emotions" are joy, anger, melancholy, anxiety, sorrow, fear and shock. The range of human emotions is of course limitless; these seven are only representative types.

These seven typical emotions are normal and healthy, enriching our daily life. It is only when they are excessive or react negatively on the person that they become pathogenetic agents. An introductory explanation of the seven emotions as internal causes of illnesses was given in Chapter 10. Chinese medical scientists have long discovered that the energies of these emotions typically react on particular organs, and they bring about characteristic reactions.

Joy typically reacts on the heart. If joy is excessive or negative, it disperses heart energy, resulting in the spirit or mind being disturbed, causing sever palpitation, insomnia, hysteria, mania, unconsciousness and even death. An example of negative joy is being pleased over the inconvenience or suffering of other people.

To say that joy reacts on the heart, does not imply that it does not react on other organs; it means the heart is the most affected by the kind of energy produced by joy. This explanation applies to all other emotions and organs in the description below.

Anger affects the liver, causing its energy to stagnate, and may result in loss of appetite, pale face, cold limbs, unconsciousness and death. A person prone to anger is usually impatient and irritable, two prevailing personality traits among those who suffer from gastrointestinal cancer. Serious stagnation of liver energy may lead to dementia (deterioration of intelligence). Anger may also cause liver energy to rise, resulting in mania or hypertension.

Melancholy affects the lungs, causing lung energy to coalesce. This may lead to depression and anxiety state, as well as coughing, vomiting, insomnia, constipation and sexual impotency. Severe cases of melancholy may lead to dementia (deterioration of intelligence), and cancer. As the lung is closely connected to the heart, melancholy which injures the lungs may also affect the heart. Because inadequacy of heart energy may lead to epilepsy, hence melancholy may sometimes cause this disease.

Negative energy from anxiety reacts with the spleen, causing spleen energy to congest. This affects the digestive system, and causes loss of appetite, chest and abdominal flatulence, blurred vision, palpitation, insomnia and loss of memory, as well as anxiety state and depression. Serious cases of anxiety may cause cancer. While western medicine believes that flatulence is caused by swallowing air, the Chinese believe it is caused by congestion of spleen energy.

Sorrow affects the lungs and the heart, causing their energies to be drained away. Thus the upper warmer, or chest cavity, becomes congested and hot. As the heart is intimately connected with other organs, sorrow would result in psychiatric and psychosomatic disorders related to other organs. Some common problems resulting from sorrow include cough, consumption, insomnia, loss of appetite, epilepsy, depressive neurosis, depressive psychosis, involutional melancholia, obsessional state, and suicidal syndrome.

Fear causes energy to sink, and affects the kidneys. This may result in psychosomatic disorders like loss of control over defecation and urination, diarrhoea, involuntarily seminal emission, and sexual inadequacy, or in psychotic disorders like anxiety state and various types of phobia. If vital energy cannot rise in severe cases of fear, schizophrenia, epilepsy or convulsion may result.

Shock affects the heart and the gall bladder, causing their energy to disperse and be chaotic. This may result in disharmony of energy and blood flow. Disorders associated with shock includes palpitation, insomnia, unconsciousness, convulsion and various types of phobia. Shock, like fear, may also affect the kidneys, causing their related disorders.

Some readers may ask, "How do the Chinese masters know that joy affects the heart, and anger affects the liver, and not the other way round, or affects other organs? How do they know that melancholy may cause dementia and cancer, and that anxiety may cause spleen energy to be congested?" These are legitimate questions.

It is like someone with little knowledge of western medical philosophy asking, "How do western experts know that depression is an internalization of aggression, and mania a defence mechanism preventing depression, and not the other way round, or some other physiological or psychological processes? How do they know that a brain defect may cause epilepsy, a certain chemical may cause cancer, and that anxiety may cause palpitation, sweating and shakiness?

Indeed, the Chinese are more "scientific" in the discovery of their knowledge. While much of the western answers to the above questions, are still speculative, all the above information of the Chinese has been gathered from centuries of empirical studies, and confirmed by equally long periods of practical application.

For example, whenever a Chinese physician examines his patients (like taking their pulse, examining outward symptoms on their body, etc.), when they are joyful, he will find that their heart system, and not the liver or other systems, is affected. And if he clears away the foreign "fire-evil" that has entered the heart system causing mania or hysteria, and restores their heart energy, his manic or hysterical patients will usually show improvements.

It is understandable that readers unfamiliar with Chinese medical thinking will find the above explanation exotic. The following concept should be even more fascinating.

According to Chinese medical philosophy, the five "zang" or storage organs are also the seats of higher powers. The heart houses the "spirit" (shen); the liver houses the "soul" (hun); the spleen houses the "will" (yi); the lung houses the "consciousness" (po); and the kidney houses the "intention" (zhi). It must be noted that this is not a metaphysical but a medical concept.

This concept further reinforces the belief that our psyche is not locked in the brain, but diffused all over the body, and specially focused at the five zang organs. This possibly explains why when some neurosurgeons — like the well known Richard Restak who exclaimed that "there is simply nothing to prove that anything exists other than the brain interacting with some aspects of external or internal reality" — operated on the brain, they could not find the mind.

Moreover, the different terms given to our psyche — spirit, soul, will, consciousness, intention — suggest the many different aspects of our mind, such as awareness, memory, intelligence, imagination, visualization, conceptualization and intuition.

Hence, while western psycho-surgeons have to operate on the brain to correct its defects (or what they think are its defects), which unfortunately are often unsuccessful, the Chinese work on neurological disorders through the meridian systems without the need for opening the brain.

For example, epilepsy can be effectively treated by clearing energy blockage at the heart and kidney systems, so that heart and kidney energies can flow to and from the brain.

Exciting new grounds may be discovered by investigating whether the brain, like what the Chinese have suggested long ago, is just a computer regulating flows of information and sensation to and from all parts of our sentient body, and not the all powerful concentration of all our emotions and intelligence.

With the exception of psycho-surgery, which is no longer popular as it often transforms patients into human vegetables, all the major modes of treatment in western psychiatry, like chemotherapy, electroconvulsive therapy, psychotherapy and behavior therapy, are found in Chinese medicine — with some important differences.

The Chinese methods do not have the weaknesses and drastic side-effects of the western treatment. Moreover, the Chinese methods are usually less expensive, more effective and faster, and they treat the patient holistically, often curing him of related psychosomatic illness. How this is done will be explained in the next chapter.

26

DISEASES CAN BE CURED IN MANY WAYS

(Treatments for Psychiatric and Neurological Disorders)

In the eyes of the patient, one who understands the patient's
feelings is a most welcomed doctor.

Ma Peng Ren and Dong Jian Hua, Practical
Chinese Psychiatry.

Differences between Chinese and Western Approaches

How could Chinese physicians treat neurological disorders when they have little knowledge of the anatomy and physiology of the brain? How could they treat psychiatric disorders when they have little knowledge of biochemistry and theories of behavior? Asking such questions, negatively, shows that we often view things from only one habitual angle, wittingly or unwittingly considering our view as the only correct one.

In a positive vein, these questions show that if the Chinese physicians have been successful, then there are other, and probably better, ways of treating psychiatric and neurological disorders.

Actually the Chinese knew about the anatomy and physiology of the brain long before the west. They also knew about biochemistry and behavior theories, although these were described in manners and terms very different from those of the west. But it is true that Chinese physicians generally have little knowledge of brain anatomy, physiology, biochemistry and behavior theories as the west know them; yet they are able to cure psychiatric and neurological disorders, probably better than currently practiced in the west. Why is this possible? The Chinese uses a different paradigm.

The philosophic framework the Chinese use for understanding psychiatric and neurological disorders, and which forms the basis of their diagnosis and therapeutic techniques, has been explained in the previous chapter. It includes five basic concepts, and the etiology of psychiatric and neurological diseases. The five basic concepts are as follows:

1. Unity of Soma and Psyche.
2. Unity of Essence, Energy and Spirit.
3. The Heart is the Seat of the Mind and Emotion.
4. Onus of Maintaining Health is on Nurturing Mind.
5. Importance of Virtue in Mind Cultivation.

The etiology of psychiatric and neurological disorders involve the following pathogenetic causes:

1. "Seven Emotions" of joy, anger, melancholy, anxiety, sorrow, fear and shock.
2. "Six Evils" of wind, cold, heat, dampness, dryness and fire.
3. "Neither-Internal-Nor-External Causes", like inappropriate food and drinks, insufficient exercise and rest, excessive sex, injuries sustained from hits and falls.

These three groups of causes of illnesses are applicable to psychiatric as well as all types of disorders. These causes as well as the diagnostic methods to find out the causes have been explained in earlier chapters.

While much of western psychiatric diagnosis is based on subjective questioning, responses and interpretation, Chinese psychiatric diagnosis is based on established principles and objective assessments. For example, as illustrated in the previous chapter, to decide whether a patient is suffering from an anxiety state, a depressive neurosis or schizophrenia, the psychiatrist has to interpret it from the patient's answers to his questions.

To the Chinese physician, terms like depressive neurosis and schizophrenia are merely convenient labels describing the conditions of the patient. What is important is not just to treat these syndromes, but to treat the patient as a whole person, including his psychosomatic illness which often accompanies his neurotic or psychotic state.

For example, from his diagnosis the Chinese physician finds, among other things, that his patient's spleen energy is congested and also that he has lost his appetite. This indicates that his psychiatric patient is suffering from an anxiety state. By clearing his energy congestion at the spleen, the physician cures both the psychiatric and psychosomatic disorders.

However if he finds his patient's energy coalesce at the lung, and that he has difficulties with his bowel movements and with sleeping at night, the physician knows more objectively than his western counterpart who depends on questioning, that the patient is suffering from depressive neurosis, as well as constipation and insomnia. By clearing the energy coalesce and employing other necessary therapeutic steps, he will be able to cure the patient's physical, psychosomatic and neurotic diseases.

If the physician finds the patient's energy sunk, his kidney system badly affected, his concept of reality distorted, and he suffers from seminal emission, the patient's psychiatric disorder is schizophrenia. He will probably have sexual problems too. Restoring his energy flow and kidney function are two of the necessary therapeutic methods to treat his disorders.

The above description mentions only the crucial points of the diagnosis. In actual practice, the diagnosis would be thorough, employing all the four principal diagnostic methods of viewing, asking, listening and feeling.

It is illuminating to note that the physician does not separate the psychiatric disorders from other kinds of illnesses both in diagnosis and in treatment. It is also significant to note that the physician does not treat the diseases, but he treats the patient as a whole person.

Even without giving labels to the diseases, by eliminating his pathogenetic conditions and restoring him to his normal self, all the disorders, psychiatric and otherwise, are cured.

Therapeutic Techniques of the Heart

The Chinese physician has a rich array of therapeutic techniques to cure psychiatric and neurological diseases, which the Chinese do not differentiate.

As the heart, which is the Chinese medical term referring to what the west would call the mind, concerns both psychiatric and neurological diseases, and the heart is also regarded as the seat of emotion, psychiatric and neurological disorders are often called "heart illness" or "emotional illness". There is a Chinese saying that "emotional illness is best cured by emotion."

Hence, besides the usual therapeutic methods applicable to all branches of Chinese medicine, like herbal medicine, external medicine, acupuncture, massage therapy and qigong therapy, the Chinese have an interesting class of curative methods which do not need medication or medical instruments for treating psychiatric disorders. These methods can be called "therapeutic techniques of the heart", and they include the following:

1. Calming the Mind.
2. Opening the Heart.
3. Overcoming Suspicion.
4. Transferring Focus.
5. Convincing Explanation.
6. Circulating Energy.
7. Interplay of Emotions.

Calming the mind refers to cultivating the mind through meditation, so that with an "expanded" or enhanced mind, the patient can now accept mental and emotional problems that he could not earlier accept.

This is in contrast with the western strategy of trying to make a nasty situation appear less unpleasant to trick the patient into accepting it. Here, the nasty situation has not changed, but the patient's mind has grown "bigger" so that the same situation is now no longer nasty. Calming the mind is explained in more detail in the next chapter.

Opening the Heart means making the patient cheerful. There are many Chinese sayings supporting the axiom that joy generates health, such as "Each time you laugh, each time you become younger; each time you frown, each time you grow older", "Whenever a person experiences a cheerful situation, his spirit is high, just as whenever the sky experiences rain, it is extraordinarily clear".

The underlying principle is that since the heart is intimately connected with all other organs, joy which affects the heart, promotes better flow of vital energy to all parts of the body.

People with mental or emotional problems are usually suspicious and lack self confidence. A hypochondriac suspects he is insidiously ill; a depressive personality suspects his own ability; and a mentally deranged person suspects the sincerity and goodwill of other people. Logically removing their suspicion and unobtrusively restore their self confidence is attacking their psychiatric and neurological disorders at their roots.

Some patients are excessively worried over their illness, thereby aggravating their conditions. A very effective method used by great masters is to transfer their focus, such as from internal suffering to an external object, form illness of internal organs to external wounds, from a concept that the illness is serious to one of recovery. A Chinese maxim teaches "transferring essence, changing energy", meaning changing the mental state of the patient which can result in marshalling his vital energy to overcome his illness.

According to Chinese medical philosophy, the source of psychiatric and neurological diseases is the heart, which is also concerned with intelligence. The patient's ignorance and misunderstanding of his illness often aggravate the disorders.

Convincing explanation is a positive step to overcome this causative factor, and is operated in four steps: inform the patient about the nature of his illness, assure him of the therapeutic principles so that he has confidence of recovery, explain to him the treatment procedure so that he can take the initiative for his own recovery, and enlighten him on specific steps that can lessen his suffering.

In Chinese medical thinking, the patient's vital energy is the basic factor for his recovery process and health. Circulating Energy refers to strengthening this vital energy and improving its harmonious flow to overcome psychiatric, neurological and other disorders. This method makes use of qigong therapy.

The Interplay of Emotions is a skilful application of the principle of five elemental processes to manipulate appropriate emotion to overcome psychiatric, neurological and psychosomatic diseases without using any medicine, acupuncture, massage therapy or any other therapeutic techniques.

The application of "fire overcoming metal" and "wood overcoming earth" in using joy to cure weak lungs, and anger to cure the emperor's queer illness, as illustrated in Chapter 6, are two examples of this interplay of emotions.

Chinese Approaches in Diagnosis and Treatment

It must be remembered that in Chinese medicine, the physician treats the patient, not the disease. His concern is to eliminate pathogenetic conditions of his patient, thus restoring him to health; not merely to prescribe stereotype medication or treatment procedure according to the label he has given to the patient's disease.

Thus, different patients suffering from what western doctors would call the same disease, may be given different treatment by the Chinese physician because the pathogenetic conditions of the individual patients are usually different. For example, two patients suffering from schizophrenia may have similar outward symptoms, and even give similar responses during consultation. But a careful diagnosis may reveal different pathogenetic conditions. For example, one patient may have congestion of liver energy, but in the other patient, his kidney energy is too weak to rise.

Treatment will therefore be necessarily different, though the two patients appear to have the same syndromes. In the first patient, the focus is on dispersing energy congestion at the liver system; whereas in the second patient, it is strengthening and promoting kidney energy flow.

Even if the main pathogenetic conditions are similar — say, both suffer from energy inadequacy at the kidney system — the precedent causes of this problem as well as related psychosomatic disorders may be different. For example, the cause of inadequate kidney energy in first patient may be due to some trouble in his lungs, whereas that of the second patient may be spleen dysfunction. Hence the first schizophrenic patient may also suffer from asthma, whereas the second patient from peptic ulcer.

How does the Chinese physician find out all these seemingly complex problems? By thoroughly diagnosing the patients as whole persons. Even if the patients exhibit schizophrenic symptoms, the Chinese physician would not allow this observation to cloud his diagnosis, least it may so affect him that he fails to discover other important pathogenetic conditions.

Because pathogenetic conditions even of the same disease may vary from patient to patient, and because eliminating these conditions is the onus of treatment, does this mean that the medical prescriptions or treatment procedures are haphazard or dependent on the arbitrary preference of the physician? No, because the numerous symptoms gathered from the diagnosis are classified into syndrome types, and while there is still great variety and flexibility in the choice of particular medicine and methods for the master, the prescriptions and procedures for various syndrome types are often generalized for the convenience of the average physician.

The rich experiences of past masters in treating typical syndromes have been recorded, and these serve as the core from which modern physicians work out their own medical prescriptions or treatment procedures which are based on their diagnosis of their patients.

In the following are described the causes and treatments for some psychiatric and neurological diseases, with an example each from herbal medicine, acupuncture, massage therapy, and qigong therapy, and two examples from "therapeutic techniques of the heart". For simplicity, only the main treatment is given, secondary treatment for related psychosomatic and other diseases is not included.

If you find the explanations of the disease and their treatments odd, please remember that Chinese medicine is based on a different paradigm; and these treatments have been proved successful in curing the respective disorders.

We may find some resemblance between Chinese therapeutic methods and western psychiatric treatment. Herbal medicine corresponds to chemotherapy or psycho-pharmacology, except that the Chinese approach treats the patient holistically and there are no drastic side effects.

The basic principle of acupuncture, massage therapy and qigong therapy is similar to that in electro-convulsive therapy, except that the Chinese use natural vital energy which invigorates the patient, whereas the west uses electric shocks which may produce frightful results. The "therapeutic techniques of the heart" correspond to psychotherapy and behavior therapy, except the Chinese methods are more extensive but less time consuming.

Herbal Medicine for Manic-Depressive Psychosis

This example is taken from the famous 18th century "Comments on Ancient and Modern Medical Case Histories" by Yu Zheng. Because of excessive melancholy, a young woman was thin and impatient. She became manic-depressive, and often laughed or cried for no reasons. Sometimes she even appeared naked, and frequently talked nonsense.

The physician, Wu Jiao Shan, found her pulse floating and uneven. He concluded that her spirit was dislodged from its seat in the heart. He asked her to boil zi he che (Placenta Hominis) into a paste, then dried it and cut into slices to be eaten randomly. Then he prescribed "Calming the Mind Decoction" to be taken in the day, and a course of "Bolus for Pacifying Intention" at night. She recovered, married, had a son the next year, and became plump and healthy.

The ingredients of "Calming the Mind Decoction" are:

> yuan zhi (Polygala tenuifolia willd)
> gan cao (Radix Glycyrrhizae)
> ren sheng (Radix Ginseng)
> dang gui (Radix Angelicae Sinesis)
> shao yao (Radix Paeoniae Alla)
> mai dong (Radix Ophiopogonis)
> da zao (Fructus Ziziphi Jujubae).

The ingredients of "Bolus for Pacifying Intention" are:

> yuan zhi (Polygala tenuifolia willd)
> ren sheng (Radix Ginseng)
> gan cao (Radix Glycyrrhiza)
> dang gui (Radix Angelicae Sinesis)
> gui xin (Plumula Cinnamomi)
> mai dong (Radix Ophiopogonis)
> shao yao (Radix Paeoniae Alla)
> fu qin (Poria)
> sheng jiang (Rhizoma Zingiberis Recens)
> da zao (Fructus Ziziphi Jujubae).

Acupuncture for Schizophrenia

According to Chinese medical thought, schizophrenia is caused by the "splitting" or "break-down" of the psyche, mainly due to severe attack on it, resulting in the spirit being dislodged from its proper place. The many types of schizophrenia may be divided into two main groups, passive schizophrenia and active schizophrenia.

Passive schizophrenia is mainly due to extreme worry or melancholy, resulting in congestion and stagnation of liver energy. This causes the production of excessive phlegm which blocks the outlets of the heart.

Some common symptoms are small and rapid pulse, light-colored tongue, thin fur on the tongue, feeling depressed and dejected, talking to oneself but seldom talking to others, laughing or crying abnormally, no appetite, being lethargic, and being deluded and illusory in sight, hearing and smell.

In treating passive schizophrenia, the main principles are to regulate energy flow, dissolve phlegm, and clear blockages. The manipulative principle of "even nourishing and even cleansing" is applied in acupuncture. The main acupuncture points for manipulation are neiguan (P 6) on the pericardium meridian, fenglong (S 40) on the stomach meridian, and renzhong (Gv 26) on the governing meridian.

Manipulating on nei guan can achieve the effects of pacifying the heart and regulating energy flow; on fenglong the effects of dissolving phlegm and detoxifying impurities; and on renzhong the effects of "cleansing yang" and opening blockages. Please see Fig 26.1 for the location of the vital points.

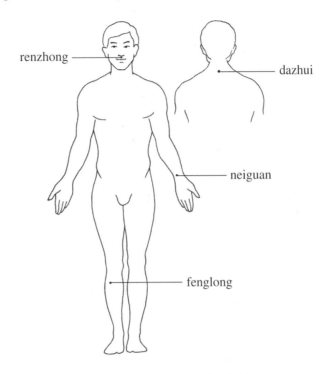

renzhong

dazhui

neiguan

fenglong

Fig 26.1 Main Acupuncture Points for Schizophrenia

On the other hand, active schizophrenia is mainly due to frustration over emotions or ambitions. Extreme anger, which injures the liver, causes liver fire and gall bladder fire to rise, and together with phlegm, disturb the spirit at the heart, causing delusions and illusions.

Patients with active schizophrenia often exhibit symptoms of smooth and terse pulse, yellow fur on tongue, flushed face and red eyes, loud and nonsensical talking, active and aggressive attitude, irresponsible and rude behavior, running wildly and shouting, damaging others' properties and hurting other people.

The therapeutic principles are dispelling fire, dissolving phlegm, and calming the spirit. The manipulative principle of cleansing is used. Main acupuncture points for manipulation are taichong (Liv 3) on the liver meridian, and renzhong (GV 26) and dazhui (Gv 14) on the governing meridian.

Manipulating on the taichong vital point (which is located just after the big toe!) can harmonize liver energy, dispel fire and clear congestion. Manipulating on renzhong can "cleanse yang" and open blockages, and on dazhui can promote physiological functions and alert the brain. Please refer to Fig 26.1.

Secondary acupuncture points that are applicable for both passive and active schizophrenia include the following. To reduce maniacal conditions, manipulate on yongquan (K 1) and daling (P 7).

To eliminate hallucinating voices, manipulate tinggong (Si 19) and tinghui (G 2). To eliminate illusory visions, manipulate jingming (B 1). To clear delusions, manipulate baihui (Gv 20). To overcome nonsensical talk, manipulate lianquan (Cv 23) and xinshu (B 15). To relieve headaches, manipulate fengchi (G 20). Please refer to Fig 26.2.

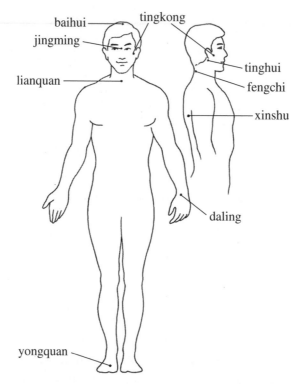

Fig 26.2 Secondary Acupuncture for Schizophrenia

Massage Therapy for Hemiplegia

Massage therapy is one of the best therapeutic methods for hemiplegia, or paralysis of one side of the body, and related neurological disorders. While western treatment of hemiplegia necessarily involves the brain, because western medical thought believes that hemiplegia is caused by an organic defect on the other side of the brain, such as a blood clot or haemorrhage in a cerebral blood vessel, the Chinese expound, and have successfully demonstrated, that it is not necessary to cut open the brain to treat hemiplegia, because even if the site of pathogenic agent is located at the brain (which itself is a debatable question), it can be removed by other means.

It is indeed unfortunate that when western doctors have the rare opportunity to come across successful cures of hemiplegia through means other than their "orthodox" medicine, all they inevitably do is to express amazement if not disbelief; apparently they are too arrogant or too busy with other work to investigate with the intention of benefiting other hemiplegia patients, especially those in western societies.

Indeed it is amazing that hemiplegia, a dreadful dehumanizing disease that mostly affects elderly people who certainly deserve more care from researchers in the younger generation, can be cured by a knowledgeable and skilful massage therapist using only his fingers! Hemiplegia may result form numerous disorders, especially head injury, brain tumour, stroke and cardiovascular diseases.

According to Chinese medical thought, hemiplegia is caused by deficiency of nutrient-energy or defence-energy, leading to disordered circulation of vital energy, often accompanied by attack of exogenous agents like "wind" or "heat".

Translated into western terms, it suggests that if the necessary neurons for neuro-transmission are insufficient, or if the defence mechanism that clears blockage in and overcome exogenous attack on the nervous system is inadequate, this will lead to a disordered flow of electrochemical impulses which transmit the necessary messages to all parts of the body.

If this natural function of our nervous system is disturbed, exogenous agents like toxic chemicals and hostile microbes (which may have been lying inside the body all the time) would have a chance to cause damage, resulting in hemiplegia. It is significant to note that the failure of natural functions or the damage by exogenous agents may or may not happen in the brain.

The therapeutic principles, which are logically developed from the pathological explanation, are improving nutrient-energy and defence-energy, and restoring the proper circulation of vital energy. If exogenous evils like "wind" and "heat" are diagnosed at certain meridians or organ systems, then the principles of clearing wind and dispersing heat are also included.

Notice that in this paradigm and if the holistic approach is used, it is not necessary to worry about the exact types of neuro-hormones that are deficient (it does not matter, for example, whether they are acetylocholine, histamine, or noradrenalin); precisely where electrochemical impulses are blocked (whether it is at some synapses in the brain or ganglia at the spinal cord); or exactly what kinds of toxins or microbes are involved (whether they are strychmine, imipramine, tubercle bacilli or meningococci).

Once the natural functions are restored, vital energy will flow harmoniously all over the body, and whatever blockages or exogenous attacks wherever they are will be cleared away. Healthy people, after all, do not have to consciously regulate their acetylocholine and histamine, nor concerned over imipramine and meningococci.

Various therapeutic techniques can be used to implement the therapeutic principles, but those from acupuncture, qigong therapy and massage therapy are most suitable. The following treatment employs massage therapy.

The specific massage treatment will be dictated by the individual pathogenetic conditions of the hemiplegia patient. The following is just a generalized example. As the patient's affected vital points and meridians are almost non-functioning, the therapist has to use more force (than is normally used on other patients) when massaging the hemiplegia patient.

Let the patient lie comfortably on his back. Using the "tui" (pushing) and "mo" (stroking) techniques, give a general massage over the affected parts, moving in the direction from his extremities to his body. This will enhance the flow of his nutrient-energy and defence-energy.

Then massage his upper limbs. Use the techniques of "qia" (piercing), "ci" (poking), "nian" (holding), and "zhen" (vibrating) on the following vital points: jianyu (Li 15), quchi (Li 11), chize (L 5), shaohai (H 3), daling (P 7), yangchi (T 4), yangxi (Li 5), and yanggu (Si 5). Use "tui" (pushing) on shousanli (Li 10) and hegu (Li 4).

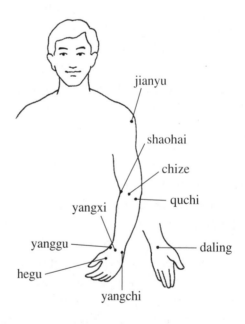

Fig 26.3 Relevant Vital Points on Upper Limb

Next massage the following vital points on his lower limbs, using the same massage techniques as for upper limbs: qichong (S 30), juliao (G 29), huantiao (G 30), fengshi (G 31), yinlingquan (Sp 9), xuehai (Sp 10), weizhong (B 40), chengshan (B 57), taixi (K 3), kunlun (B 60), jiexi (S 41). Use "tui" (pushing) for zusanli (S 36).

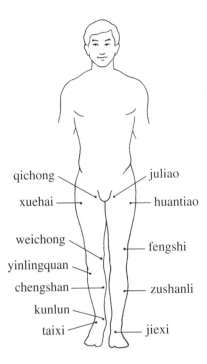

Fig 26.4 Relevant Vital Points on Lower Limb

Massage the face with the "mo" (stroking) and "rou" (rotating) techniques. Use the "tui" (pushing) and "na" (gripping) techniques for the following vital points: taiyang (G 1), cuanzu (B 2), jingming (B 1), yifeng (T 17), jiache (S 6), and dicang (S 4).

The patient should supplement the massage therapy with physiotherapy exercises, like moving and bending his arms and legs, and turning and rotating his head. He should use his healthy hand to help himself with the exercise.

Qigong Therapy for Epilepsy

Epilepsy, a disorder characterized by convulsion and seizure, is another good example illustrating the typically different approaches and considerations the west and the Chinese have for this disease. Western medicine is still unsure about the cause and treatment for epilepsy. Much effort is concentrated on its pathophysiology, attempting to find out at the smallest possible units the electrochemical conditions of the brain cells at the onset of the disease.

The different kinds of epilepsy are divided into two broad groups, namely idiopathic epilepsy in which there is no evidence of any organic brain disorder, and symptomatic epilepsy where the attack is a symptom of organic brain disease, which is thought to be caused by fever, cerebral tumour, lack of oxygen, presence of toxins or excessive sugar, or drug withdrawal.

As the causes are uncertain, western medicine is quite at a loss regarding the treatment for epilepsy, which is principally chemotherapy to suppress seizure. This treatment by drugs is further aggravated by the need to prescribe different types of drugs for different types of seizure, for example, phenytoin or phenobarbital for generalized seizures, ethosuximide or valproate for absence seizures, carbamazepine or primidone for partial seizures, and corticosteriods or clonazepam for myoclonic epilepsy. All these drugs possess powerful toxic effects.

In contrast, the Chinese forget about the leaves and branches, and focus on the forest: they are not worried about the minute details of its pathophysiology and biochemistry, but consider the epileptic patient as a whole person.

Chinese medical scientists believe that the source of epilepsy is fear or shock, which was experienced at an early age, or more significantly while the foetus was in the mother's womb. The negative energies generated by fear or shock caused the patient's vital energy to sink and be chaotic, affecting the heart and the kidneys. The deficiency of kidney energy and heart energy in turn affects the liver and the spleen. Inadequacy of the liver and the spleen systems generates "wind" and produces phlegm, which flow up and cause blockages in various parts of the body, resulting in convulsions and seizures.

As expected, those not familiar with Chinese medical philosophy may find the above explanation strange, even ludicrous; just as those uninformed about western medical theory may find such concepts as sugar in the brain or erratic discharge of neurons outrageous. But what is important is that, while western medicine is at a loss in this matter, the Chinese etiology of epilepsy, which is confirmed by their diagnosis, provides effective therapeutic principles and treatment for the disease.

The therapeutic principles are to restore the harmonious vital energy flow of the heart, kidney, liver and spleen systems, and to disperse "wind" and dissolve phlegm. Qigong therapy, acupuncture and herbal medicine provide useful therapeutic techniques to accomplish these principles.

There are two aspects in qigong treatment for epilepsy. One is to stop the convulsions and seizures when the disease occurs; and the other aspect is to cure the patient by eliminating his pathogenetic conditions, through qigong practice during the absence of the epileptic attack.

When the patient is under convulsion and seizure, first assure him that the attack can be brought under control and ask him to relax as much as he can. Loosen his clothing and take off his shoes. Open his vital points of baihui (Gv 20), shenque (Cv 8), dazhui (Gv 14) and mingmen (Gv 4) on his body by gently rotating a finger on them. Please see Fig 26.5 for the locations of these points. Then open some vital points on his arms and legs, such as those points used in massaging a hemiplegia patient, as illustrated in Fig 26.3 and Fig 26.4 above.

If the patient has clenched his fingers or toes, massage and straighten them, holding them straight with one hand and stroking them downwards with the other. Transmit vital energy into the patient through his mingmen vital point.

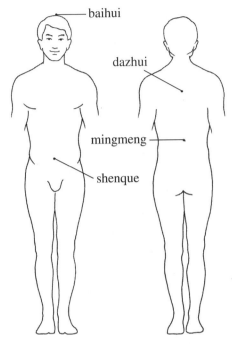

baihui

dazhui

mingmeng

shenque

Fig 26.5 Relevant Vital Points on the Body

When the patient is not under attack, teach him qigong exercises to restore his harmonious energy flow. He has to practice the exercises twice a day for a few months. Qigong is the most holistic of the Chinese therapeutic methods. Almost all general qigong exercises can achieve the effect of harmonizing energy flow. The Five-Animal Play explained in Chapter 22, and Abdominal Breathing and Golden Shower in Chapter 24 are excellent examples.

For faster, but not necessarily better, result, special qigong exercises that work on the heart, kidney, liver and spleen systems may be practiced in place of general qigong exercises.

Curing Depressive Psychosis and Phobia

One of the most interesting and effective ways of curing psychiatric illnesses is the special group of treatment procedures collectively called "therapeutic techniques of the heart". There was once a scholar with a pretty wife. Unfortunately the wife died soon after marriage, leaving the scholar extremely sad and depressed. No doctors could cure him of this depressive psychosis until one day the master physician, Zhu Zhen Heng, treated him.

After asking the patient about his complaints and taking his pulse, the physician felt the patient's stomach. Then he said, "You have lost your appetite, and have no urge for food nor drinks. This is a clear sign that you are pregnant with a baby!"

Hearing this ridiculous diagnosis, the scholar roared with laughter. Since then, each time he met his friends, he would tell them, "That great fool, Zhu Zhen Heng, is suppose to be a great physician. He diagnosed that I am pregnant with a baby!" And they all would laugh and make a fool of Zhu Zhen Heng.

About half a month later, the scholar's depressive psychosis was gone — virtually without his realizing it. The great physician used the therapeutic technique of "Opening the Patient's Heart", i.e. making him cheerful so that his vital energy will flow harmoniously.

The next case history was that of the Yuan Dynasty physician, Zhang Zi He, employing the technique of "Transferring Focus". A merchant and his wife, together with other guests, were robbed in a hotel during a business trip. The robbers made so much noise banging tables and doors that the woman was scared stiff and hid under a bed. When they returned home she developed a phobia. Her psychotic condition was so serious that she would become terrified by the slightest noise in her house. Many physicians had prescribed expensive herbs, acupuncture and other treatment procedures to pacify her mind, but all to no avail.

The famous physician, Zhang Zi He, used an extraordinary yet simple method. He asked the woman to sit on a chair with two strong servants holding her. Then he gently hit the table in front of the woman with a stick. She was scared, but she could not move away as she was being held. "It's only a table. Are you afraid of the table?" he asked gently. "No," the woman replied, though she still trembled.

The physician continued hitting the table with the stick, softly at first, but gradually working to a loud din. Meanwhile he transferred the woman's unknown fear to the table in front, eliciting responses from her that she was not afraid of the table. Later he hit the door and other parts of the house real hard and loud, yet the woman was not afraid, even when the servants had released their hold.

At night, while the woman was sleeping, he asked servants to make a lot of noises and hit her bedroom door. But she was not disturbed; her phobia was gone. This method may appear simple, but only a master could have thought of it and use it artfully. The physician had transferred the focus of her inner unknown fear to the external table, and changed the mental state of the patient to marshal her vital energy to overcome her problem.

Chinese medicine has much to offer the west. Many disorders commonly considered incurable in western medical thinking can be, and have been, cured by using Chinese medical methods.

The benefits are not just acquiring some useful therapeutic techniques, as is often done by some enterprising western doctors, but more importantly, I believe, in understanding Chinese medical philosophy, which is so different from that in western medicine and which can help medical scientists to view their current seemingly unsolvable problems from a different perspective so that they can come up with answers, still using western conventional treatments, for the many medical problems afflicting western societies today.

27

PATH OF GREATEST ACHIEVEMENT
(Meditation in Medicine)

The Greeks seem not to have distinguished Man's divine nature from his human one, and managed to include soul and spirit as well as mind within him. Decartes put Mind and Body asunder. Darwin diminished Man's divinity severely. Freud and his school started the process of putting mind back into human affairs, and lowered the divine part of humanity still further. As in the past, the religious aspects, here the soul and spirit, were simply ignored. The emphasis on sexuality in Freud seemed to debase Man even more.

Prof. Philip Rhodes, The Value of Medicine.

Man as a Unity of Essence, Energy and Spirit

The difference in the concept of health between the west and the Chinese lies beyond pathological principles and therapeutic techniques. To the Chinese, to be healthy is not just being free from disease; it includes physical, emotional, mental and spiritual well-being. A person cannot be said to be healthy, if, even when he is free from physical illnesses, he is easily irritated, has little concentration power, or beset with vice and wickedness.

The Chinese believe that man is an organic unity of essence, energy and spirit. Essence (jing) is the physical substance of the person; energy (qi) is the life force; and spirit (shen) is the mind, soul or consciousness. Health means well-being of all these three aspects of man.

Infectious diseases, as when a person is attacked by hostile microbes, are disorders of jing or essence; physiological dysfunction, as when certain vital organs are not functioning properly, are disorders of qi or energy; psychic illnesses, like when a patient has frightful hallucinations, is a disorder of shen or spirit.

This division, nevertheless, is only for the sake of convenience; when any one aspect is inflicted with sickness, the other two aspects are also involved, because these three aspects of jing, qi and shen are not three different parts but three intimately related aspects of the same organism.

In western medical thought, mind may be different from spirit, but in Chinese, because of cultural and linguistic differences, mind, spirit, soul and consciousness may sometimes be used inter-changeably. Hence, psychiatric or psychic disorders may sometimes be interpreted as spiritual disorders.

It is interesting to note that modern westerners are probably the only people in the whole history of mankind who have alienated the spirit from the body in medicine and health.

All known peoples of the world's greatest civilizations, like the ancient Egyptians, Mesopotamians, Indians, South Americans, Arabs as well as the Chinese, viewed health holistically, taking into consideration man's spiritual besides his physical needs. It was no historical coincidence that most of the ancient physicians of the world civilizations, with the notable exception of the Chinese, were also priests.

This wholesome attitude is still prevalent in modern time amongst many highly civilized peoples. For example, Dr. Vasant Lad says that Indian medicine "views health and disease in holistic terms, taking into consideration the inherent relationship between individual and cosmic spirit, individual and cosmic consciousness, energy and matter."

Shaykh Hakim Moinuddin Chishti, a modern Muslim healer, says that "there must be a knowledge and consideration of the physical, mental and spiritual planes of existence for there to be true health."

In the past, western people too regarded the spirit as an essential part of the body. It was only in the Middle Ages that the dichotomy formally started, with doctors of theology looking after the spirit and doctors of medicine looking after the physical body, though spiritual healing in various forms has continued to play a significant role in western culture, albeit indifference if not disdain from many orthodox medical doctors.

This failure to understand or appreciate the holistic view of spirit and body, probably more than anything else, has led many modern western scholars to regard ancient medical systems as superstitious practices, although these systems were successfully practiced by highly civilized peoples.

Happily, as more and more western doctors are placing greater and greater importance on the mind in medical matters, there is recently also a return to the concept of the spirit.

Francis MacNutt, the world renown Christian healer, says, "The `Anointing of the Sick' is now for the professed purpose of healing the whole man and is no longer primarily a preparation of the soul for death." Does it work for physical and emotional sickness? "In the past eighteen years I think I can safely say that I have seen thousands of healing take place through prayer," answers MacNutt, who has healed in more than 30 countries.

Spirituality is Universal

Since the Chinese have always considered the spirit and the body as one unity, why were ancient Chinese physicians, unlike most of their counterparts in other great ancient civilizations, not priests too? This was because the Chinese did not (and do not) insist on any particular religious practice in attaining spiritual health.

Although the Chinese are spiritual, i.e. they believe in the reality of the spirit that transcends the physical body, they are not specifically religious. In other words, the Chinese believe that spiritual health can be realized through any religion, or even without a formal religion. Thus, the discussion on spiritual health in this chapter is strictly non-religious.

Nevertheless, as spiritual health is closely related to religious development, much of what is discussed here is often found in mysticism and metaphysics rather than in medicine proper. A brief discussion on the spiritual development in the world's greatest religions is, therefore, relevant.

Although the world's greatest religions appear to be strikingly different in their ritualistic aspects, their basic teachings are amazingly similar! This is evident from the following simple experiment. Quoted below are the fundamental aims of the world's greatest religions as taught by their greatest teachers, with their give-away terms like "God" and "Brahman" replaced by the neutral term "Supreme Reality". Can you tell the religions from the quotations?

> Avoid doing all forms of evil, practice all forms of goodness; ultimately let your heart return to the Supreme Reality.

> There is one Supreme Reality and Source of all mankind, who is Lord of all, works through all, and is in all.

> The Supreme Reality is all. From the Supreme Reality come appearances, sensations, desires, deeds. But all these are merely name and form. To know the Supreme Reality one must experience the identity between him and the Self.

> The Supreme Reality exists before heaven and earth, and has no form nor appearance. It is forever changing; and its constant transformation gives rise to form and appearance of everything in the universe.

> Every scripture and every prophet from the first have said the same thing: that we are created by the Supreme Reality, and that the special purpose of our existence is to endeavor to work our way back to Him.

The first quotation was from Zhi Yi, a Buddhist master. "Supreme Reality" here should be replaced by "Void". The second quotation was from the Bible. "Supreme Reality" and "Source" should read "God" and "Father" respectively. The third was quoted from the Upanishads, the scared books of the Hindus.

"Supreme Reality" here should be "Brahman". The fourth quotation was from Lao Tzu in the Tao Te Ching. "Supreme Reality" should read "Tao". The fifth was from Shaykh Hakim Moinuddin Chishti, a Muslim master. "The Supreme Reality" should be replaced by "a wise and loving Creator".

Not only their aims, but also the ways to realize them are also similar. The following is the gist of the methods taught by their greatest masters to attain spiritual fulfilment. Can you tell the religions from which these quotations are taken?

> It is preventing the heart from thinking of anything whatsoever, keeping it free from all vain thoughts.

> Intro-version concentrates the mind on its own deepest part in what is seen as the final step before the soul finds Reality.

> The basic technique of internal viewing is silence of the heart, and its application the termination of all thoughts.

> It is the filling of the mind with God to the exclusion of all else.

> The mind enters into the sphere of the Great Seal of clear light devoid of dualistic elaborations.

The method in the first example was described by Mir Valiuddin, a Muslim master. The second is the Christian method of spiritual fulfilment taught by Saint Augustine. The word "Reality" in this example should be replaced by "God". The third example was taught by Liu Hua Yang, a Taoist saint. The fourth was by Swami Paramananda, a Hindu master. The fifth method is from Vajrayana Buddhism, taught by His Holy Highness the Dalai Lama himself.

Many readers may have difficulty in matching the quotations with their respective religions because basically they are similar in their aims as well as the methods to realize them. The apparent differences in their outward rituals and ceremonies are due to historical, geographical, cultural, linguistic and other factors.

Fundamentally, the aims of the world's great religions are to return to or be united with the Supreme Reality, known by various names like God, Brahman, Tao and Buddha. Their methods, as taught and practiced by their greatest teachers at the highest level, and which may be unfamiliar to most common followers, are through meditation. Meditation (sometimes called contemplation, concentration or introversion) refers to the training of the mind (spirit, soul or consciousness) to achieve different and deeper (or higher) levels of reality.

Some readers may wonder what has this discussion on the universality of spiritual development to do with Chinese medicine or any healing system. There are two good reasons.

One, according to Chinese medical philosophy, health is the wholesome well-being of essence, energy and spirit as one united organism in relation to the whole cosmos; or in western terms, health is not only physical but also emotional, mental and spiritual well-being individually as well as universally.

Two, the similarity in the basic aims and methods of the different religions demonstrates that spirituality is universal; hence, the meaning of and practice to attain spiritual health explained in this chapter is non-religious, i.e. it can be followed by people of any religious conviction and also by those who claim to profess no religion.

Spiritual Illness and Spiritual Health

Because of cultural and religious differences, different people may have different ideas of what constitute spiritual illness and spiritual health. The following, therefore, is only a suggestion.

As morality is the basis of every great religion, it can be safely said that any form of immorality is a symptom of spiritual illness. For example, a person is sick if he or she is involved in, or even harbours thoughts of wittingly causing grievous physical or emotional harm, stealing others' properties or spouses, and obvious wicked acts like killing, raping, torturing and forcing males or females into slavery and prostitution.

A person who has no love or respect for himself and others, who lacks confidence and a sense of responsibility, who feels lost or drifting meaninglessly in life, who meddles in black magic and appeases lesser spirits for personal gains, and who fears ghosts and devils, is spiritually unhealthy.

Spiritual health includes a feeling of inner peace, a zest for living, and a cosmic awareness that there is more to physical life. A spiritually healthy person is generous, charitable, loving and kind to all beings, irrespective of race, culture and religion, and irrespective of whether the beings are human, astral or otherwise.

Moral or religious education is an excellent preparation for spiritual health as well as for curing spiritual sickness.

Nevertheless, spiritual realization is an intuitive, not an intellectual, experience. While intellectual understanding is very helpful, to realize our spiritual self we have to experience it directly.

This is what Lao Tzu meant when he says, "The Tao that can be named, is not the real Tao." Someone who has experienced Tao, or the Supreme Reality, may describe it exactly, but because of the limitation of language and our lack of direct experience, we still will not know what it is despite his excellent description, just as one who has never eaten an orange will not know how it tastes no matter how accurate the description may be.

Similarly, Jesus says, "The Kingdom of God is within you." No matter how well a description of the Kingdom of God is, we will not know it unless we experience it directly. To experience the Kingdom of God, or Tao, or Buddhahood, or be united with Brahman, or to return to Allah, or to attain any form of spiritual fulfilment, the timeless, golden path is meditation.

Holistic Health and Spiritual Realization

Some people may have the impression that meditation is sitting cross-legged with the eyes close. This is only one of numerous outward forms of meditation. Meditation may take any outward form, but the essential point is to train the mind or spirit to attain different states of awareness, and at the highest or deepest states, the meditator attains spiritual realization. Deep prayers and recitation of religious verses are forms of meditation. Meditation is the paramount path to mental and spiritual health.

Recalling his experience at "a small conference of scientists all of whom practiced meditation on a daily basis", Lawrence LeShan explains that meditation is "like coming home ... to find, to recover, to come back to something of ourselves we once dimly and unknowingly had and have lost without knowing what it was or where or when we lost it."

Brugh Joy, M.D., who gave up his highly successful orthodox medical practice to teach transformational process, says that "meditation is the journey to everywhere of the entire universe, to the nowhere of the infinitesimal point at the centre of the individual consciousness."

Meditation is a general term. There are countless techniques to attain a meditative state of mind. Summarizing the countless meditation techniques in an interesting way, and quoting Joseph Goldstein, Daniel Goleman says, "All meditation systems either aim for One or Zero — union with God or emptiness. The path to the One is through concentration on Him, to the Zero is insight into the voidness of one's mind."

At the most advanced level, the One and the Zero are the same, referring to the only One and no other undifferentiated, timeless, spaceless Supreme Reality devoid of any phenomena as experienced in ordinary consciousness.

Sri Dhammananda, a Buddhist master, sums up the benefits of meditation succinctly: "The immediate purpose of meditation is to train the mind and use it effectively and efficiently in our daily life. The ultimate aim of meditation is to seek release from the wheel of Samsara — the cycle of birth and death."

To anyone irrespective of his religious conviction, the last sentence may be modified to read: The ultimate aim of meditation is to seek spiritual realization.

At a lower, more prosaic level, meditation is an effective mean for curing and preventing illnesses! It is well know that meditation masters are not only emotionally matured, mentally fresh and spiritually peaceful, but also radiant in physical health. Many people may accept that meditation can cure spiritual, mental or emotional disorders; but how does it cure physical diseases, like a viral infection or an organic dysfunction?

As meditation is the process of training the mind and spirit, logically it is effective for correcting emotional, mental and spiritual ills, which are after all the consequences of a weak mind or spirit.

In line with Chinese medical philosophy, curing such disorders using meditation is treating the patient as a whole person and attacking the disease at its root cause. Your mind or spirit is considered by many philosophers as the "permanent" Real You, while all your physical self is constantly changing.

Some philosophers, like the Theravada Buddhist, regard even the mind as "transient". This great truth is now acknowledged by modern science. The renown biologist Prof. E.J. Ambrose says:

> A most notable feature of living organisms, whether composed of single cells as in bacteria or of assembles of diverse cell types as in mammals, is that molecules are continuously entering organisms from the environment, while other simple and closely related molecules are continuously being eliminated from the cells. This flow of matter through the organism is a universal phenomenon observed in all life ... So the organism has no material permanence.

Your whole physical body, including all the current cells of your diseased organs as well as the microbes inside you, will be totally changed at the most in seven months, some parts even within a few seconds! A meditation master can actually influence the rate and nature of this change.

Why is it that when a person progresses in his meditation practice, he gradually discards his negative traits like envy, jealousy, arrogance and malice, and develops positive attitudes like compassion, courtesy, tolerance and kindness? This is because his spirit is an expression and integral part of the Universal Spirit, called by various names like God, Brahman, Tathagata, and Tao. This divine spark in him, which manifests only good qualities, has been veiled by layers of defilement, shrouded by illusions of gross sense perceptions. As he advances in meditation, he approaches spiritual realization, which links him organically to the Universal Spirit, thereby overcoming and tearing down the layers of defilement and illusions, and manifesting his intrinsic divine qualities.

Speaking on spiritual healing by the laying one's hands on his patients, which he terms "bio-energotherapy", and which is similar to one aspect of Chinese qigong therapy, the famous Russian psychologist who is also a former champion at rowing and volleyball, Dr. Victor Krivorotov, explains the following which is akin to Chinese medical thinking, and which may open rewarding avenues for western medicine, although initially some western doctors may oppose it vehemently.

> A disease is that state of the system in which full spiritual potential is unrealized. Deformations inside any one of a person's subsystems are reflected in the state of the other systems and the whole, and lead to a drop in spiritual potential. Given this definition of disease, what does effective treatment consist of? Treatment consists in stimulating the patient's spirit, which affects all the systems, bringing them into a harmonious state.

> The stimulation of the spirit may be accomplished in one of two ways: either directly or by correcting the subsystem which is the initial source of the disease. For the most part, modern medicine effects somatic corrections.

> Consequently, treatment can be successful only in those cases where the initial source of the disease is in the body. But for modern man, the primary source of disintegration has become a negative system of conditioning (manifesting egotism, arrogance, vanity, envy, jealousy, etc), the system of values, and world-view.

Hence, when a patient suffers from a viral infection, an organic dysfunction, or any physical, emotional or mental disorder, his spirit is also affected. In Chinese medical terms, illness at the essence and the energy dimensions also affects the spirit dimension, and vice versa. This hampers full spiritual realization.

The disease can be cured in two ways: working at the spiritual level, as in meditation; or working at the essence and the energy levels, as in herbal medicine, acupuncture, massage therapy and other therapeutic approaches.

But how does working at the spiritual level cure disorders of the essence and of the energy dimensions? Or, put in another way, how can meditation cure diseases like measles and hepatitis B, or diabetes and peptic ulcers? Before we laugh at the answer whatever it may turn out to be, because the question, according to the orthodox western medical paradigm, seems so ludicrous, let us not forget that at present, western medicine can offer no cure for viral infections and organic diseases, and it appears unlikely that any cure may be found in the near future if western medicine persists in its current mechanical and reductionist perspective.

It may come as a great surprise to many people to be aware of the fact that most if not all healing involves the spiritual or mind dimension. Viruses of all types, many of which are probably still unknown to us, attack us all the time; wear and tear, residues and toxins of various forms constantly affect all our organs. Yet, we are normally healthy, because of the wonderful, almost unbelievable work performed by our myriad and minute units of consciousness which the Chinese collectively called the spiritual dimension that maintains what western science call the feed-back, immune, defence and other natural systems of our body. Without the spirit, the physical body is merely a heap of meat and bones, which micro-organisms can easily reduce to carbon, nitrogen, oxygen, hydrogen, calcium and other elements.

Meditation, which is a development of our mental and spiritual powers, can enhance all these natural abilities of our body for our survival and meaningful living. In meditation, if we have the skill and know the techniques, we can literally channel vital energy to where it is needed, repair wear and tear, clear away residues and toxins, contain hostile microbes, as well as accomplish other astonishing tasks (like mind projection and distant healing) that many people dare not believe they are possible, and which some would ridicule as fakery.

All these fantastic feats, like controlling physiological functions and applying psychic abilities, have been demonstrated by yogis, psychic healers, qigong masters and other people. It was not for no reasons that William James, the father of American psychology, considered the mind as the most powerful force in the world.

However, to achieve high levels of meditation whereby such incredible abilities are possible, demands much time and great effort. When they are sick, most people find it easier to seek the help of western doctors, Chinese physicians or other healers.

Yet, even if you are not interested in or ready for applying meditation to cure illnesses or perform fantastic feats, practicing meditation is very beneficial, such as helping you to manage stress, improve your mental concentration, promote clarity of thought, and perhaps most significantly provide mental and spiritual health. When you are ready, it will set you on the golden path to the greatest achievement any person could ever have, namely spiritual realization.

Achieving Mental and Spiritual Health

There are literally hundreds of mediation techniques. When we make allowance for personal preference and variations, it is true to say that there are as many meditation techniques as there are meditators. These numerous techniques can be classified into major groups, and then into sub-groups. The more important major groups are as follows.

1. Using the breath.
2. Focusing on an external object.
3. Focusing on various parts of the body.
4. Focusing on a vision.
5. Using sound (including reciting scriptures).
6. Using numbers (including using rosary).
7. Concentrating on a thought.
8. Meditating on the void.

The following example uses breathing as a technique to enter into a deep meditative state of mind so as to reach the spirit. It is bafflingly simple, but the benefits, if you have the discipline to practice regularly and consistently for a few months, will probably be more than what you would expect.

Sit in any comfortable position. The best choice is the double lotus position, where you sit cross-legged with both feet placed at your thighs and both soles facing upwards. This is a difficult posture for most untrained people. The next best position is the single lotus, where only one sole is placed on the thigh and facing upwards. You can place your palms on your knees, or one on top of the other in front of you on your folded legs, or in any comfortable position you like. Please see Fig 27.1.

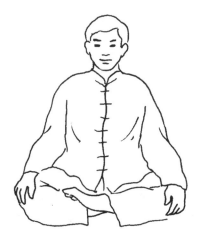 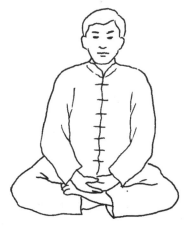

Fig 27.1 Double Lotus and Single Lotus for Meditation

A much easier posture is the simple upright sitting position, where you sit upright on a hard seat with your thighs almost horizontal to, and your feet firmly on the ground. Place your two palms comfortably on your thighs.

Instead of sitting, you may stand comfortably upright with feet fairly close together and arms hanging loosely on both sides. For the sitting and standing positions, the body should be comfortably upright and relaxed, and the head tilted slightly forward. Please see Fig 27.2.

Those who are too old or weak may practice mediation lying down on a bed or a couch. Throughout the meditation practice, the eyes should be gently closed or half close.

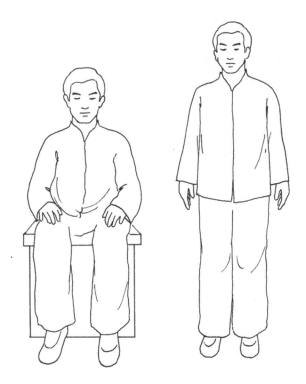

Fig 27.2 Simple Sitting and Standing Positions

Be totally relaxed. Smile from your heart. Then be gently aware of your breathing. There is no need to breath consciously. Follow your breath gently each time your breathe in, and follow your breath gently each time you breathe out. Continue this seemingly simple procedure for about five minutes.

This is virtually all you need to do for the meditation practice, but it is a mistake to think this is easy. Focusing the mind is one of the most difficult tasks to accomplish, though it can be done with determination and practice. In this case, we use breathing as the mean to focus our mind.

Irrelevant thoughts will start entering your mind. Discard them firmly as soon as they enter, and carry on focusing on your breathing in and out. If you lose track of your breathing, resume your focus as soon as you realize it. Sometimes you may feel drowsy, or you may have actually slept in your meditation. As soon as you recover your awareness, resume your focus on your breathing.

Do not be disappointed if you find that the total time you can successfully follow your breaths adds up to less than a minute. Indeed, if you can successfully focus your mind on your breath for one minute, i.e. achieving a one-pointed mind for one minute, you would have done remarkably well.

After practicing this meditation technique for about five minutes, rub your two palms together to warm them. Place the center of your palms on your eyes, dab your eyes to warm them as you open them. Then gently massage your face and head. Get up from your posture and walk about briskly for about thirty steps. This completes the whole meditation exercise.

Other meditation teachers may suggest a longer period of meditation practice per session. In the school of meditation I am trained in, namely Shaolin, we emphasize on quality rather than quantity.

We believe that achieving a one-pointed mind (or "void" in a different kind of meditation practice) continuously for a minute in a five minute session, is better than sitting in mental chaos for half an hour with occasional flashes of mental one-pointedness, though these separate bits of flashes may add up to more than a minute.

Later, as you progress, as you find that you can more easily focus your mind on your breathing for longer time, you can gradually increase the time of practice per session. Practice twice a day, preferably a session in the morning and another at night.

As you progress, you may experience certain odd sensations. You may, for example, feel as if your mind or physical body is revolving, or you have lost certain parts of your body, or you have become very big or small in size. These are normal signs of your progress, but you should not place any special importance on them, neither should you hope that these sensations would happen.

However, if you experience any frightful visions or sounds or any unpleasant sensations like headaches, palpitation and fear, firmly order these unwelcome experiences to dissolve, and assure yourself that these bad experiences cannot harm you because they were merely tricks of your mind or perhaps psychic expressions of your own thoughts or emotions.

If these unpleasant experiences frequently trouble you, you should stop your meditation practice, at least for the time being.

Using the Mind or Spirit in Healing

After you have acquired the skill to control your mind, you can apply some useful techniques to cure illnesses or accomplish other wholesome tasks. The following are some examples. Go into a meditative state of mind. See in your mind's eye, your diseased part, then see that your own regenerative processes cure the diseased part. Hold this self-healing vision as long as you comfortably can.

Let say you have a peptic ulcer or a kidney failure. First visualize your stomach with the ulcer, or your kidneys not functioning as they should. Then visualize the injured cells in your stomach or kidneys being replaced by healthy, normal cells.

Hold this vision of your recovery as long as you comfortably can. It is very important that you must not force your vision. If you lose the vision, rest for a short while, still in your meditation poise, then resume the visualization gently.

At a later stage, start your visualization straight away with vision of your healthy stomach or kidneys, and hold the healthy vision. All this time you are in a meditative, or subconscious, state. You will enhance your self-curing processes if you also believe and feel during your ordinary consciousness that you are cured.

Later when you go for a medical examination, your doctors will be surprised that tests show you are actually cured.

For some diseases, like insomnia or diabetes, it may not be easy to localize the sickness to visualize it. In such cases, use visions that explicitly demonstrate you are cured, like visualizing that as soon as you go to bed you sleep soundly, or that you have discarded your insulin tablets or injection, yet you can drink tea or coffee with sugar and without any ill effects.

Some people may find it hard to visualize; they may, during their meditation, gently and subconsciously think of their recovery processes or situations indicating that they have recovered.

The regenerating and self-curing processes in your visualization are real, not imaginary. They are our natural abilities, performed by us unconsciously all the time. For some reasons, these natural functions partially fail, resulting in peptic ulcer, diabetes or other diseases. Visualizing (or thinking of) these processes working as they should in our meditation, restores and enhances their natural functions.

Millions of cells are being replaced in our body every second; holding an appropriate vision during our meditation, acts like providing a master blue-print for healthy and normal cell reproduction.

Although this truth is little known (or appreciated) by most modern medical scientists because most of the time they are too pre-occupied with the reductionist mechanics of cells and enzymes to consider the holistic functioning of the patient as a whole person, the influence or control of the mind over the body was long recognized by ancient masters, and is now demonstrated by such occasions as spiritual healing and bio-feedback.

How does the mind influence or order the body to produce the right cells to heal the peptic ulcer, or to restore the natural production of the right hormones to overcome diabetes? It does so in the same way as it orders your mouth to eat your dinner, or your eyes to read this writing.

The physical body, without the mind or spirit, is lifeless matter; it is the mind or spirit that is responsible for all physiological and psychological activities. For example, someone who lacks the mental ability or whose mind is not focused, will not understand what he reads, although his physical eyes and all relevant muscles and nerves are structurally and functionally intact.

The numbers of successful spiritual healing in various religions throughout history as well as in our present time are too large and wide-spread for any sensible person to dismiss their success as placebo effect or coincidence.

Although there are bogus healers in spiritual healing as in all other kinds of healing, the situations and the standing of many spiritual healers are such that to suggest their cures are faked, is ridiculous, if not downright disrespectful. Most patients who seek spiritual healing do so as a last resort, after trying many other forms of healing to no avail.

How sensible, then, is it to suggest that thousands of patients all over the world who have suffered many years of so-called incurable diseases, conspire with highly religious masters whom many patients may have never met before, and who may not charge them any money, to fake cures to mislead other people?

If some modern scientists feel uncomfortable to believe that divine forces are involved in spiritual healing, then my explanation above, which was based on the influence of mind over body, may provide an alternative answer.

However, I personally think, the two explanations are ultimately similar, because when we reach our own spirit in deep meditation we become intimately, organically linked to the Universal Spirit. This mind-over-body theory may also explain what many doctors find puzzling, namely spontaneous remission.

This observation, of course, never implies that physical medicine — whether western, Chinese or others — is inferior to spiritual healing. For most people, most of the time, curing their illnesses by swallowing pharmacological drugs, drinking herbal decoction, having acupuncture needles inserted into their body, or taking any other appropriate therapeutic measures is easier, and probably more effective, than curing by meditation or by travelling half the world to seek genuine spiritual healers. But the observation provides at least three good points for thought and action.

One, for those who believe in mind-over-matter and who have the self-discipline to practice meditation, visualizing the recovery processes in a meditative state of mind, will speed up whatever physical or psychiatric treatment they are undergoing.

Secondly, for the few unfortunate people who suffer from so-called incurable illnesses, there is still much hope. They may cure themselves through their own spirit in meditation, or through the Universal Spirit in spiritual healing. They can derive a lot of confidence from the fact that since these two methods have worked for thousands of other people, they can also work for them.

Thirdly, for the brave medical scientists who dare to be ahead of their mediocre colleagues, yet working within the principles and practice of their training, the ideas discussed above may provide a conceptual framework for research leading to some medical breakthroughs.

TOWARDS HOLISTIC HEALTH

(Possible Chinese Contribution to the West)

The weight of scientific evidence has disprove the doctrine of specific etiology which has dominated medical thought for the past century. Looking back, the doctrine was merely a fad in the course of medical history, a fad fueled by unbridled faith in the reductionist approach to illness which followed in the wake of Pasteur's germ theory. The new medicine has returned us to our roots in Hippocratean theory.

Melvyn Werbach, M.D., 1986.

Strength and Weakness of Western Medicine

Dr Werback's observation above is typical of a growing reaction against the exceedingly reductionist and mechanical approach of modern western medicine. Dr Stephen Fulder reminds us Hippocrates,

> believed that health was restored by equilibrium — crasis — within the fluid essences — humours — of man. In his view, the healing process was designed only to aid the body's own self-healing capacities ... modern medicine has only dominated medical practice for the last 100 years. It may represent no more than a swing of the pendulum from Hygieia (whereby good health is the result of man's understanding of how to live) to Aesculapius (whereby disease is healed by correcting imperfections); indeed there are already signs that medicine is beginning to move back from the scientific extreme.

Prof. John W. Thompson, commenting that there is a large and growing number of people who wish to find out more about alternative medicine, says,

> Conventional medicine does not hold all the answers to the problems of disease and that is why it is so important to find out what positive contributions can be made by complementary medicine. The best of both systems then need to be brought to work together for the greater benefit of the human race.

Two significant points should be noted. All the quotations above as well as similar quotations elsewhere in this book are made by experts eminently qualified in western medicine; many are authorities in their fields.

Secondly, all these experts are fully aware of the great contribution of western medicine to world health; their dissatisfaction is not due to any pessimism or lack of confidence, but due to their sincere concern for correcting certain setbacks in western medicine for the benefit of all humanity. Their courage and care for the progress of their profession is the more admirable when we realize that throughout western medical history, such farsightedness has always been vehemently opposed by the mediocre majority. For example, Harvey, who discovered blood circulation for western medicine, and Pasteur, the father of germ theory himself, were severely ridiculed; Wilhelm Reich, the founder of bioenergetics, and Ruth Drown, one of the pioneers of radonics, spent many years in prison for their discoveries.

It must be stressed again that the constructive criticism of western medicine should not distract us from its other marvellous achievements. There is no doubt that western medicine has made, and will continue to make, a tremendous contribution to humanity. The accomplishments of western medicine especially in curing or immunizing against infectious diseases is awe-inspiring.

For me personally, the discovery of Paracetamol is a pharmacological wonder. Imagine someone in the past with an excruciating headache; he would probably be willing to pay a lot of money to get his pain removed. Yet with Paracetamol costing less than a dollar, now he merely has to swallow two tablets with some water and a little rest, to have his pain relieved.

On the other hand, if readers are impressed with the profundity and effectiveness of Chinese medicine as explained in this book, they should also be aware that unlike western doctors who have to be properly qualified before they are permitted by the medical authority of their respective countries to practice, in many societies almost anyone can practice various forms of Chinese medicine. Because of this lack of control, some Chinese practitioners may not be properly qualified.

It is also a mistake to think that most Chinese know much about Chinese medicine. In fact, the average Chinese are as ignorant of Chinese medical philosophy and practices as they are ignorant of Chinese poetry, kungfu or the I Ching; and ironically enough, many of them believe that Chinese medicine is primitive and unscientific! After all, it was only recently in China that knowledge of arts and science ceased to be the exclusive privilege of the elite.

The role of western medicine in overcoming former killer-diseases, like cholera, malaria, smallpox and tuberculosis, fills us with awe and gratitude. For us lucky to be living in the twenty first century when these killers are completely under control, we may not fully appreciate the terror and suffering these diseases brought.

In the past, more soldiers were killed by diseases than actual fighting even during times of war. The Franco-Prussian War of 1870-1 was the first time in history when more solders died in fighting than of diseases. Of the 300,000 crusaders who left Western Europe in 1096, only 20,000 reached their destination. More South Americans died of smallpox, which they regarded as a whiteman's disease, than from fighting the invaders during the Spanish conquest. Typhus killed 300,000 French soldiers in the Peninsular War and decimated Napolean's Moscow campaign.

During peace times, something like a third of the total population of Europe was wiped out by epidemics! In the cholera epidemic of 1830-2, 60,000 people in Britain died between 1931-2, and this figure was low when compared to other European countries.

In Britain the death ratio was 1 in 131 people, in Poland it was 1 in 32, Austria 1 in 30, in Russia 1 in 20! Paul Hastings gave a vivid, morbid picture of epidemics: "Moral ties vanished. In the wild scramble for safety mother fled from child, brother from brother, and husband from wife. Villages were deserted, some never to be reoccupied, and grass grew in the streets."

In 1832 the cholera epidemic spread to America. The people were so terror-stricken that "in Pennsylvania several persons suspected of infection were murdered along with the men who sheltered them. Armed Rhode Islanders turned back New Yorkers fleeing across Long Island Sound, while at Ypsilanti local militia fired upon the mail-coach from cholera-stricken Detroit. Despite such efforts only Boston and Charleston of America's major cities escaped."

Against such a background, we can understand the great admiration and respect the first half of the twentieth century gave to western medicine. The euphoria was probably highest in the 1970s when Paul Hastings said, "Today a man of seventy can justly claim that more medical progress has been made in his life-time than in all previous history."

Probably, with the grim picture of the European epidemics in mind, Paul Hastings was comparing the effectiveness of modern chemotherapy with cupping and blood-letting, which were the standard therapeutic methods of the nineteenth century.

It was also likely that he was unaware of the tremendous achievements made in Chinese medicine in previous centuries. Epidemics had threatened China earlier, but the Chinese could satisfactorily contain them. It is sobering to reflect whether many lives could be saved had Chinese medical knowledge and practices been available to the west then.

While western medicine has successfully overcome deadly infectious diseases, other groups of sickness, especially cardiovascular illnesses, cancer and psychiatric disorders, have now reached epidemic proportions in western societies.

In its fight against infectious diseases, the basic philosophy of western medicine was to isolate and identify the particular disease-causing agents, then to prescribe specific drugs against them. In time this philosophical perspective has made western medicine to be exceedingly reductionist and mechanical in its approach.

While this approach is effective against infectious diseases, it is not suitable for organic and psychiatric disorders, where the patient as a whole person as well as his mental or spiritual aspects have to be considered.

In this respect, Chinese medicine has much to offer the west, not only in treatment methods, but also in background theory and empirical knowledge that has been gathered over many centuries. Information on Chinese medicine has been scarce; whatever little that manages to reach the west is often inadequate or, worse still, misleading.

This is understandable, for a good writer for this purpose need not only be well versed in both Chinese and western medical knowledge, but, perhaps more significantly, he must also be able to present his material in a way that western readers can readily comprehend and enjoy reading.

Because of cultural, linguistic and other factors, meaningful and poetic medical writings in Chinese, if poorly translated, can become very dry and even appear foolish, as has been demonstrated many times in this book, with the inevitable result that many interested western readers would be put off.

This book is a modest but conscious attempt to overcome these difficulties to present a comprehensive introduction of Chinese medicine to the west, with the earnest hope that some enterprising researchers may investigate the claims made in this book, so that if the claims are verified they can be widely used to overcome pressing medical problems troubling the world today.

Is Chinese Medicine Primitive and Unscientific?

The adjectives "modern" and "traditional", with their connotations of "scientific" and "primitive", that are frequently used to describe western medicine and Chinese medicine respectively are misleading. Is Chinese medicine primitive and unscientific as many uninformed people would think?

It is safe to say that anyone who has read even some of the material presented in this book would be amazed at the very advanced principles and practices in Chinese medicine.

In herbal medicine, for example, the Chinese physician does not merely prescribe a certain herb or herbal mixture for a particular complain. After a thorough diagnosis to find out not just the disease, but the pathogenetic conditions of the patient as a whole person, and planning a systematic therapeutic program which takes into consideration such factors as the relative strength of the patient's natural resistance against the disease, the location and developmental stage of the illness, and the most suitable mode of eliminating the pathogenic agents, the physician prescribes not just herbs to overcome the patient's major and secondary ailments but also look after his other needs like promoting relevant physiological processes, neutralizing possible side effects, and guiding the medication to where it is needed.

In massage therapy, a self-contained healing system in Chinese medicine that can be used to cure almost all kinds of diseases, a therapist can use thirty different major types of massage techniques and hundreds of energy points to accomplish medical tasks that would appear incredible to the laymen.

For example, a master massage therapist can increase the amount of antibodies in our immune system, strengthen our defence system to fight infectious diseases, regulate the supply of acids and other chemicals in our muscles, influence the functions of our vital organs to cure degenerative diseases, and calm our heart or mind so as to better handle psychiatric problems.

By any standards, no responsible critic can say such a medical system, even basing on accomplishments in herbal medicine and massage therapy alone, as primitive.

The next question is whether Chinese medicine is scientific. There is much difference in opinions as what constitutes a science. Many lay persons consider western medicine scientific, and Chinese medicine unscientific because the former makes extensive use of technological instrumentation like blood test, x-ray, electroencephalography, computerized transaxial tomography (CATT scan), and isotope ventriculography, whereas the latter does not use even a simple stethoscope.

Some people ask, "How can Chinese physicians treat patients successfully if they do not even have basic scientific equipments for blood tests and x-rays?" The answer, as has been demonstrated in this book, is that these equipments are not necessary (though many modern Chinese physicians will gladly use them if they are available), because Chinese medicine uses different methods.

Indeed many western experts are presently concerned that western medical practice is becoming too impersonal and over dependent on instruments. The well known neurologist, Sir John Walton, laments that "there is an unfortunate tendency in some centers to submit all patients to a routine series of disturbing, irrelevant and often expensive laboratory or radiological studies."

The much respected western expert, Prof. Norman Cousins, reminds doctors that "the practice of medicine, as it has been emphasized over the centuries by almost every great medical teacher — from Hippocrates to Holmes, from Galen to Cannon, from Castiglione to Osler — calls first of all for a deeply human response by the physician to the cry of the patient for help." Listening and talking to machines, instead of listening and talking to patients, is unlikely to bring out the deeply human response of a physician.

Hence, the application of technological instrumentation is not a valid criterion to judge whether a healing system is scientific. Science refers to a discipline or field of study where its body of knowledge has been acquired empirically, arranged systematically into suitable classes, and principles or laws are generalized.

Aristotle is often regarded as the father of science because of this philosophical perspective. This was actually the way how the huge body of Chinese medicine has been acquired, classified and generalized throughout the ages.

A Chinese herbalist prescribes an appropriate mixture of da huang (Radix et Rhizoma Rhei), huang lian (Rhizoma Copti-dis) and huang ling (Radix Scutellariae) for stomach infections because this treatment has been found effective not just for decades, but for centuries.

A massage therapist, employing the principle of "wood creates fire", manipulates the liver meridian system of a patient to treat his heart disease, not because the therapist is inclined to metaphysics, but because from their long years of experience and study, past masters have generalized such effective treatment methods into the theory of five elemental processes represented here by wood and fire.

These treatment methods, like all other Chinese therapeutics, are predictable and repeatable — two significant features of a science. In other words, the above Chinese physicians can accurately predict the effect of da huang (Radix et Rhizoma Rhei), huang lian (Rhizoma Coptidis) and huang ling (Radix Scutellariae) on the patient with a stomach infection, or the effect of massaging the liver meridian on the heart patient. The effects, given the same conditions, can be repeated in Beijing, Washington or anywhere, tomorrow, three months later or anytime.

Yet, the success of medicine in curing patients' illnesses lies more in its art than its science. Science provides the theory and knowledge; it is the art of the western doctor, Chinese physician or any healer that is mainly responsible for successfully diagnosing the patients' illness and prescribing the appropriate treatment amongst a range of many possibilities, even if the data upon which he makes his decision are provided by scientific instruments.

In medical research too, art has a very important part to play. It is the art of the scientific researcher in visualizing problems and possible solutions from different angles, in formulating imaginative research programs, as well as in persuading both his sponsors and his colleagues to support his daring projects, that is probably more crucial than the mechanics and technology of science to bring about medical breakthroughs. In all these exciting tasks for the sake of humanity, the philosophy and methods of Chinese medicine have much to offer the west.

Rich Body of Empirical Knowledge

There are at least three areas where Chinese medicine can be very useful to western medical practice and research: its huge body of empirical knowledge which are hitherto exotic to the west; its medical theories and principles with their emphasis on emotional, mental and spiritual besides physical health; and its extensive range of treatment methods which are economical, effective and easily available. All these can be incorporated into western medicine without disrupting current western practices.

When we compare the history of western medicine with Chinese medicine (Chapters 1 to 4), we can readily find so many discoveries where the Chinese preceded the west, often by a few centuries.

This fact should inspire us, if we can free ourselves from provincial thinking and misplaced pride, to investigate what the Chinese presently know in medical matters that the west still does not, with the intention of testing it, and if it is valid, incorporating whatever is useful and feasible into our own system.

Needless to say, no western doctors should feel any sense of inadequacy or inferiority to learn from the Chinese or any other people. After all, the Chinese and virtually the whole world have learnt, and are still learning, from the west, and have benefited tremendously. A medical system that has been successfully practiced by the world's largest population for thousands of years certainly has much to teach us.

Indeed there is so much useful knowledge in Chinese medicine still unknown to most other peoples, that the following is only a random suggestion.

The meridian system, evolved by the Chinese through thousands of years, is one rich area promising great rewards for the scientific investigator. Once we understand the meridian system, which links every part of our body meaningfully, many of the successful therapeutic methods which previously appeared irrational, now become sensible.

We can also understand, for example, why practicing qigong or Taijiquan can prevent and cure degenerative diseases, why strengthening the kidneys can improve one's sexual performances and enjoyment, why by feeling the pulse or examining eyes or mouth, a Chinese physician can have a good idea of the conditions of his patient's internal organs.

When Russian scientists discovered in 1960 the existence of meridians and energy points precisely where the Chinese had known them for centuries, and Dr Kim Bong Lan of North Korea discovered in 1963 that the skin cells along a meridian are structurally different from other skin cells, the world scientific body realized their importance and rightly honoured these scientists.

Yet these discoveries are only a very small part of the comprehensive meridian theory of the Chinese. Perhaps in the past such Chinese knowledge was little known in the west, but today the situation is different. It is not difficult now for western researchers, with the cooperation of Chinese masters, to study more deeply these meridians and open a whole new field of hope and possibilities for western medicine.

Another rewarding area for study is the Chinese understanding of the relationship between different emotions and particular organs, resulting in psycho-somatic as well as psychiatric and neurological disorders.

We need to suspend our western knowledge on these matters, at least for the time being, if we are to derive some meaning and benefits from the Chinese, because the Chinese and the west use totally different paradigms.

This paradigm shift is worthwhile if we bear in mind that while psychosomatic, psychiatric and neurological diseases have posed great problems to western medicine, the Chinese have satisfactorily cured them.

It is not just novelty, but to many people the difference between suffering and well-being, to learn that according to Chinese medical knowledge, degenerative diseases, like cardiovascular disorders and hardening of the liver, are closely related to negative emotions, and their curative (not just palliative) treatments are possible by other methods besides taking drugs. Heart and liver problems, for example, can be cured by treating the small intestine and the spleen systems respectively, using acupuncture, qigong therapy and other methods!

Chinese medical case histories record many examples of curing diseases like liver infections, liver hardening, lung infections and kidney swelling not by tending to the afflicted organs, but by way of the spleen-stomach system.

The Chinese provide fascinating or outlandish explanations — depending on whether one understands their working — for psychiatric and neurological disorders. While emotions play a major part in their pathogenesis, psychiatric disorders are traceable to the relevant vital organs, which the Chinese believe house various kinds of consciousness!

For example, those suffering from depression often has stagnation of spleen energy, while those suffering from schizophrenia has energy blocked in their liver. This information suggests that if we promote energy flow at the spleen and the liver system respectively, we can alleviate the depressive and schizophrenic emotions of the patients.

While western medical philosophy believes that neurological diseases like epilepsy and dementia are probably caused by organic brain defects, the Chinese teach that the cause of these disorders, which may or may not be located in the brain, is energy blockages due to exogenous agents like "wind" and "fire", or endogenous agents like excessive shock and melancholy. Hence, neurological diseases can be cured by removing their root cause, without having to operate on the brain!

Medical Principles and Theories

The second area where Chinese medicine can enrich western medicine concerns medical principles and theories, which actually represent the generalization into concise statements and concepts the successful practice of the Chinese over thousands of years. Again, the wealth of knowledge is so much that the following examples are suggested randomly.

Much of the operation of Chinese medicine can be explained by the principles of yin-yang and of five elemental processes. In their simplest forms, yin-yang refers to the two opposing yet complementary aspects of reality, be it expressed in objects or ideas.

The five elemental processes refer to five archetypal groups of processes with characteristic behavior, into which all the countless actions and reactions in the universe are generalized, ranging from the infinitesimal subatomic level to the infinite scale of galaxies. These two principles, like some mathematical formulae, may be simple in form and concept, but their manifestations can be exceedingly varied and profound.

For example, Chinese medical philosophers use the yin-yang principle to explain that for health to be possible, both the structure and the function of man's vital systems, and the psychological and the physiological aspects of all operations, or his internal and his external environments, must be in harmony.

This explains why degenerative diseases are a great problem to western medicine, because most of its instruments measure only structural and not functional defects; why modern living in western societies generates so much sickness, because emotional stress can be translated into physical diseases; and why despite physical well-being many people still feel sick, because they have failed to react efficiently to environmental, climatic or cosmic influences. Chinese medicine does not merely provide the theory, but also supplies numerous methods to restore yin-yang harmony.

Western scientists can draw much inspiration from the concept of the five elemental processes to formulate research programs to investigate hitherto seemingly random or disorderly operation in man or in nature.

Can this principle of the five elemental processes be used to unlock the mystery of hitherto apparently unpredictable behavior of both useful and hostile bacteria and viruses inside man's body; of the arrangement of adenine, guanine, thymine, and cytosine in the DNA; of man's reaction to his physical and social environments; and of the invisible but undeniable effects on our body and mind from outer space?

There are a lot of intriguing examples found in Chinese medicine, many of which have been explained in this book.

At the physical level, Chinese masters have found that the characteristic tastes of herbs have predictable, distinctive effects on the electrochemical reactions in our body.

At the psychological level, Chinese masters have successfully employ this principle of five elemental processes to cure emotional and mental diseases. Indeed, there is sufficient explanation and examples given in this book to justify the claim that if no progress is made by modern research in this direction, it is due not to lack of background information but to want of trying.

Another fundamental principle of Chinese medicine which the west would find beneficial to investigate is holistic treatment of the patient as a whole person. There are already hopeful signs that western medicine, after a century of localistic pathology and therapeutics that necessitate a reductionist, mechanical approach, is moving back to the holistic spirit of Hippocrates' humourism, which actually dominated the greatest proportion in western medical history, and which is also characteristic of most of the medical philosophies of other great peoples.

How sensible is it to presume that a patient's health can be restored by a somatic correction of his minute, isolated parts, with an almost total neglect of all his other parts, and an alienation of his psychic dimension?

Related to this holistic treatment of the whole person is the Chinese belief that we are all healthy by nature and that we can cure ourselves of all kinds of diseases so long as our natural abilities are functioning properly.

Given the extremely hostile environment man is in, with millions of deadly microbes, constant radioactive bombardment, and continuous wear and tear inside and outside his body, if not for this self-curative and regenerative principle, humanity would not be able to survive even for a short while.

Of course, if the disease-causing agent is unreasonably excessive, like someone wearing himself out with severe grief, or contaminating the environment with excessive radioactive material, it ceases to be a question of medicine but one of committing suicide or murder. Dr Morton Glasser, with more than thirty years of clinical experiences, expresses this self-curing aspect succinctly:

> To those grateful patients who have made me responsible for the cause of their recovery, I say, 'You cured yourselves.' Regardless of whether or not I treated them, I am convinced that the majority of my patients would get well. Admittedly, I sometimes hasten my patients' recovery or relieve their pains through medication or therapy, but most would improve on their own.

This principle, as has been discussed elsewhere in this book, has crucial effects on our concept of patho-genesis and therapeutics. So many diseases, ranging from the simple cold and numerous other viral infections to degenerative diseases like cancer and heart problems, are considered to be incurable in western medicine, because, I believe, of the implicit western premise that since diseases comes from outside, it is necessary to find the exact cause before effective treatment is possible.

Partly because the unknown factors are limitless, and partly because of its reductionist and mechanical approaches, the causes of these diseases have continued to elude western medicine. The sobering fact is not that these diseases are incurable; it is that western medicine has not found the cures because it cannot find the causes. The noble endeavor of western medical researchers, despite much time, efforts and money spent on it, is greatly hampered by a doubtful premise, which necessarily dictates the direction and nature of their research development.

The outlook can be easily changed if we are willing to try a different philosophical perspective. This perspective has been found valid and effective in Chinese medicine for centuries, namely health will be restored if we can successfully restore the natural abilities of the patient. The change, which promises so much benefit for humanity and which costs comparatively little risk, can be made so easily that it becomes a great irony that we find it so hard to make the change.

What will the outlook be if we can gather enough courage and effort to make the philosophical shift? Suddenly, as if by the wave of a magic wane or the Grace of God, the term "incurable" becomes irrelevant. Since we can cure all kinds of diseases when our natural abilities function as they should, there is no such things as incurable diseases.

If a particular disease in a particular patient is not cured — in fact, if the disease ever occurs at all — it is because one or more of his natural functions were not operating properly. The logical task is to find out which function or functions are involved, then restore them. Chinese medicine provides ample examples in both theory and practice if we adopt such a philosophical perspective.

In this philosophical perspective, our task becomes so much easier, because we are dealing with comparatively known factors, as the workings of the human mind and body is relatively well known.

Let us take for simple illustration, an analogy of an automobile, an example well suited for a reductionist, mechanical modality. If you wake up one morning and find your car not working, what do you or your mechanic do to get it going again? Do you analyze the surrounding air, and the petrol you just pumped in, to see if they cause your car to fail. You probably don't.

Even if the air or petrol is polluted, within reasonable limits, the filters of your car would have cleansed the input. Neither would you examine the mileage your car travelled the previous week, nor the passenger load it took. Unless you have gone out of your senses, in all probability you will examine the parts of the car itself, like the spark plugs, the car battery and also the air and oil filters.

Why then, when you wake up one morning and find yourself with diabetes or a heart disease, instead of finding out why your natural systems have failed to neutralize the excess sugar or cholesterol you normally take, you or your doctor start worrying about your food, your drink, your exercise and your weight even though you have not drastically changed your life style recently?

Just as your automobile breaks down because of its malfunction, you become sick because your natural systems fail to function properly. The onus, therefore, is to find out why your natural systems which have worked perfectly before, now cannot react efficiently to external factors; rather than to find out what external factors which do not cause any illness to normal people, cause your natural systems to fail.

Perhaps this philosophical shift in looking at disease may lead to finding a cure for AIDS. AIDS is unknown in traditional Chinese medicine. It is not clear whether the ancient Chinese were ignorant of AIDS though it happened in the past, or because it never happened at all in ancient China.

If it had occurred under different names, then it is possible that Chinese physicians might have cured it! Of course they did not know it was AIDS, nor it was caused by the human immuno-deficiency virus (HIV), but they probably would have treated the patient as one who suffered from excessive yin deficiency.

As emphasized many times in this book, the concept of incurable diseases does not occur in Chinese medicine. In theory, at least, AIDS is curable; those who are found to be HIV positive do not necessarily develop AIDS. Of the many approaches in Chinese medicine, qigong is the most effective in improving a person's immune system. This follows that qigong prevents immune deficiency, and even cures immune deficiency if it is unfortunately acquired!

Extensive Range of Therapeutic Techniques

The third area where Chinese medicine can offer much help to western medicine is the extensive range of effective Chinese therapeutic techniques.

Presently this is the area where interested western doctors are most actively involved, because it is probably easier and more practical to learn a few useful techniques to be incorporated into their own medical practices, than to study esoteric theories and principles which were not readily available in the first place.

However, even if these supplementary techniques are useful, when applied without understanding their underlying principles, they are at best superficial, and may at times be harmful.

For example, fang feng (Radix Ledebouriellae) is a common, effective herb for relieving colds, fevers, headaches, and joint pains. But, because of insufficient knowledge, if this herb is given to a patient whose symptoms like the above are caused by yin inadequacy, it will have adverse effects.

Manipulating energy points like qihai (Cv 6), zhaohai (K 6) and zusanli (S 36) with acupuncture or massage therapy to enhance the patient's vital energy is effective for stopping his vomiting if it is an "empty illness" (i.e. illness caused by the weakening of natural functions).

However, if the vomiting is a "solid illness" (i.e. illness caused by exogenous pathogens), enhancing energy through these points would aggravate his suffering.

A more rewarding approach is to transfer the theory and practices of useful Chinese therapeutic techniques into western medicine, instead of merely using these techniques in a haphazard, ad-hoc manner. For example, the profundity of Chinese herbal prescription can be applied to western chemotherapy.

Instead of just prescribing specific pharmacological drugs for specific complaints on a one drug to one complaint basis, western medical scientists may investigate the possibility and benefit of assessing the many complaints of the patient holistically, examining the relationship and mutual influence of the complaints, then categorizing them into major syndromes, so that a medication combination as a system instead of individual drugs can be administered.

The next developmental step is to classify the drugs according to their principal function in the medication combination, such as one class for strengthening the natural systems of the patient, another for attacking exogenous pathogens, a third for neutralizing expected side-effects, and the fourth for acting as catalysts or guides to bring the medication to where it is needed.

This classification is based on the function of the drugs in this particular combination, not based on its general behavior. Hence, the same drugs may be classified into different classes according to their function in different medications. Of course, the favorable and unfavorable inter-reaction of different drugs when used together, must be studied.

The above suggestion could bring much excitement to researchers as well as clinicians. Besides searching for more and more drugs, they can now also search for better and more profound uses of known drugs in different combinations. For the clinician, prescribing medicine is no longer a dull stereotype of giving drug A for disease X. Like the Chinese physician, he acts like a general, planning a strategy of treatment as if manoeuvring an army for battle. Chinese medicine provides many interesting examples of such war games.

On the other hand, for those who prefer a general to a thematic approach, lessons from qigong therapy supply a contrasting alternative. How would you like a few treatment methods that can cure almost all ailments, including the so-called incurable diseases like cardiovascular disorders, cancer and psychiatric illnesses? Some readers may think I am joking; the less tolerant may even consider suing me for making false claims.

The claims, although may appear wild to many people, are made in sincerity and good faith. Despite having been ridiculed many times before, often by people who should have known better, it is my earnest wish to make known to more people that suffering from so-called incurable diseases can be relieved through qigong.

Of course, whether these people would take advantage of this wonderful practice is their prerogative.

It is understandable that those not familiar with qigong find it hard to believe that a combination of a few qigong exercises can cure a wide range of illnesses, just as those unfamiliar with genetics find it hard to believe that just four basic units of DNA can build a countless variety of living creatures ranging from bacteria and tadpoles to elephants and humans. Just as the range of creatures is extremely wide, the quality and kinds of qigong can be vastly different too.

Yet, it can be safely said that almost any type of qigong, if performed correctly, is beneficial to health, although if the type is elementary it may not be powerful enough to cure "incurable" diseases. And if you wish to practice advanced qigong, you must learn it from a master or a qualified instructor.

As discussed earlier, "incurable" diseases are irrelevant in Chinese medical philosophy, which expostulates that man, by nature, is healthy and is capable of overcoming all illnesses.

Qigong, which makes use of cosmic energy in the universe and vital energy in man, is probably the most natural of all therapies. It works on the principle that life is a meaningful exchange of energy, and its fundamental purpose is to ensure that this meaningful energy flow is continuously harmonious, or to restore its harmony if for any reason this flow is disturbed. Its concern is not just physical, but also emotional, mental and spiritual health.

Predicting that the next greatest medical breakthrough of the world will be made through qigong, Prof. Qian Xue Sen, the father of the Chinese rocket, says:

> Qigong is the stepping stone to open the door to the science of man, to arrive at its great hall of achievement. Why is it so? Qigong therapy is neither a therapy of medication nor a therapy of physical exercise. It employs man's consciousness to harmonize his natural functions. It directly involves the consciousness, reflecting the central philosophy in the science of man.

Moreover, the concept of equilibrium of man's functions is derived from qigong practice. In the qigong (or meditative) state of mind, man becomes aware of the equilibrium of his natural systems.

Even in Chinese medicine, when we think of illness we cannot directly see the equilibrium of man's systems. We have to start from qigong. Qigong constitutes a breakthrough in research in the science of man. If we can understand this point, it will greatly help us in our work.

Qigong, which was kept as a top secret in the past, is possibly the best gift from Chinese medicine to the west. It can help to solve the many and varied ills prevalent in western societies today.

More significantly, we need not have to be sick to enjoy the benefits of qigong. Qigong is practiced not just for curing or preventing illnesses; it adds more years to our life and more life to our years. It is the best approach in Chinese medicine that provides physical, emotional, mental and spiritual health.

BIBLIOGRAPHY

Chapter 2.
1. Dr.Andrew Stanway. Alternative Medicine. Ridby Ltd., Adelaide. 1979. pp. 9-10.
2. Stephen Fulder. The Handbook of Complementary Medicine. Coronet Books, London. 1989. p. 16

Chapter 3.
1. Stephan Palos. The Chinese Art of Healing. Bantam Book, New York, 1971. pp. X-xi

Chapter 5.
1. The six evils of cold, heat, etc are quite different from the five climatic conditions of cold, heat etc, though they are closely related. Climatic cold and heat, for example, are realistic terms; whereas the evils of cold and heat are symbolic. Pathogenic micro-organisms are symbolized as fire evil.

Chapter 7.
1. Nanjing Chinese Medical College. Commentary and Explanation on the Classic of Difficult Topics. People's Health Publishing House, Beijing. pp77-79.

Chapter 8.
1. Modern science calls them proton, electron and neutron.
2. Lao Tzu. Tao Te Ching (The Classic of the Way and Virtue), Section 42. In Chinese.
3. Cheng Yi Shan. Ancient Chinese Philosophies on Energy. Hupei People's Publication. 1986. p.111. In Chinese.
4. Ibid. p.20. In Chinese.

Chapter 10.
1. Wyngaarden and Smith (ed). Cecil Textbook of Medicine. W.B.Saunders Company, Philadelphia. 1985. p.6.
2. Pearson and Shaw. Life Extension: A Practical Scientific Approach. (Taiwan Edition). Imperial Book Company, Taipei. 1982. p.83.

Chapter 19.
1. Yang De An. Introduction to a Study of Practical Acupuncture. Tianjin Science and Technology Publication. 1986. pp.170-1. In Chinese.
2. Ibid. pp.229-30.

3. Ibid. pp.182-4.

Chapter 21.
1. Wang Fu. Massage Therapy for Everybody. People's Health Publishing House, Beijing. 1984. p.10. In Chinese.
2. Ibid. pp.10-6. In Chinese.
3. Ibid. pp. 60-4. In Chinese.

Chapter 22.
1. Liang Shi Feng. Marvelous Arts of Dynamism and Tranquility. Guangdong Higher Education Publication, China. 1985. pp.49-62. In Chinese.

Chapter 23.
1. Dr. Julian M.Kenyon. 21st. Century Medicine. Thorsons Publishers Ltd., Wellingborough. 1986. p.22.

Chapter 24.
1. Guy Lyon Playfair; Medicine, Mind and Magic; Aquarian Press, Wellingborough, 1987.
2. Quoted from Experiencing and Explaining Disease, Open University Press, 1985, p.30.
3. Cited in Ernst Baumler, Cancer: A Review of International Research, The Queen Anne Press, London, 1968, pp.198-9.
4. Reported in the Star Newspaper, Malaysia, August 2, 1993.
5. Frederick B. Levenson, the Causes and Prevention of Cancer, Sidgwick & Jackson, London, 1985, p. 99.
6. Baumler, op.cite., p.81.
7. Baumler.
8. Baumler, p.118.
9. William A Creasey, Cancer: An Introduction, Oxford University Press, New York, 1981, p. 121.
10. Frederick B. Levenson, the Causes and Prevention of Cancer, Sidgwick & Jackson, London, 1985, pp.19-20. Explanation in brackets, my own.
11. Levenson, op.cite., p.17.

Chapter 25.
1. Robert Priest and Gerald Woolfson, Handbook of Psychiatry, William Heinemann Medical Books, London, 1986, p.139.
2. Elton B. McNeil, The Psychoses, Prentice-Hall, New Jersey, 1970, p. 142.
3. Donald A. Bakal, Psychology and Medicine, Springer Publishing Company, New York, 1979, p.179.

4. Elton B.McNeil, op.cite., p. 140.
5. Elton B.McNeil, op.cite., p. 168.
6. Richard Restak, The Brain, Bantam Books, Toronto, 1984, p.343.

Chapter 27.
1. Dr. Vasant Lad. Ayurveda: The Science of Self Healing. Lotus Press, Santa Fe, New Mexico. 1985. p.18.
2. Shaykh Hakim Moinuddin Chisti. The Book of Sufi Healing. Inner Traditions International, New York. 1985. p.16.
3. Francis MacNutt, "Healing Prayers", in Church and Sherr (ed), The Heart of the Healer, Signet Book, New York, 1987, p. 191.
4. Ibid., p. 196.
5. Lawrence LeShan, How to Meditate, Bantam Books, Toronto, 1988, p.1.
6. Daniel Goleman, The Meditative Mind, Jeremy P. Tarcher, Inc., Los Angeles, 1988, p.xvii.
7. K.Sri Dhammananda. Meditation: The Only Way. Buddhist Missionary Society, Kuala Lumpur. 1987. p.33.
8. Edmund Jack Ambrose, The Nature and Origin of The Biological World, Ellis Horwood Ltd., Chichester, 1982, pp.18-9.
9. Victor Krivorotov, "Love Therapy: A Soviet Insight" in Church and Sherr (ed), The Heart of the Healer, Signet Book, New York, 1987, pp. 185-6.

Chapter 28.
1. Stephen Fulder, Complementary Medicine, Coronet Books, London, 1989, pp.12-3. In brackets, my own.
2. Ibid, Forward.
3. Paul Hastings, Medicine: An International History, Ernest Benn, London, 1974, p.41.
4. Ibid., p.106.
5. Sir John Walton, Essentials of Neurology, Pitman, London, 1984, p.33.
6. Norman Cousins, "Changing Fashions in Disease" in Church and Sherr (ed), The Heart of the Healer, Signet Book, New York, 1989, p.37.
7. Morton Glasser, MD and Gretel H.Pelto, PhD, The Medical Merry-Go-Round, Redgrave Publishing Co., Pleasantville, NY, 1980, p.2.
8. Qian Xue Sen and Chen Xin, "The Science of Man is a Major Part in the System of Modern Science and Technology." in Ming Zhen (ed), Reports of Yan Xin's Qiqong Experiments, New China Publications, Hong Kong, 1988, p.14. In Chinese.

SUGGESTED READING

1. Alternative Medicine. Ridby Ltd., Adelaide. Dr.Andrew Stanway.
2. The Handbook of Complementary Medicine. Coronet Books, London. Stephen Fulder.
3. The Chinese Art of Healing. Bantam Book, New York, 1971. Stephan Palos.
4. Nanjing Chinese Medical College. Commentary and Explanation on the Classic of Difficult Topics. People's Health Publishing House, Beijing.
5. Tao Te Ching (The Classic of the Way and Virtue), Lao Tzu.
6. Ancient Chinese Philosophies on Energy. Hupei People's Publication. 1986. Cheng Yi Shan.
7. Cecil Textbook of Medicine. W.B.Saunders Company, Philadelphia. 1985. Wyngaarden and Smith (ed).
8. Life Extension: A Practical Scientific Approach. (Taiwan Edition). Imperial Book Company, Taipei. 1982. Pearson and Shaw.
9. Introduction to a Study of Practical Acupuncture. Tianjin Science and Technology Publication.1986. Yang De An.
10. Massage Therapy for Everybody. People's Health Publishing House, Beijing. 1984. Wang Fu.
11. Marvelous Arts of Dynamism and Tranquility. Guangdong Higher Education Publication, China. 1985. Liang Shi Feng.
12. 21st. Century Medicine. Thorsons Publishers Ltd., Wellingborough. 1986. Dr. Julian M.Kenyon.
13. Medicine, Mind and Magic; Aquarian Press, Wellingborough, 1987. Guy Lyon Playfair.
14. Experiencing and Explaining Disease, Open University Press, 1985.
15. Cancer: A Review of International Research, The Queen Anne Press, London, 1968. Cited in Ernst Baumler.
16. The Causes and Prevention of Cancer, Sidgwick & Jackson, London, 1985. Frederick B. Levenson.
17. Cancer: An Introduction, Oxford University Press, New York, 1981. William A Creasey.
18. Handbook of Psychiatry, William Heinemann Medical Books, London, 1986. Robert Priest and Gerald Woolfson.
19. The Psychoses, Prentice-Hall, New Jersey, 1970. Elton B. McNeil.
20. Psychology and Medicine, Springer Publishing Company, New York, 1979. Donald A. Bakal.
21. The Brain, Bantam Books, Toronto, 1984. Richard Restak.
22. Ayurveda: The Science of Self Healing. Lotus Press, Santa Fe, New Mexico. 1985. Dr. Vasant Lad.

23. The Book of Sufi Healing. Inner Traditions International, New York. 1985. Shaykh Hakim Moinuddin Chisti.
24. The Heart of the Healer, Signet Book, New York, 1987. Francis MacNutt, "Healing Prayers", in Church and Sherr (ed).
25. How to Meditate, Bantam Books, Toronto, 1988. Lawrence LeShan.
26. The Meditative Mind, Jeremy P. Tarcher, Inc., Los Angeles, 1988. Daniel Goleman.
27. Meditation: The Only Way. Buddhist Missionary Society, Kuala Lumpur. 1987. K.Sri Dhammananda.
28. The Nature and Origin of The Biological World, Ellis Horwood Ltd., Chichester, 1982. Edmund Jack Ambrose.
29. "Love Therapy: A Soviet Insight" in Church and Sherr (ed), The Heart of the Healer, Signet Book, New York, 1987. Victor Krivorotov.
30. Complementary Medicine, Coronet Books, London, 1989. Stephen Fulder.
31. Medicine: An International History, Ernest Benn, London, 1974. Paul Hastings.
32. Essentials of Neurology, Pitman, London, 1984. Sir John Walton.
33. "Changing Fashions in Disease" in Church and Sherr (ed), The Heart of the Healer, Signet Book, New York, 1989. Norman Cousins.
34. The Medical Merry-Go-Round, Redgrave Publishing Co., Pleasantville, NY, 1980. Morton Glasser, MD and Gretel H.Pelto, PhD.
35. "The Science of Man is a Major Part in the System of Modern Science and Technology." in Ming Zhen (ed), Reports of Yan Xin's Qigong Experiments, New China Publications, Hong Kong, 1988. Qian Xue Sen and Chen Xin.

USEFUL ADDRESSES

MALAYSIA

Grandmaster Wong Kiew Kit,
81 Taman Intan B/5,
08000 Sungai Petani, Kedah, Malaysia.
Tel: (60-4) 422-2353
Fax: (60-4) 422-7812
E-mail: shaolin@pd.jaring.my
URL:http://shaolin-wahnam.tripod.com/
  index.html
  http://www.shaolin-wahnam.org

Master Ng Kowi Beng,
20, Lorong Murni 33,
Taman Desa Murni Sungai Dua,
13800 Butterworth, Pulau Pinang,
Malaysia.
Tel: (60-4) 356-3069
Fax: (60-4) 484-4617
E-mail : kowibeng@tm.net.my

Master Cheong Huat Seng,
22 Taman Mutiara,
08000 Sungai Petani, Kedah, Malaysia.
Tel: (60-4) 421-0634

Master Goh Kok Hin,
86 Jalan Sungai Emas,
08500 Kota Kuala Muda, Kedah,
Malaysia.
Tel: (60-4) 437-4301

Master Chim Chin Sin,
42 Taman Permai,
08100 Bedong, Kedah, Malaysia.
Tel: (60-4) 458-1729
Mobile Phone: (60) 012-552-6297

Master Morgan A/L Govindasamy,
3086 Lorong 21, Taman Ria,
08000 Sungai Petani, Kedah, Malaysia.
Tel: (60-4) 441-4198

Master Yong Peng Wah,
Shaolin Wahnam Chi Kung and Kung Fu,
181 Taman Kota Jaya,
34700 Simpang, Taiping, Perak, Malaysia.
Tel: (60-5) 847-1431

AUSTRALIA

Mr. George Howes,
33 Old Ferry Rd, Banora Point,
NSW 2486, Australia.
Tel: 00-61-7-55245751

AUSTRIA

Sylvester Lohninger,
Maitreya Institute,
Blättertal 9,
A-2770 Gutenstein.
Telephone: 0043-2634-7417
Fax: 0043-2634-74174
E-mail: sequoyah@nextra

BELGIUM

Dr. Daniel Widjaja,
Steenweg op Brussel 125,
1780 Wemmel, Belgium.
Tel: 00-32-2-4602977
Mobile Phone: 00-32-474-984739
Fax: 00-32-2-4602987
E-mails: dan widjaja@hotmail.com,
daniel.widjaja@worldonline.be

CANADA

Dr. Kay Lie,
E-mail: kayl@interlog.com

Mrs. Jean Lie,
Toronto, Ontario.
Telephone/Fax: (416) 979-0238
E-mail: kayl@interlog.com

Miss Emiko Hsuen,
67 Churchill Avenue, North York,
Ontario, M2N 1Y8, Canada.
Tel: 1-416-250-1812
Fax: 1 - 416- 221-5264
E-mail: emiko@attcanada.ca

Mr Neil Burden,
Vancouver, British Columbia.
Telephone/Fax: (250) 247-9968
E-mail: cosmicdragon108@hotmail.com

ENGLAND

Mr. Christopher Roy Leigh Jones,
9a Beach Street, Lytham, Lancashire,
FY8 5NS, United Kingdom.
Tel: 0044-1253-736278
E-mail: barbara.rawlinson@virgin.net

Mr. Dan Hartwright,
Rumpus Cottage, Church Place,
Pulborough, West Sussex RH20 1AF, UK.
Tel: 0044-7816-111007
E-mail: dhartWright@hotmail.com

GERMANY

Grandmaster Kai Uwe Jettkandt,
Ostendstr. 79,
60314 Frankfurt, Germany.
Tel: 49-69-90431678
E-mail: Kaijet@t-online.de

HOLLAND

Dr. Oetti Kwee Liang Hoo,
Tel: 31-10-5316416

IRELAND

Miss Joan Brown,
Mullin, Scatazlin, Castleisland, County,
Kerry, Ireland.
Tel: 353-66-7147545
Mobile Phone: 353-87-6668374
E-mail: djbrowne@gofree.indigo.ie

ITALY

Master Roberto Lamberti,
Hotel Punta Est Via Aurelia, 1
17024 Finale Ligure (SV), Italy.
Tel: ++39019600611
Mobile Phone: ++393393580663
E-mails: robertolamberti@libero.it

Master Attilio Podestà,
Via Aurelia 1,
17024 Finale Ligure (Savona), Italy.
Tel/Fax: +39 019 600 611
E-mail: attiliopodesta@libero.it
OR
Hotel Punta Est Via Aurelia 1,
17024 Finale Ligure (Savona), Italy.
E-mail: info@puntaest.com
Web-site: www.puntaest.com

Mr. Riccardo Puleo,
via don Gnocchi, 28,
20148 Milano, Italy.
Tel: 0039-02-4078250
E-mail: rpuleo@efficient-finance.com

LITHUANIA

Mr. Arunas Krisiunas,
Sauletekio al.53-9,
2040 Vilnius, Lithuania.
Tel: +3702-700-237
Mobile Phone: +370-9887353
E-mail: induva@iti.lt

PANAMA

Mr. Raúl A. López R.,
16, "B" st., Panama City,
Republic of Panama.
OR
P.O. Box 1433, Panama 9A-1433.
Tel: (507) 618-1836
E-mail: raullopez@cwpanama.net
        taiko@hotmail.com

PORTUGAL

Dr Riccardo Salvatore,
Tel: 351-218478713

SCOTLAND

Mr. Darryl Collett,
c/o 19A London Street, Edinburgh,
EH3 6LY, United Kingdom.
Mobile phone: 0790-454-7538
E-mail: CollDod@aol.com

SPAIN

Master Laura Fernández,
C/ Madre Antonia de París, 2 esc. izq. 4° A,
Madrid - 28027 – Spain.
Tel: 34-91-6386270

Javier Galve,
Tai Chi Chuan and Chi Kung Instructor
of the Shaolin Wahnam Institute
C/Guadarrama 3-2°A-28011-Madrid,
Spain.
Phone: 34-91-4640578
Mobile Phone: 34-656669790
E-mail: shaolin@inicia.es

Master Adalia Iglesias,
calle Cometa, n° 3, atico,
08002 Barcelona, Spain.
Tel: 0034-93-3104956
E-mail: adalia@xenoid.com

Master Román Garcia Lampaya,
71, Av. Antonio Machad,
Santa Cruz del Valle,
05411 Avila, Spain.
Tel: 34-920-386717, 34-915-360702
Mobile Phone : 34-656-612608
E-mail: romangarcia@wanadoo.es

Master José Díaz Marqués,
C/. del Teatro, 13
41927 Mairena del Aljarafe / Sevilla,
Spain.
Tel: + 34-954-183-917
Mobile Phone: 34-656-756214
Fax: + 34-955-609-354
E-mail: transpersonal@infotelmultimedia.es

Dr. Inaki Rivero Urdiain,
Aguirre Miramon, 6 – 4° dch.,
20002 San Sebastian, Spain.
Tel: + 34-943-360213
Mobile Phone: 34-656-756214
E-mail: psiconet@euskalnet.net
Web-site: www.euskalnet.net/psicosalud

Master Douglas Wiesenthal,
C/ Almirante Cadarso 26, P-14
46005 Valencia, Spain
Tel/Fax: +34 96-320-8433
E-mail: dwiesenthal@yahoo.com

Master Trini
Ms Trinidad Parreno,
E-mail: trinipar@wanadoo.es

SOUTH AFRICA

Grandmaster Leslie James Reed,
312 Garensville, 285 Beach Road, Sea
Point,
Cape Town, 8000 South Africa.
Tel/Fax: 0927-21-4391373
E-mail: itswasa@mweb.co.za

SWITZERLAND

Mr. Andrew Barnett,
Bildweg 34, 7250 Klosters,
Switzerland.
Tel/Fax: +41-81-422-5235
Mobile Phone: +41-79-610-3781
E-mail: andrew.barnett@bluewin.ch

USA

Mr. Anthony Korahais,
546 W147th Street, Apt. 2-DR,
New York, New York, 10031, USA.
Tel: 917-270-4310, 212-854-0201
E-mails: anthony@korahais.com,
anthony@arch.columbia.edu

Mr. Eugene Siterman,
299 Carroll St., Brooklyn,
New York,11231.
Tel: 718-8555785
E-mail: qipaco@hotmail.com

INDEX